Transforming Pharmaceutical Research With Artificial Intelligence

Miltiadis D. Lytras
Effat University, Saudi Arabia

Sarah A. Alajlan
Almaarefa University, Saudi Arabia

IGI Global
Scientific Publishing
Publishing Tomorrow's Research Today

Vice President of Editorial — Melissa Wagner
Managing Editor of Acquisitions — Mikaela Felty
Managing Editor of Book Development — Jocelynn Hessler
Production Manager — Mike Brehm
Cover Design — Phillip Shickler

Published in the United States of America by
IGI Global Scientific Publishing
701 East Chocolate Avenue
Hershey, PA, 17033, USA
Tel: 717-533-8845
Fax: 717-533-7115
Website: https://www.igi-global.com E-mail: cust@igi-global.com

Library of Congress Cataloging-in-Publication Data

LCCN: 2024052976 (CIP Data Pending)
ISBN: 979-8-3693-6270-9
EISBN: 979-8-3693-6271-6
British Cataloguing in Publication Data
A Cataloguing in Publication record for this book is available from the British Library.

Table of Contents

Detailed Table of Contents

This chapter explores the profound impact of artificial intelligence (AI) on pharmaceutical research, particularly focusing on its integration into drug discovery, development, and clinical trial processes. The narrative details how AI-driven methodologies like predictive modeling, virtual screening, and machine learning revolutionize the identification and validation of drug targets and compounds. Additionally, the chapter discusses the application of AI in optimizing clinical trial designs, enhancing patient recruitment, and monitoring trial data in real-time. Ethical considerations including data privacy, bias, and the need for transparency in AI applications are critically analyzed to underscore the necessity for ethical guidelines and regulatory compliance in the evolving landscape of AI-driven pharmaceutical research. The comprehensive overview provided by the authors demonstrates how AI technologies not only accelerate drug development processes but also improve their efficacy, safety, and cost-efficiency.

The application of artificial intelligence in the design and conduct of patient recruitment in clinical trials is targeted at addressing some of the key inefficiencies, including longer timelines and the lack of some participant characteristics. This chapter presents readers with the opportunities and advantages of using AI to make protocols more specific and execute patient recruitment more efficiently. This chapter integrates thorough discussions that explain how predictive analytics, machine learning, and other tools such as natural language processing can be used to identify participants and refine the design of trials. Moreover, this chapter contains a description of the use and results of AI implementation with the help of the provided case studies. In this way, it is possible to learn how to increase the efficiency of a trial, the number of sourced participants, and recruitment issues using AI technology. Ethical and regulatory issues are also discussed in this chapter, which provides an overview of the role and functions AI can play in the process of clinical trials.

This chapter discusses the transformational role of artificial intelligence (AI) across real-world evidence (RWE) analysis throughout health care. It shows how AI (through Machine learning and Natural language processing) is powerful enough to help deal with voluminous, heterogeneous amounts of semantic-rich healthcare data; full-text records coming from clinical notes. Most notably, AI applications such as predictive models, risk stratification and pattern analysis, or adverse event detection (ADE) are reviewed to underscore how new technologies could enable improved data accuracy along with meaningful information extraction in patient care personalization. Importantly, this complete review highlights the promise of AI to modernize health analytics in a truly meaningful sense and achieve better clinical results.

The usual use of artificial intelligence (AI) in drug research and discovery is poised to usher in a revolutionary era for the pharmaceutical sector. This chapter examines the significance of artificial intelligence in pharmaceutical engineering, emphasising significant developments and approaches that are transforming the discipline. AI is also accelerating the time-to-time market and cutting costs in clinical trials by optimising patient selection, providing real-time monitoring, and designing adaptive studies. This chapter also explores the regulatory environment, ethical issues, and the potential applications of AI in the pharmaceutical industry. This chapter intends to educate and motivate researchers, business experts, and legislators to fully use AI's promise to transform pharmaceutical engineering by offering a thorough review of the technology's role in drug discovery and development.

The KSK approach to BP patient healthcare monitoring, which is powered by AI and IoT, has the potential to completely transform the way hypertension is treated. It makes it easier for healthcare providers to make decisions based on exact information, as well as to monitor patients accurately and in real time, customise treatment plans, and empower patients. We anticipate a major improvement in the management of hypertension and other chronic disorders with additional technological developments. Three measures are used to evaluate classifier performance. Accuracy, precision, and recall are all measured. The KSK technique used in the BP healthcare industry currently achieves an accuracy rate of 89% to 93% for each condition.

This research paper demonstrates role of QSP modeling efforts in Rifampicin development program via empirical pharmaceutical research, which were selected to cover a wide range of mathematical modeling methods including agent-based modeling, partial differential equation modeling, and ordinary differential equation modeling. Other applications of systems modeling include evaluation of new target pathways; optimization of compound physicochemical properties; characterization of efficacy and toxicity mechanisms of action; recommendation of treatment posology of monotherapies and combination therapies by balancing efficacy and toxicity; and guidance of study subject stratification strategies based on clinical responder features. Particularly, quantitative systems modeling plays a critical role in predicting clinical hematological toxicity risks by translating preclinical data obtained from micro-physiological systems (MPS). The analysis of Rifampicin as personalized medicine in MPS data is routinely performed to simulate clinical outcomes under various dosage regimens.

Because of their qualities, medicinal plants are essential to both traditional and modern medicine. In this work, we suggest employing machine learning to identify therapeutic plants. The collection of data, feature extraction, model training, and prediction are some of the essential elements of the suggested system. First, a large collection of photos of medicinal plants is collected from databases. Then, using image processing techniques, pertinent elements like leaf form, texture, and color are retrieved from the photos. Following the extraction of features, ML methods like Convolutional Neural Networks (CNNs) are used to train a classification model. From input photos, the trained model can then correctly identify therapeutic plants. A user-friendly interface might be created to encourage user participation, enabling users to submit photos and get instant identification results.

Medication adherence remains a significant challenge within healthcare systems globally, especially among groups with chronic illnesses like diabetes, hypertension, and asthma. Despite universally accessible, low-cost Artificial Intelligence (AI) technologies to adherence, an information crevice exists on the utilization of this innovation and its effect on medicine self-efficacy and pharmaceutical adherence in therapeutically underserved populations with an assortment of persistent sicknesses. AI-enabled smartphone applications have surfaced as an encouraging remedy, presenting innovative methods to monitor patient behaviors, verify medication consumption, and deliver personalized reminders. By utilizing real-time monitoring, tailored communication, and behavioral nudges, AI can tackle the various barriers to medication adherence through creative solutions, including forgetfulness, lack of motivation, and insufficient health literacy, while fostering improved health outcomes, particularly among individuals with chronic conditions.

Abstract: Natural products (NPs) are mostly understood to be unique structures that interact with therapeutic protein targets. Their unique characteristics and structural diversity continue to astound scientists with their capacity to produce medicines that are modeled after naturally occurring products, even if the pharmaceutical industry has mostly given up. Nowadays, a lot of sectors and research domains use artificial intelligence (AI) because of developments in computer technology, storage capacity, software accessibility, and affordable online education. Two subfields of artificial intelligence (AI), natural language processing and machine learning algorithms, have evolved in recent decades to address challenges in NP drug discovery and open up new options. This chapter looks at and discusses the practical applications of artificial intelligence (AI) methods developed to aid in the discovery of bioactive natural products (NPs) and to determine the molecular "patterns" of these favored structures for target selectivity or combinatorial design.

The pharmaceutical supply chain is fraught with challenges, including counterfeit drugs, lack of transparency, and stringent regulatory compliance. Blockchain technology offers a transformative solution to these issues through its decentralized, immutable, and transparent nature. This chapter explores the implementation of blockchain in pharmaceutical supply chains, detailing the technology's fundamentals, types, and the specific challenges it addresses within the industry. Case studies illustrate successful blockchain applications, highlighting enhanced traceability, reduced counterfeiting, and improved regulatory compliance. Furthermore, the chapter discusses the practical aspects of blockchain implementation, including feasibility studies, stakeholder involvement, technical integration, and data privacy concerns. Finally, it delves into future prospects, emphasizing the integration of emerging technologies like IoT and AI, and predicting trends that will shape the future of blockchain in the pharmaceutical industry.

This chapter provides an overview of the history and impact of artificial intelligence on businesses, with a specific focus on the pharmaceutical industry and research. It discusses the basic principles of pharmacoeconomics, explores ways AI can enhance business processes, and examines various applications of AI in pharmaceutical research, such as drug development, digital therapy, personalized treatment, clinical trials, epidemic forecasting, and supply chain management. The chapter also addresses challenges and considerations related to ethics, safety, data privacy, and liability in AI implementation. Finally, the discussion provides insights into AI's economic opportunities and implications in pharmaceutical research.

Preface

In Transforming Pharmaceutical Research with Artificial Intelligence book we offer an in-depth exploration of how artificial intelligence (AI) is revolutionizing every aspect of pharmaceutical research, from drug discovery to patient care. As AI continues to make significant strides, it's reshaping the way the pharmaceutical industry operates, driving efficiencies, enhancing research, and improving patient outcomes. At the core of this change is AI's function in hastening drug discovery and lowering expenses. By examining extensive quantities of biological and chemical data, AI can forecast how various compounds will engage with biological systems, thus speeding up pinpointing potential drug candidates. This not only diminishes the time and costs that have traditionally been linked with introducing new drugs to the market, but it also creates avenues for finding innovative therapies more efficiently is taking on a crucial role in clinical trials, enhancing the design process and boosting patient recruitment by aligning patients with trials based on intricate datasets. This results in more precise, quicker, and cost-efficient trials, delivering essential treatments to patients more rapidly. Additionally, AI assists in evaluating real-world evidence, which facilitates a deeper understanding of how treatments function beyond the clinical environment, thereby informing more accurate therapeutic approaches. The incorporation of AI with precision medicine is another significant element of the book. Through digital biomarkers and AI-driven analytics, pharmaceutical research can now progress toward more customized treatments designed for individual patients. These technologies hold the potential to enhance drug effectiveness while reducing adverse effects, resulting in improved health outcomes. The book further explores the groundbreaking convergence of AI and IoT technologies, where AI-driven systems monitor and manage chronic diseases, like blood pressure, in real-time. This functionality greatly improves patient care and adherence to treatment plans, guaranteeing enhanced management of long-term health concerns.

Additionally, Transforming Pharmaceutical Research with Artificial Intelligence discusses the growing significance of AI in the creation of natural products and herbal medicines. By utilizing AI to assess the therapeutic properties of plants, researchers are unearthing new potential remedies sourced from nature, thereby broadening the horizons of pharmaceutical advancement. The use of AI in drug modeling and pharmacokinetics is also investigated, with AI assisting in the refinement of drug behavior assessment within the body, especially for conditions such as tuberculosis. These sophisticated models facilitate more tailored treatments and improved results for patients, customizing therapies to meet individual requirements. Besides its influence on drug creation, the book analyzes the wider implications of AI within pharmaceutical supply chains and medication adherence, illustrating how AI can enhance supply chain management through reliable, transparent systems like blockchain. AI is also vital in bolstering patient compliance with prescribed medications, which is crucial for improved treatment results and lower healthcare expenses.

Furthermore, the book reviews the economic landscape melded by AI in pharmaceutical research, emphasizing both the advantages and challenges that AI brings regarding cost reduction, new revenue opportunities, and possible disruptions in the sector. Transforming Pharmaceutical Research with Artificial Intelligence serves as a thorough resource for comprehending how AI is transforming the pharmaceutical industry. Through its insights into the varied applications of AI, the book provides readers with a guide for navigating the future of pharmaceutical research, where AI not only advances the discovery of new medications but also enhances patient care, boosts efficiencies, and opens new avenues in healthcare.

Transforming Pharmaceutical Research with Artificial Intelligence fits squarely at the intersection of two rapidly evolving fields: artificial intelligence and healthcare. In today's world, the pharmaceutical industry is under immense pressure to innovate faster, reduce costs, and improve patient outcomes. Traditional methods of drug discovery and development, while effective, are often slow, resource-intensive, and costly. As the global healthcare landscape becomes more complex. This is where artificial intelligence comes in.AI is already transforming various sectors, but its impact on pharmaceuticals is particularly profound. With the ability to process and analyze vast amounts of data at lightning speed, AI is enabling pharmaceutical companies to accelerate drug discovery, optimize clinical trials, and create personalized treatment plans that were once unimaginable. This shift is not just about improving the speed and efficiency of research; it's also about ushering in a new era of precision medicine that tailors treatments to the individual characteristics of each patient, rather than relying on a one-size-fits-all approach. Additionally, as the healthcare industry moves towards more integrated, patient-cantered care, AI is playing a critical role in improving patient monitoring, medication adherence, and real-time decision-making. The rise of AI-powered tools, such as wearable devices and digital health platforms, is empowering both patients and healthcare providers to better manage chronic conditions and optimize treatment regimens. At a global level, the intersection of AI and pharmaceutical research is also being driven by the growing importance of data. The proliferation of electronic health records, genetic sequencing, and other forms of big data is creating new opportunities for AI to identify trends, predict disease outbreaks, and even discover new treatments hidden within vast datasets. AI is also enabling better drug safety monitoring and more accurate predictions of adverse drug reactions, which has the potential to save lives and reduce healthcare costs. With the increasing complexity of global health challenges and the need for faster, more effective drug development, the role of AI in pharmaceutical research is more vital than ever. As technology continues to advance, the book highlights how AI can help bridge the gap between the promises of science and the realities of healthcare, driving breakthroughs that will shape the future of medicine and improve lives worldwide. In this context, Transforming Pharmaceutical Research With Artificial Intelligence is an essential contribution to understanding how AI is not just a technological trend but a powerful force reshaping the very foundation of pharmaceutical research and healthcare delivery today. It serves as a guide for industry professionals, researchers, and policymakers looking to navigate the rapidly changing landscape of AI in healthcare, providing both a snapshot of current innovations and a vision for the future of Pharma.

CHAPTER OVERVIEW

Ch1. The Dawn of AI in Pharmaceutical Research

This chapter is vital in providing a foundational understanding of how artificial intelligence (AI) has transformed pharmaceutical research. It explores how AI is integrated into drug discovery, development, and clinical trial processes, accelerating the pace of innovation. The chapter emphasizes the power of AI-driven techniques like predictive modeling and machine learning, which enable better identification of drug targets, more efficient clinical trials, and improvements in drug efficacy and safety. The inclusion of ethical considerations around AI, such as bias and data privacy, highlights the importance of responsible AI implementation, making this chapter crucial for understanding both the potential and the challenges of AI in the pharmaceutical industry.

Ch2. AI in Clinical Trial Design and Patient Recruitment

Focusing on the intersection of AI and clinical trials, this chapter discusses how AI is revolutionizing clinical trial designs and patient recruitment. By using predictive analytics and machine learning tools, AI helps in creating more precise trial protocols and overcoming common challenges like patient recruitment delays. Through case studies, the chapter illustrates how AI enhances the efficiency of trials, making them faster and more cost-effective. The exploration of ethical and regulatory issues provides an essential framework for understanding the complexities of using AI in such critical areas of healthcare, underlining the importance of its responsible application.

Ch3. Real-world Evidence and AI in Healthcare Analytics

This chapter highlights the transformative role of AI in analyzing real-world evidence (RWE) and its potential to change healthcare analytics. It demonstrates how AI technologies, including machine learning and natural language processing, can extract meaningful insights from vast amounts of unstructured data in clinical settings. By focusing on predictive models, risk stratification, and adverse event detection, this chapter shows how AI can improve the accuracy of healthcare data and personalize patient care. The comprehensive review presented underscores AI's potential to enhance healthcare outcomes, making this chapter crucial for understanding the future of evidence-based medicine.

Ch4. Revolutionizing Pharmaceutical Engineering

This chapter examines how AI is driving significant changes in pharmaceutical engineering, from drug discovery to production. AI's role in optimizing patient selection, real-time monitoring, and designing adaptive clinical studies is highlighted as a means to reduce costs and time in the development process. By focusing on the regulatory environment and ethical challenges, it offers readers a nuanced view of how AI technologies are reshaping the pharmaceutical sector. This chapter is crucial for understanding how AI is not just a tool, but a catalyst for a fundamental shift in the way pharmaceutical research and development are conducted.

Ch5. Drug Design and Discovery through Artificial Intelligence: Concept of Drug Target Interactions

The chapter explores the application of AI in drug design, particularly its ability to analyze drug-target interactions efficiently. It delves into how AI, through deep learning and data digitization, enhances the discovery of new compounds and improves the drug design process. By addressing the complexity of handling large datasets, the chapter illustrates AI's potential in overcoming traditional challenges in drug discovery and development, offering a clear vision of the future of pharmaceutical research.

Ch6. Exploring the Role of Digital Biomarkers and Artificial Intelligence in Precision Therapeutics

This chapter examines the critical role of digital biomarkers and AI in advancing precision therapeutics, where treatments are tailored to an individual's unique biomarker profile. The integration of AI with data from wearable technology allows for more accurate disease monitoring and personalized treatment plans. The chapter's in-depth analysis of clinical applications, such as using MRI for Parkinson's disease management, highlights the real-world impact of these innovations, making it an essential read for understanding how AI and digital biomarkers are reshaping personalized medicine.

Ch7. AI-Powered-IoT (AIIoT) Based Decision Making System for BP-Patient Healthcare Monitoring

This chapter presents the innovative combination of AI and the Internet of Things (IoT) to monitor and manage blood pressure in hypertensive patients. By focusing on real-time data collection, personalized treatment plans, and decision-making accuracy, it demonstrates how AI-IoT systems are enhancing hypertension management. The chapter's practical examples and performance metrics emphasize the potential of this technology to transform chronic disease care, making it a valuable resource for understanding the intersection of AI, IoT, and healthcare.

Ch8. Mechanism-Based PKPD Models for Rifampicin Evaluation - Quantitative Systems Pharmacology through Pharmacometrics

In this chapter, the role of quantitative systems pharmacology (QSP) in drug development, specifically in evaluating Rifampicin, is explored through various modeling approaches. By focusing on mathematical modeling techniques and how they optimize drug efficacy and safety, the chapter provides a deep dive into the importance of QSP in personalized medicine. It showcases how AI-driven models predict clinical outcomes and help tailor treatments to individual patients, offering readers critical insights into the future of pharmacometric modeling.

Ch9. Leveraging AI to Identify Medicinal Herbal Plants' Properties

This chapter introduces the use of AI, particularly machine learning, in identifying and classifying medicinal plants. By integrating image processing and feature extraction techniques, AI can be used to enhance the identification of plant species with therapeutic properties, a tool that could revolutionize traditional medicine research. The chapter's practical approach to building classification models using Convolutional Neural Networks (CNNs) demonstrates AI's potential to bridge the gap between natural remedies and modern medicine, making it an essential read for researchers in the field of ethnopharmacology.

Ch10. Harnessing AI to Improve Medication Adherence

This chapter addresses the global challenge of medication adherence, particularly in chronic disease management, and how AI can offer innovative solutions. By focusing on AI-enabled applications that track patient behavior, deliver personalized reminders, and improve patient engagement, it outlines how AI can overcome barriers like forgetfulness, low motivation, and health literacy. The discussion on AI's impact on adherence, especially for underserved populations, emphasizes its potential to improve health outcomes and reduce healthcare costs, making it a key resource for those interested in the intersection of AI and patient care.

Ch11. Cognizing Nature: The AI Frontier in Natural Product Drug Discovery

Focusing on the application of AI in natural product drug discovery, this chapter explores how AI can aid in identifying bioactive compounds from nature. By using machine learning and natural language processing, AI systems can analyze vast datasets to uncover new therapeutic agents, making the process of drug discovery more efficient. The chapter emphasizes the role of AI in reimagining how natural products can contribute to modern pharmacology, providing readers with a comprehensive view of this evolving research area.

Ch12. From Concept to Reality: Implementing Blockchain Solutions in Pharmaceutical Supply Chains

Blockchain's potential to revolutionize pharmaceutical supply chains is the focus of this chapter, which highlights how the technology can address critical issues such as counterfeiting, transparency, and regulatory compliance. By exploring case studies and practical implementation strategies, the chapter provides a clear understanding of how blockchain can enhance the pharmaceutical supply chain's efficiency and security. The discussion of integrating AI and IoT with blockchain points to future advancements, offering a roadmap for how these technologies will shape the future of pharmaceutical logistics.

Ch13. The Economic Implications of AI in Pharmaceutical and Research

This chapter offers an in-depth exploration of the economic impact of AI on pharmaceutical research and development. By examining AI's role in enhancing business processes, improving drug development timelines, and increasing cost-efficiency, it highlights both the opportunities and challenges associated with AI in the industry. Additionally, the chapter addresses the ethical, safety, and data privacy concerns that arise as AI becomes more integrated into pharmaceutical research. This discussion is critical for stakeholders looking to understand the broader economic implications of AI's role in the pharmaceutical sector.

Our target audience is professionals, researchers, and students in the fields of pharmaceutical sciences, healthcare, biotechnology, and artificial intelligence. It will be especially valuable for pharmaceutical researchers, clinical trial experts, data scientists, AI developers, and healthcare providers looking to understand how AI can optimize drug development processes and enhance patient care. Additionally, policymakers and regulatory professionals interested in the ethical, legal, and economic implications of AI in healthcare will find key insights to guide decisions in this rapidly evolving space. The book is also accessible to anyone with an interest in the future of healthcare and technology, including tech enthusiasts, entrepreneurs, and individuals curious about how AI is transforming the pharmaceutical and healthcare industries. Whether you're a medical practitioner, business leader, or student, this book also offers valuable insights into the ways AI is reshaping medicine, drug discovery, and healthcare delivery on a global scale.

Transforming Pharmaceutical Research With Artificial Intelligence provides a timely and crucial contribution to the fast-changing integration of artificial intelligence and pharmaceutical research. By examining the various methods AI is being incorporated into drug discovery, clinical trials, personalized medicine, and healthcare systems, the book underscores both the transformative possibilities and the challenges that accompany this technological shift. It acts as a thorough resource for professionals in the pharmaceutical, healthcare, and technology fields, equipping them with the understanding and insights needed to effectively utilize AI in their work.

The book's thorough investigation of AI's applications offers specific examples of how these technologies are not only enhancing research efficiency and accuracy but also resulting in breakthroughs in treatment development, patient monitoring, and healthcare delivery. Through its extensive analysis, it presents a clearer perspective on how AI can address some of the industry's most urgent issues, from decreasing costs and timelines in drug development to facilitating more personalized and effective treatments. By tackling both the opportunities and the ethical, regulatory, and economic obstacles AI presents, Transforming Pharmaceutical Research With Artificial Intelligence ensures that readers are not just aware of the latest innovations but also prepared to navigate the complexities of implementing AI in practical situations. The book's emphasis on both the technical and human elements of AI integration establishes it as an essential resource for influencing the future of pharmaceutical research and healthcare. In this way, it contributes significantly to the ongoing discussion on how AI can be utilized to enhance human health, making it an important addition to the literature on AI in the life sciences.

Miltiadis D. Lytras
Effat University, Saudi Arabia

Sarah M. Alajlan
Almaarefa University, Saudi Arabia

Chapter 1
The Dawn of AI in Pharmaceutical Research:
AI Transforming Pharma – Ethics, Trials, and Beyond

Abdullah Saeed
https://orcid.org/0000-0002-2021-1089
Ministry of Health, Saudi Arabia

Sarah A. Alajlan
https://orcid.org/0000-0003-0050-4164
Almaarefa University, Saudi Arabia

ABSTRACT

This chapter explores the profound impact of artificial intelligence (AI) on pharmaceutical research, particularly focusing on its integration into drug discovery, development, and clinical trial processes. The narrative details how AI-driven methodologies like predictive modeling, virtual screening, and machine learning revolutionize the identification and validation of drug targets and compounds. Additionally, the chapter discusses the application of AI in optimizing clinical trial designs, enhancing patient recruitment, and monitoring trial data in real-time. Ethical considerations including data privacy, bias, and the need for transparency in AI applications are critically analyzed to underscore the necessity for ethical guidelines and regulatory compliance in the evolving landscape of AI-driven pharmaceutical research. The comprehensive overview provided by the authors demonstrates how AI technologies not only accelerate drug development processes but also improve their efficacy, safety, and cost-efficiency.

DOI: 10.4018/979-8-3693-6270-9.ch001

1. CHAPTER SUMMARY

Artificial Intelligence (AI), a bundling of multiple technologies capable of reasoning, learning from experience, and rendering valuable insights, has paved its way into pharmaceutical research with beneficial contributions. AI-driven tools and their extensive utilities are selling points that lead to a surge of activity including negotiations for business partnerships, mergers, and acquisitions. Startups are able to raise a hundred-thousand-dollar investment as they scaffold AI as the mainstay aiding in drug discovery, which was impossible to reach in previous years. Pharmaceutical research and development, being a costly and time-consuming course, is expected to shell out about 2.8 trillion USD—estimated to mature by 2024; furthermore, the cost of creating a viable new drug stands at 2.6 billion USD. With this evaluative approach, AI strategies are phenomenal in brands looking to mature its drug discovery paradigm and bring precision medicine to the limelight in drug development. AI approaches to drug discovery are creating tremors in the political landscape and economic forums.

Although the incurrence of expenditures via AI resourcing has its own challenges with respect to the implementation of additional financial overheads, it is staunchly believed that DCs would register long-term efficiency and cross-functional benefits when appropriately tailored and integrated into drug discovery strategies. AI is foraying into pharmaceutical landscapes in every stage of the drug development process. This chapter bites down on the endless potentials of AI that hold economic and marketable promises in clinical and tangible applications. With a peek into the historical orientation of AI/ML in matching the blocks of pharmaceutical research, the chapter tracks the evolution of AI tools adopted from the realms of academia into the real-world pharmaceutical environment with a spotlight on the recent successes and plummeting failures. The reign of AI tools and the immense enthusiasm it has sparked with the startup culture, mergers with big pharma, and acquisitions have been intracranially scanned to produce judicial inferences set against the existing horizon of claims, potential, and promise. Could AI be the right fit on the bedside table shadowing the development of precious drugs within the white sheets of pharmaceutical innovation?

2. INTRODUCTION TO AI IN PHARMACEUTICAL RESEARCH

The vision of discovering new drugs through computers in a fraction of the time needed for traditional drug development is fast becoming a reality. Thanks to the integration of artificial intelligence and machine learning, this process can now be transformed, making it significantly faster and more efficient. In the field of pharmaceutical research, AI technologies are expected to contribute significantly to solving complex issues. These include not only the diversification of drug discovery targets but also the advancement of regenerative medicine and the creation of useful and personalized health data. With AI, the possibilities are endless, and the potential for groundbreaking discoveries in the field of drug development has never been greater. AI-powered systems can analyze vast amounts of data, identify patterns, and predict the efficacy and safety of potential drugs with unprecedented accuracy. This opens up new opportunities for designing innovative and targeted therapies, revolutionizing the way we approach medical treatments. Furthermore, AI can assist in the manufacturing process, optimizing drug production, and ensuring quality control. As we continue to unlock the full potential of AI, the future of drug discovery and development looks incredibly promising. With each passing day, we are getting closer to a world where life-saving medications are developed faster, more efficiently, and with greater precision. The collaboration between humans and machines in the pharmaceutical industry promises to redefine healthcare and improve countless lives worldwide. Together, we are on the cusp of a new era in medicine, where AI will play a pivotal role in bringing us closer to the cures we seek (Blanco-Gonzalez et al., 2023).

Most AI technologies make use of AI, which refers to a computer system that performs human-like thinking activities and represents a set of constraints within which AI performs functions and tasks. Machine learning is a method for implementing AI. In contrast to conventional programming, in which the functions that the computer performs are manually written and implemented, machine learning methods enable computers to automatically learn patterns, associate functions, and make decisions based on data. In this chapter, the main focus is on the use of machine learning because of the key role it plays in pharmaceutical advancements and drug discovery. AI natural language processing and deep learning are also discussed in the different stages of the drug discovery process (Selvaraj et al., 2021). Pharmaceutical advancements and drug discovery have greatly benefited from the use of machine learning techniques. Machine learning, being a subfield of artificial intelligence (AI), has revolutionized the way computer systems can emulate human-like thinking and reasoning. These AI technologies utilize complex algorithms and models to perform various tasks and functions, enhancing the efficiency and accuracy of the drug discovery process. Machine learning techniques enable computers to automatically learn and adapt from data, unlike traditional programming methods where tasks and functions are manually coded. By analyzing large datasets, machine learning algorithms can identify patterns, develop associations, and make informed decisions. This ability to learn from data has significantly contributed to the success of pharmaceutical advancements (Patel & Shah, 2022). In the field of drug discovery, machine learning plays a pivotal role in various stages. It aids in the identification of potential drug targets, prediction of compound efficacy, analysis of molecular structures, and optimization of drug properties. By leveraging AI natural language processing, computers can extract valuable information from scientific literature, patents, and clinical trial reports, helping researchers navigate the vast amount of data available. Deep learning, another branch of AI, has also found applications in the drug discovery process. By utilizing neural networks with numerous layers, deep learning algorithms can uncover intricate relationships and representations in data, leading to valuable insights. This advanced approach has shown promising results in tasks such as image recognition, virtual screening, and predicting molecular properties (Pandey et al.2022). The integration of machine learning, AI natural language processing, and deep learning in the field of drug discovery has accelerated the pace of advancements. These technologies enable researchers to analyze vast amounts of data efficiently, identify potential drug candidates, and optimize drug development processes. With continued advancements in AI, the future of pharmaceutical advancements and drug discovery looks brighter than ever before. (Dara et al.2022)

Conceptually, a clear logical distinction exists between AI and humans, in which AI conducts pattern-cognition tasks based on statistical data to understand complex activities and make inferences based on probability and possibility through machine learning and image recognition. The development of AI in new drug development is expected to revolutionize traditional methods. Such a concept may require much less time and effort than conventional procedures, as drug candidates could be deciphered through data analysis. The minimum time span for drug development, from the discovery of new targets to the confirmation of effectiveness, is approximately 25 years. However, many cases end up in failure, and it is estimated that the probability of success is less than 10%. Therefore, the primary motivation for introducing AI is to reduce the risk of development (Schlander et al.2021).

3. AI-DRIVEN METHODOLOGIES IN DRUG DISCOVERY

The application of AI-driven methodologies at all stages of drug discovery can greatly enhance the efficiency and effectiveness of the drug discovery process by accelerating the identification and efficacy testing of drug candidates. In particular, there are various AI-driven methodologies that focus on identifying potential compounds to act as a starting point for novel drug discovery. These include machine learning algorithms that can analyze vast amounts of data to generate correlation and predictive models to identify molecular interactions between target proteins and small molecules. At its core, the goal of such programs is to optimize late-stage clinical trials by selecting the most promising drug candidates to progress to the efficacy testing phase. In order to achieve this, a plethora of innovative AI-based methodologies focused directly on speeding up the drug discovery process has been developed. This includes large-scale computer simulations of biological phenomena and the incorporation of experimental bioinformatics data in order to design and optimize promising compounds for the first time. These cutting-edge AI-driven approaches have revolutionized the field of drug discovery, allowing researchers to explore a wider range of potential drug candidates and significantly reducing the time and cost associated with traditional drug development methods. By harnessing the power of artificial intelligence and machine learning, scientists can now expedite the identification, synthesis, and testing of drug molecules, ultimately leading to the discovery of new and more effective treatments for a variety of diseases and conditions. The integration of AI into drug discovery processes has opened up new avenues of research and innovation, paving the way for personalized medicine and targeted therapies. With the continuous advancements in AI technology, the future of drug discovery holds immense potential for groundbreaking discoveries and transformative advancements in healthcare (Jiménez-Luna et al.2021).

Moreover, artificial intelligence (AI) has been extensively utilized as a fundamental tool for the selection of the most promising drug candidates that are generated in silico. These candidates are then synthesized and subjected to laboratory testing, effectively streamlining the initial stages of drug discovery. The generation of such data to develop these models, as well as the validation of the models in the design of new compounds, often creates a bottleneck for the application of these methods. Consequently, there is a pressing need to develop new bioinformatic methods that can adequately assess the performance of these compounds. (Selvaraj et al., 2021) Within this realm, numerous methods have emerged with a primary focus on optimizing existing methodologies by integrating new topics and addendums into standard simulation techniques. It is understandable that a significant portion of these assessments revolves around molecular dynamics and the success of docking techniques. However, there exist several challenges and limitations when implementing these methodologies (Nayarisseri et al.2021). One of the key challenges is ensuring the quality of the data used in these AI-driven approaches. It is crucial that the inputs are reliable, accurate, and comprehensive. Additionally, the sharing of data between different research groups and institutions poses a challenge, as it requires the establishment of standardized protocols and platforms for efficient collaboration. Another challenge lies in aligning AI-driven methodologies with the established good practices and workflows of drug discovery. The field of drug discovery is heavily regulated, and there are stringent guidelines and constraints that must be adhered to. Integrating AI approaches into this framework necessitates careful consideration to ensure compliance with regulations without compromising the efficacy and safety of the drug design process (Avacharmal et al.2023). To address these challenges and demonstrate the potential benefits of AI-driven drug discovery, successful case studies and their applications are imperative. These case studies serve as powerful illustrations of the immense time-saving potential, with estimates suggesting at least a ten-year reduction in the extensive drug design process. In summary, the integration of AI in drug discovery has revolutionized the early stages of the process. However, it also presents several obstacles that must be overcome for its successful implementation. Overcoming these challenges requires the development of robust bioinformatic methods, ensuring data quality and sharing, and aligning AI-driven methodologies with existing good practices and regulatory requirements. Nonetheless, the potential timesaving and advancements offered by AI in drug design serve as strong motivation to persist in overcoming these obstacles.

4. AI APPLICATIONS IN DRUG TARGET IDENTIFICATION AND VALIDATION

AI applications in drug target identification and validation represent one of the key technological leaps that will significantly shape the landscape of pharmaceutical research and development in the upcoming years. These groundbreaking applications can be observed within a wide range of areas such as predictive modeling, advanced machine learning techniques, and sophisticated data mining processes. With the integration of AI, researchers have unlocked the potential for a more comprehensive and robust analysis of diverse genomic and proteomic data, revolutionizing the field. The power of AI-driven drug target prediction studies is evident in their ability to accurately identify and pinpoint highly promising targets. When compared to traditional strategies, these AI-powered approaches have demonstrated unparalleled precision and enhanced efficiency in uncovering potential drug targets. This breakthrough holds immense promise for accelerating the development of innovative therapies and treatments. Furthermore, the implementation of AI-driven target validation techniques has proven to be a game-changer in expediting the validation phase of potential target involvement in specific pathologies. By harnessing various computational and IT-driven solutions, researchers can simulate and explore the effects of over- or under-activity of a target. These simulations, whether based on rule-based algorithms or machine learning algorithms, provide invaluable insights and assist in a more thorough understanding of the complex interactions within biological systems. By leveraging AI in drug target identification and validation, researchers are better equipped with the tools necessary to unravel the intricate nature of diseases and develop precision-targeted treatments. The transformative impact of AI in this domain is poised to revolutionize not only the speed and accuracy of drug discovery, but also the overall optimization of healthcare outcomes. As AI continues to evolve and advance, it holds the potential to open up new frontiers in pharmaceutical research and shape a future where personalized medicine is truly within reach (Huang et al.2024).

Several AI-driven drug target identification case studies provide strong evidence on the potential for the use of these technologies in quickly generating target hypotheses. These studies have demonstrated the accuracy and reliability of screening methods to predict hits from the outset. Furthermore, there is a profound correlation between the compounds that have entered the validation process, and the value attributed to these targets. In the aforementioned study, a fascinating inverse relationship was observed between the number of targets introduced in a specific year and the number of drugs emerging from these targets and making their way into the market years later. It appears that by reducing the number of targets within the system, a remarkable increase in terms of relevance can be achieved (Han et al., 2023). Examples of drugs that have been developed with the support of computational methodologies, partially employing AI, can be found throughout the pharmaceutical landscape. One noteworthy instance involved a drug development project that commenced as far back as 1993. The data gathered from this endeavor vividly depicts how AI drastically reduced the overall development time, while simultaneously elevating the success rate. This breakthrough, however, also brings attention to the potential regulatory considerations associated with AI approaches. As these technologies heavily rely on datasets, it becomes crucial to acknowledge and address any implicit or explicit built-in biases they may carry. Hence, it is imperative to exercise caution and thorough scrutiny when utilizing predictive aging datasets, for they possess an exceptionally high probability of containing biases. It is prudent to refrain from drawing conclusive and detailed regulatory prospects from such datasets at this relatively early stage. Instead, a promising future awaits, where AI in collaboration with pharmaceutical industries and competent regulatory authorities will foster a platform for the exchange of valuable experiences, consolidating wide-ranging conclusions. In this manner, the most recent advancements and developments in the field can be effectively taken into consideration (Mhlanga, 2021). With respect to target validation, the utilization of advanced techniques, often rooted in physics or system biology, can yield invaluable discriminatory power, significantly impacting the outcome of the validation process. The experts surveyed overwhelmingly affirm the positive influence of predictive approaches on target identification. Such approaches have expedited the recognition of consequential factors and have facilitated the swift elimination of inadequate targets that have progressed to phase 2 of development. The data obtained from phase 2 trials plays a pivotal role in determining the prediction of "overall survival." Demonstrating the relevance and clinical significance of a phase 2 trial is primarily gauged by the extent to which "overall survival" is established. The stronger the association between the prediction of survival and the satisfactory results obtained, the greater the assurance of the effectiveness of future phase 3 developments (Oladoyinbo et al.2024). Another noteworthy aspect of predictive aging involves the inclusion of multiple survival curves for diverse diseases. By stratifying patients based on gender, age range, co-morbidities, smoking habits, prior therapies, HLA phenotype, genetic background, performance status, and biological markers, it becomes possible to estimate the clinical success of phase II trials and registration trials for new drugs. This stratification becomes particularly crucial in the context of multiple clinical trials conducted to combat serious diseases, such as cancer, which demand a greater level of confidence in the inferences drawn regarding the prognosis. The partitioning of such stratification provides a robust measure to evaluate the effectiveness of personalized medicine. Naturally, in studies pertaining to overall survival, which persist for an average of at least five years for diseases with a positive prognosis or preferably at least six months for rare diseases, the definitions and assessments can only be made through frequent updates. These updates are executed throughout the entire study, enabling a more expeditious conclusion towards a therapeutic course (Baron et al.2023).

5. AI IN CLINICAL TRIAL OPTIMIZATION

Although deep learning and other machine learning algorithms are not widely used in clinical research, there are a number of ways in which AI methodologies could optimize clinical trial performance and maximize enrollment of carefully selected groups of patients. One way is to predict enrollment challenges ahead of time. For instance, these algorithms could search for variables that have historically been especially difficult to accommodate in clinical trials and screen out patients if the trial recruitment rate has started to slow. They can also predict an individual patient's risk of having a headache, and if it is very low, may leave that patient out of a control arm of a trial comparing whether or not a medication is likely to trigger a headache. Given that nearly half of clinical trials are permanently halted before they are completed due to slow recruitment, these methodologies may be used to considerably reduce the morbidity and the economic costs due to the inefficiency stemming from participant dropouts in trials. The accelerated time to market due to the implementation of these technologies may also result in significant savings. Using the same models, clinical trials may be monitored more accurately in real time and may also be designed with adaptive elements. Studies with adaptive designs have improved participant care and reduced the size and cost of clinical trials. However, ethical considerations are also involved. While AI can be used to identify patients for clinical trials, it can also be used preemptively to impede access to a trial for fears of a negative outcome, and patients may not provide informed consent if these additional exclusion/warning criteria are kept confidential. Nonetheless, these technologies promise to further the future of an otherwise slow-moving and traditionally conservative field. By leveraging the power of AI and machine learning, clinical trials can potentially revolutionize the healthcare industry, enabling more precise and effective treatments to be developed and brought to market faster. With the ability to predict and address enrollment challenges, closely monitor the progress of trials, and optimize patient selection, AI methodologies have the potential to greatly improve the efficiency, accuracy, and cost-effectiveness of clinical research. This transformative shift could lead to better patient outcomes, reduced healthcare costs, and a more streamlined and productive research process. By embracing AI technologies, the field of clinical research has the opportunity to usher in a new era of innovation and advancement that has the potential to benefit both (Uzzan et al.2023).

6. ETHICAL CONSIDERATIONS IN AI-DRIVEN PHARMACEUTICAL RESEARCH

Given the scale and potential of AI technologies in pharmaceutical research and drug development, responsible innovation is absolutely essential. The ethical considerations that accompany AI are of utmost importance, as they address concerns regarding privacy, consent, and the ethical and equitable practices of data-sharing and management. It is crucial to recognize that AI algorithms are only as good as the data they are based on and the individuals who create and train them. Consequently, these algorithms can reflect human biases, which is why it is imperative to encourage transparent AI processes in order to foster trust among all stakeholders involved. Furthermore, the utilization of AI in pharmaceutical marketing and sales applications is not without controversy, as it raises legitimate concerns about patient well-being and equal access to healthcare for all individuals. The immense power of AI technologies in drug development decision-making continues to evolve, with the potential to greatly impact health outcomes and streamline patient stratification decisions. However, maintaining transparency in AI decision-making processes is of the utmost importance. While achieving accountability can be challenging due to the inherent 'black box' nature of AI, it is crucial to establish internal life sciences standards and governance protocols. This will define the extent to which AI is integrated into scientific decision-making processes and establish internal guidelines. We fully acknowledge the need for extensive ethical deliberation in the development of AI technology, particularly in terms of promoting stakeholder input, especially from patients themselves. This survey serves as an important reminder of the necessity to engage policymakers in order to standardize approaches, particularly at the country level. Additionally, it is crucial to streamline discussions and definitions between regulatory agencies to effectively govern the use of AI in drug development. Finally, we strongly encourage industry to strike a delicate balance between innovation and regulation. Regulators should also serve as valuable sources of information regarding the implementation and impact of ethical AI principles in drug development, drawing upon their extensive practices and responsibilities. Furthermore, the attainment of these goals may necessitate additional research in areas such as ethical considerations and patient involvement in the development and application of AI. We firmly believe that a proactive approach, combined with a careful balance between risk and ethical concerns, the interests of all stakeholders, and scientific considerations, is absolutely necessary in order to effectively address and overcome these barriers and pave the way for responsible and impactful AI integration in pharmaceutical research and drug development (Kumar et al., 2023).

7. REGULATORY COMPLIANCE AND GUIDELINES IN AI RESEARCH

Existing regulatory requirements are designed to ensure the safety, reliability, and efficacy of interventions in clinical practice. Ensuring compliance with these regulations is crucial in all AI applications in pharmaceutical research. In the current regulatory environment, algorithms are used as a medical product, just like the pharmaceutical products they support, whether used in basic research, the discovery phase, or employed as decision support tools in clinical programs. At the same time, this is an evolving field with regulatory agencies across the globe working tirelessly to provide clear and comprehensive guidelines on AI-related research, with limited intervention to test only to date. As technology continues to advance at a rapid pace, it is essential for regulatory bodies to stay updated and adapt their frameworks, accordingly, ensuring that AI-driven solutions in the pharmaceutical industry adhere to the highest standards of quality, safety, and effectiveness. Furthermore, collaborative efforts are being made by governments and industry leaders to promote international harmonization in regulatory approaches, fostering a globally unified approach to AI implementation in healthcare. By doing so, we can ensure that AI technologies not only accelerate medical advancements but also enhance patient care and outcomes on a global scale (Bhattamisra et al.2023).

The relevance and expanded regulatory access lie in the oversight role taken by regulators in governing AI-driven drug development processes through accelerated approval of, for example, AI trial designs, AI data acquisition systems using digital endpoints, and AI-based modeling for submission across numerous domains. As this trend continues, there will be increased scrutiny of algorithms themselves, including their software, data, and even human-algorithm interfaces. One of the key challenges in applying established medical product regulations to AI research may be ambiguity and inconsistency in the guidelines across different regulatory environments and communities. The evolution of scientific and regulatory guidelines is also slow compared to the rapid pace of AI innovation. Furthermore, we experiment and develop our AI in real time; while complying with the lack of automated or clear recall guidelines, the operation of any AI or learning system is at an arm's length from immediate intervention. It is important to evaluate that your system is conducting its experiments in a way that meets regulatory standards for the study conditions you are running it in. This is also a universal requirement across all regulatory relevant domains (Gadade et al.2024). In order to ensure compliance and adherence to regulations, it is of utmost importance to have a thorough and all-encompassing comprehension of the intricate and complex nature of AI-driven drug development processes. The expansion of regulatory access becomes indispensable and absolutely essential, as it not only empowers and enables regulators to possess a more profound and extensive level of involvement but also grants them an enhanced and augmented capacity to exercise stringent oversight throughout these multifaceted processes. By possessing a crystal-clear and unambiguous understanding of the intricacies and nuances of AI trial designs, regulators are equipped with the necessary tools and knowledge to effectively and meticulously evaluate and assess the safety, efficacy, and reliability of ground-breaking and innovative drugs that are meticulously formulated and developed through the utilization of AI technology (Meskó & Topol, 2023). Furthermore, the utilization of artificial intelligence data acquisition systems utilizing digital endpoints provides regulators with highly valuable and insightful information on the overall performance and effectiveness of these pharmaceutical drugs. By thoroughly analyzing the data generated by AI, regulators can effectively detect and pinpoint any potential risks or adverse effects that might be correlated with the consumption of these drugs, thus enabling them to enforce and establish enhanced safety protocols and precautionary measures that aim to safeguard the well-being and welfare of individuals. The utilization of AI-powered data acquisition systems acts as a game-changer for regulators, as it equips them with a comprehensive understanding of the intricate nuances and complexities surrounding these medications, thus empowering them to proactively address any emerging concerns and ensure the utmost safety and efficacy of such pharmaceutical products. (Padmanaban2023) Additionally, the implementation of AI-based modeling systems in various domains presents regulators with an incredibly potent instrument that aids in the meticulous evaluation of drug development data quality and reliability. The utilization of these advanced AI models empowers regulators to thoroughly scrutinize the submitted data, guaranteeing that the entire drug development process is carried out with utmost precision and adherence to scientific principles. With the assistance of AI, regulators can make informed decisions based on the accuracy and validity of the data, thereby promoting a more robust and trustworthy drug development landscape (Larson et al.2021). However, as the role and involvement of AI in drug development processes continue to expand and grow exponentially, there is an undeniable and pressing need for increased scrutiny and diligent analysis of the algorithms themselves. Regulators must undertake comprehensive and meticulous assessments of the intricate software and meticulously examined, and thoroughly scrutinized data utilized within AI systems in order to guarantee their utmost integrity, credibility, and trustworthiness. Furthermore, it is imperatively crucial to meticulously and meticulously scrutinize and carefully examine the human-algorithm interface to holistically comprehend the magnitude of human involvement and its profound potential impact on the comprehensive and all-encompassing drug development process as a whole. This critical evaluation and exhaustive exploration are essential to ensure the seamless progress and advancement of the pharmaceutical industry and the continuous improvement of drug discovery and development methodologies (Mak et al.2024). A significant challenge in applying established medical product regulations to AI research is the ambiguity and inconsistency in guidelines across different regulatory environments and communities. This lack of harmonization can lead to confusion and hinder the efficient regulation of AI-driven drug development. Efforts should be made to establish clear and standardized guidelines that can be universally applied, ensuring a cohesive and effective regulatory framework for AI research. It is crucial for regulatory bodies and stakeholders to collaborate and address this challenge in order to foster innovation, promote patient safety, and enhance public trust in the development and deployment of AI technologies in healthcare. By developing comprehensive and robust guidelines, regulatory authorities can streamline the evaluation and approval processes for AI-based medical products, facilitating their timely access to the market. This will contribute to advancing medical research, improving patient care, and ultimately benefiting society as a whole. In addition, the establishment of clear guidelines will also provide clarity and predictability for AI-driven drug development companies, enabling them to navigate the regulatory landscape with greater ease and certainty. By promoting consistency and harmonization in regulatory guidelines, we can create an environment that fosters responsible innovation, while ensuring the safety and efficacy of AI-driven medical products. With the rapid advancements in AI technology, it is essential to adapt regulatory frameworks to keep pace with these developments and leverage the full potential of AI in healthcare. By doing so, we can harness the power of AI to transform healthcare delivery, enhance diagnostics, personalize treatments, and improve patient outcomes. However, it is important to strike a balance between regulation and innovation, ensuring that regulatory frameworks do not stifle creativity and hinder the progress of AI research. Collaboration between regulatory bodies, researchers, industry leaders, and other stakeholders is key to achieving this balance and overcoming the challenges associated with regulating AI in medicine. With a clear and standardized regulatory framework in place, we can create an environment where AI-driven medical products are developed, evaluated, and deployed in a responsible and beneficial manner, ultimately benefiting patients and society as a whole (Díaz-Rodríguez et al.2023). Furthermore, it is crucial to acknowledge that the slow evolution of scientific and regulatory guidelines, in comparison to the lightning-fast pace of AI innovation, brings forth yet another challenge in the realm of AI-driven drug development. With AI technology progressing at an unparalleled rate, it becomes imperative for regulations to stay abreast in order to guarantee the utmost safety and efficacy. To overcome this challenge, an ongoing and robust collaboration between regulatory bodies and scientific communities is of utmost importance. Through this collaboration, the gap between innovation and regulation can be effectively bridged, allowing for the seamless integration of AI in drug development while ensuring compliance with safety protocols and standards. Ultimately, this collaborative effort will serve as the cornerstone for the successful and responsible implementation of AI-driven advancements in the field of medicine and pharmaceuticals (Suriyaamporn et al.2024). Moreover, in the rapidly evolving field of artificial intelligence, the real-time experimentation and development of AI systems pose unprecedented challenges when it comes to ensuring compliance with recall guidelines. As AI operates independently and autonomously, there may be minimal opportunities for immediate intervention in the event of a malfunction or error. Hence, it becomes absolutely essential to thoroughly validate and verify that AI systems are carrying out experiments in a manner that strictly adheres to regulatory standards and study conditions. This critical requirement applies universally across various regulatory relevant domains, serving as a cornerstone for upholding the integrity and reliability of AI-driven drug development processes (Benjamens et al., 2020). In conclusion, the expansion of regulatory access plays a vital role in governing AI-driven drug development processes. Through accelerated approval, robust oversight, and scrutiny of algorithms, regulators can safeguard the safety, efficacy, and quality of AI-based drugs. Harmonization of guidelines and continuous collaboration between regulatory bodies and scientific communities are essential to address challenges and ensure effective regulation in an era of rapid AI innovation.

Research communities and international bodies concerned with harmonization are actively discussing the recommendations for responsible and beneficial development and deployment of AI in pharmaceutical research, and they advocate the substitution of well-developed guidelines to govern AI-based research within the pharmaceutical enterprise. In this discussion, a vision was provided for a one-size-fits-all AI and data-specific framework or guideline to exist under the International Council for

Harmonization of Requirements for Pharmaceuticals for Human Use, known as ICH AI, based on the accepted norm of human and automated model development and deployment. International regulatory collaboration in the elaboration of such frameworks is, therefore, crucial. In the context of global regulatory expectations of ICH AI, a suitable number of guidelines and several official channels are planned to initiate discussion of this content, and preparation in partnership with other ICH AI working groups, so that content is available for the next ICH meeting in the spring. This would also be applicable to the subset of AI involved in the development and validation of disease or other pharmaceutical AI, and, if not, how should they differ (Mirakhori & Niazi, 2024). The rapid advancement of artificial intelligence (AI) in pharmaceutical research has attracted significant attention and interest from research communities worldwide as well as international organizations that focus on harmonization and standardization efforts. This widespread interest has spurred active discussions within these circles regarding the responsible and advantageous development and utilization of AI in the field of pharmaceutical research. To address the various challenges and concerns associated with AI-based research in the pharmaceutical sector, experts propose the establishment of comprehensive guidelines that encompass regulations specifically tailored to AI and data-driven methodologies. The aim of these guidelines would be to provide a standardized framework that governs and guides the development, deployment, and overall implementation of AI technologies in pharmaceutical research. To achieve these objectives, the International Council for Harmonization of Requirements for Pharmaceuticals for Human Use, commonly known as the ICH AI, would play a central role in overseeing the development and implementation of these guidelines. Creating and implementing such a comprehensive framework hinge on building upon the existing best practices and experiences gained from both human-driven and automated model development and deployment. By learning from these experiences, it becomes possible to establish a robust, adaptive, and efficient regulatory system that effectively addresses the unique challenges posed by AI in pharmaceutical research (Gornet & Maxwell, 2024). Given the increasingly interconnected and rapidly evolving landscape of pharmaceutical research and the widespread implementation and utilization of cutting-edge AI technologies, fostering robust and seamless international regulatory collaboration has become an imperative and indispensable endeavor of utmost significance. The construction and establishment of these all-encompassing and intricate frameworks undeniably require dynamic engagement, proactive participation, and harmonious cooperation of regulatory bodies, esteemed research organizations, leading pharmaceutical companies, and a multitude of other key stakeholders, all operating on a truly global stage. It is through such multifaceted international collaboration that the incorporation of diverse perspectives, expertise, and novel insights can be effectively achieved and harnessed, ultimately culminating in the formulation of comprehensive and authoritative guidelines that are not merely efficacious and efficient, but also universally embraced, adhered to, and championed within the ever-evolving realm of pharmaceutical research and development (Desai et al.2024). In conclusion, the increasing prominence of AI in pharmaceutical research highlights the need for comprehensive guidelines to govern and facilitate its responsible and beneficial development and deployment. By adopting these guidelines, the pharmaceutical sector can leverage the power of AI while ensuring necessary regulations are in place. International regulatory collaboration is vital for successfully creating these frameworks, as it brings together the collective expertise and experiences of various stakeholders from around the world, ultimately driving the advancement and harmonization of AI in pharmaceutical research. Considering the immense global regulatory expectations of the International Council for Harmonization of Technical Requirements for Pharmaceuticals for Human Use (ICH), an array of comprehensive guidelines and official channels are currently being strategically planned to expedite and foster meaningful discussions surrounding this immensely crucial and pertinent topic. The ultimate objective is to diligently prepare and equip ourselves in close collaboration with other ICH AI working groups, ensuring that the content is conveniently accessible for meticulous scrutiny and thoughtful contemplation during the highly anticipated ICH meeting slated for the blossoming season of spring. These extraordinary discussions and meticulously crafted guidelines encompass not only the realm of state-of-the-art AI applications fervently driven towards the development and meticulous validation of pharmaceutical therapies but also transcend the boundaries of traditional medical research by ingeniously incorporating AI methodologies in the realm of disease elucidation and groundbreaking explorations of pharmaceutical-related fields. The overarching aim is to craft and establish an unparalleled unified approach to the impeccable governance of AI technologies in these groundbreaking areas, and furthermore, any potential discrepancies in the regulatory landscape will be examined with utmost scrupulousness, effectively addressed, and thoughtfully harmonized to foster unparalleled synchronicity and flawless standardization (Bade & Tomomewo, 2024).

8. IMPACT OF AI ON DRUG DEVELOPMENT PROCESSES

Artificial Intelligence (AI) has the incredible potential to meaningfully accelerate, improve, and transform the intricate and multifaceted drug discovery and development process at all stages. This encompassing process starts from the crucial drug target identification, progresses through pre-clinical drug development and meticulous clinical trials, and extends all the way to post-marketing surveillance. Harnessing the power of AI in this realm can yield remarkable outcomes by significantly reducing the time and cost associated with the arduous task of developing new drugs. Studies have revealed the extraordinary advantages of incorporating AI in drug discovery projects. Research indicates that projects employing AI exhibit a greater likelihood of advancing to clinical trials compared to those not utilizing this groundbreaking technology. As AI technology continually progresses and matures in the ever-evolving drug discovery market, the potential for remarkable precision medicines and targeted interventions aligned with the individual patient's genetic and lifestyle profile expands exponentially. This promising development has the potential to revolutionize the field of medicine by delivering highly personalized and tailored treatments to patients, maximizing the efficacy and optimizing the outcomes (Raparthi et al.2022). Endowed with its vast computational capabilities, AI can revolutionize the process of drug discovery and development by expediting and enhancing the understanding of complex biological systems. By scrutinizing extensive datasets and identifying intricate patterns that might otherwise go unnoticed, AI algorithms can unlock invaluable insights, enabling researchers to make informed decisions and advancements. Furthermore, AI can aid in the prediction of drug safety, potential adverse effects, and drug interactions, facilitating a more comprehensive understanding of the potential risks and benefits associated with specific medications. This augmented understanding empowers healthcare professionals to make sound and evidence-based choices that prioritize patient safety and well-being. Moreover, the integration of AI in drug discovery holds considerable potential for streamlining the entire research and development pipeline. By automating tedious and time-intensive tasks, AI technology can free up researchers' invaluable time, enabling them to focus on more intellectually demanding endeavors and critical decision-making processes. This accelerated workflow, combined with the incredibly insightful analysis provided by AI, has the power to revolutionize the pace and efficiency of drug development, potentially leading to the expedited introduction of life-saving medications to those in dire need (Vatansever et al.2021). In conclusion, the implementation of AI in the drug discovery and development process represents a monumental leap forward in transforming the field of medicine. From expediting drug target identification to optimizing clinical trials and beyond, AI offers unprecedented avenues for progress and innovation. The remarkable potential of AI to reduce time, costs, and risks associated with drug development and to usher in an era of personalized medicine is both awe-inspiring and incredibly promising. As AI technology continues to flourish and evolve, its capacity to guide the creation of novel and targeted interventions will undoubtedly shape the future of healthcare, benefiting countless patients worldwide.

The AI can also assist with selecting the right patients for clinical trial participation, thereby improving trial results. The appropriate use of big data and AI in clinical trial design could reduce total trial costs significantly. People are critical of applying AI, knowing that it can be amoral, dehumanizing, and can cause programming errors or biases, and then firms take it and use it in places it was not designed for. It is good to see that the top pharmaceutical companies are slowly getting into collaborations with companies that specialize in advanced technologies to integrate them with their complex business models, thereby using the integrated processes across the entire drug journey more effectively. For workflow considerations, further change is needed in terms of training and HR policies. AI companies need to provide overall shift readiness training to staff changing roles and help them establish a lifecycle of work and continuing education. Reinforcement of learning AI should be encouraged. It enhances our ability to understand complex software systems as they involve algorithms for which machine learning will always underpin their accuracy and usefulness. It's clear that the industry agrees that AI has potential (Vasey et al.2022).

9. AI'S ROLE IN PERSONALIZED MEDICINE

Personalized medicine tailors treatments individually to patients, optimizing the benefits of a therapeutic approach while minimizing adverse effects. The potential impact of Artificial Intelligence (AI) in such an approach is nothing short of revolutionary. In this context, AI enables the interrogation of diffuse data sets in silico, spanning fields such as genomics, imaging, high-throughput phenotyping, and electronic health records. By doing so, it identifies unique features of individuals that have the potential to predict their response or resilience to different therapies. The power of machine learning models comes into play as they can be trained to make alternative treatment choices. This is especially crucial when disease presents itself in unusual and hidden ways. By analyzing complex disease-associated datasets, these models can extract features that have the capability to predict patients' responses. Furthermore, through network training, we can even identify biomarkers of diseases prior to the manifestation of any phenotypic traits. Perhaps the most significant aspect is that the predictions generated by AI at each of these intersecting points can be subjected to prospective validation in clinical trials. This ensures that the efficacy and reliability of these predictions are thoroughly evaluated before being implemented in clinical practice. The potential for AI in the field of personalized medicine is truly groundbreaking, offering a glimpse into a future where treatments are tailored to the specific needs of each patient, resulting in improved outcomes and enhanced patient care (Janosevic et al., 2024).

The wide-ranging and extensive utilization of data in the structuring of health care services, coupled with the highly advanced dynamic system design implemented to comprehensively cover nearly all aspects of health care, gives rise to a multitude of profound implications. One such implication is the potential necessity for consent that extends well beyond the realm of traditional research scenarios and surpasses the specific utilization of individual data. This consent will not only encompass areas of health care delivery that do not involve the dissemination or examination of novel treatments, but it will also expand to cover various other domains. Furthermore, the preservation of data privacy is poised to gain increasing significance in the eyes of people, prompting health care professionals to grapple with predictable and scientifically-derived concerns regarding the potential exploitation of predictive data in areas such as discrimination within credit and insurance markets, among others. Notably, certain projects entail collaborative research endeavors involving artificial intelligence (AI) systems and individual participants, their joint efforts aimed at showcasing the efficacy of functioning AI systems in the domain of personalized medicine. The pivotal role of these projects lies in their provision of user-friendly interfaces for clinic staff, thus facilitating the utilization of crucial disease maps that effectively integrate clinical cells with biological insights (Abulibdeh et al., 2024).

Artificial intelligence (AI) in personalized medicine has the immense potential to greatly support and assist physicians in their clinical practice. By offering positive and invaluable advice, AI can guide and counsel healthcare professionals towards the most effective interventions within their own clinics and practices. Additionally, AI empowers physicians by providing them with highly insightful intraclinic economic analyses and assessments, granting them the ability to comprehensively evaluate and analyze the various potential benefits and advantages derived from AI-based interventions and treatments. This transformative and groundbreaking integration of AI interventions can be further augmented, enhanced, and customized through modified AI-driven predictions, which accurately and meticulously forecast and anticipate likely patient responses and outcomes based on advanced digital biomarkers. This remarkable and exceptional capability serves as a truly transformative and revolutionary approach to stratify and categorize patients for appropriate interventions and treatments, effectively shifting and transforming the existing paradigm of passive patients to becoming actively engaged and involved participants in their own healthcare journey. Through this remarkable and cutting-edge utilization of AI technology, the future of personalized medicine becomes even more promising and exciting, with physicians and healthcare providers at the forefront of a new era of healthcare innovation and advancement (Alowais et al., 2023). Undoubtedly, the ultimate success and realization of personalized medicine's full potential will necessitate a robust and synergistic partnership between the tenets of good clinical practice and the limitless opportunities presented by AI. Through this profound collaboration, a new era of healthcare can emerge, where the benefits of personalized medicine are seamlessly harnessed and amplified by the indomitable power of AI-driven advancements. Together, these forces will shape the future of medicine, revolutionizing patient care and propelling the boundaries of human health and well-being to unprecedented heights. In this extraordinary union, the convergence of personalized medicine and AI will unlock boundless possibilities never before envisioned by mankind. The blend of their distinctive capabilities will not only enhance the precision and effectiveness of diagnosis and treatment but also spawn innovative approaches that transcend the current boundaries of medical science. As personalized medicine and AI join forces, a symbiotic relationship will gradually unfold, bolstered by the rich tapestry woven from the integration of genetic data, advanced algorithms, and machine learning. This amalgamation of cutting-edge technologies will propel the evolution of medical practices, igniting a revolution that transcends conventional models of healthcare. The transformative power of personalized medicine, when united with the inexorable force of AI, will bring forth a new dawn in patient care. The synergistic alignment of these two revolutionary pillars will harness the potential to elucidate intricate patterns, develop tailor-made treatments, and forecast disease progression with unparalleled accuracy. The walls that confine traditional healthcare will crumble, allowing for individualized interventions that address the precise needs of patients, paving the way for unprecedented levels of wellness and vitality (Arin, 2023). While the horizon shimmers with the promise of personalized medicine and the limitless realm of AI, it is essential to recognize the critical role that comprehensive clinical practice and ethical considerations play in this collaboration. The embrace of rigorous research, harmonized regulations, and meticulous oversight will consolidate the groundbreaking opportunities offered by the fusion of personalized medicine and AI, ensuring the protection of patient rights and the preservation of ethical standards. In this momentous symphony that harmonizes personalized medicine and AI, the orchestra of science and technology will rise to crescendo, enveloping the field of healthcare in an awe-inspiring melody. Our journey towards an era where each treatment is intricately tailored, and each patient's journey is amplified by the omnipotent capabilities of AI, holds within it the potential to redefine the boundaries of human health and well-being. May we march forward with unwavering determination, propelled by the pioneering collaboration between personalized medicine and AI, towards a future where the harmonious symphony of science and technology orchestrates a world of boundless possibilities. A world where every individual receives the precise care they need, and the transformative potential of personalized medicine flourishes, augmented by the extraordinary power of AI-driven innovations (Osasona et al.2024).

10. ARTIFICIAL INTELLIGENCE (AI) IN GENE THERAPY

In gene therapy, an innovative approach that has shown extraordinary promise, there has been a remarkable enhancement in precision and efficacy when administering treatments. This cutting-edge technology has been further revolutionized by the integration of AI, which has transformed the way therapeutic interventions are delivered, surpassing previous levels of accuracy and efficiency. As a result, treatment plans are optimized to a degree where they can be precisely tailored to individual patients' specific genetic profiles, thus leading to the creation of personalized and highly effective gene therapy interventions that hold immense promise for the future (Zeb et al., 2024). Furthermore, AI in gene therapy not only facilitates personalized treatment approaches but also paves the way for innovative discoveries and breakthroughs. By leveraging AI, researchers are able to identify novel gene targets and gain a deeper understanding of complex genetic mechanisms. The ability to analyze and interpret intricate genetic data sets opens new avenues for the development of advanced gene therapies, offering hope for previously untreatable diseases and conditions. In addition to its impact on treatment strategies and scientific advancements, AI in gene therapy also plays a vital role in enhancing patient care and outcomes. Through AI-powered systems, healthcare professionals can monitor patients' genetic profiles in real-time, enabling early detection of potential genetic risks and promptly adjusting treatment plans accordingly. This proactive approach to patient care not only improves the chances of successful treatment outcomes but also enhances overall patient experience and satisfaction (Rasool et al.2024). As the field of gene therapy continues to evolve, the integration of AI will undoubtedly be instrumental in driving progress and expanding our understanding of genetic diseases. The combination of AI's analytical capabilities and genetic expertise holds the potential to revolutionize the diagnosis, treatment, and prevention of a wide range of genetic conditions, marking a paradigm shift in healthcare as we know it (Ozcelik et al.2024). In summary, it can be said that the integration of artificial intelligence (AI) in gene therapy has brought about a revolutionary transformation in this field. By significantly enhancing precision, efficacy, and personalized care, AI has proven to be a valuable tool. Its remarkable ability to analyze vast genetic datasets empowers healthcare professionals to make targeted decisions and develop optimized treatment plans. The incorporation of AI in gene therapy research has also presented the potential to uncover significant discoveries that were previously unforeseen, thereby opening new avenues for the treatment of untreatable diseases. Looking ahead, with further advancements, AI will undoubtedly continue to reshape the landscape of gene therapy, driving progress, and ultimately leading to improved patient outcomes (Eskandar, 2023).

Artificial intelligence (AI) has indisputably and remarkably transformed the domain of pharmaceutical research by affording the opportunity for expedited and exceedingly precise drug discovery procedures. Such an advancement has paved the way for accelerated and methodical breakthroughs, offering immense potential for revolutionizing medical treatments. The integration of AI in pharmaceutical research has revolutionized the industry, propelling it into a new era of efficiency and innovation. With AI-powered algorithms analyzing vast amounts of data, drug discovery has become faster and more accurate than ever before. This technological leap has opened doors to groundbreaking discoveries and enhanced treatment options for patients worldwide. By leveraging AI's computational power, researchers can navigate complex molecular structures, predict drug interactions, and identify potential targets with unprecedented precision. These advancements not only save valuable time but also reduce costs and resources required for traditional trial-and-error methods. The ability of AI to rapidly analyze and process vast quantities of data has also accelerated the identification of potential drug candidates that may have previously gone unnoticed. This has led to the discovery of novel compounds and therapeutic approaches, some of which have already shown promising results in clinical trials. Moreover, AI has also played a crucial role in personalized medicine, tailoring treatments to individual patients based on their genetic makeup and specific healthcare needs. By analyzing genetic data and patient records, AI algorithms can identify patterns and predict optimal treatment strategies, providing targeted therapies that maximize effectiveness and minimize side effects. In addition to drug discovery, AI has also revolutionized other aspects of pharmaceutical research, such as drug repurposing and adverse event detection (Patel & Shah, 2022). By mining databases and analyzing real-world patient data, AI can identify existing drugs that could be repurposed for new therapeutic applications, saving time and resources in the drug development pipeline. Furthermore, AI-powered algorithms can detect and predict adverse events or potential drug interactions, enabling early intervention and improved patient safety. The integration of AI in pharmaceutical research has not only expedited the drug discovery process but has also enhanced our understanding of disease mechanisms and paved the way for new treatment paradigms. With AI's continuous development and refinement, we can expect even more significant advancements in the future, changing the landscape of healthcare and improving patient outcomes on a global scale (Yadav et al., 2024).

REFERENCES

Abulibdeh, A., Zaidan, E., & Abulibdeh, R. (2024). Navigating the confluence of artificial intelligence and education for sustainable development in the era of industry 4.0: Challenges, opportunities, and ethical dimensions. *Journal of Cleaner Production*. https://doi.org/10.1016/j.jclepro.2023.140527

Alowais, S. A., Alghamdi, S. S., Alsuhebany, N., Alqahtani, T., Alshaya, A. I., Almohareb, S. N., Aldairem, A., Alrashed, M., Bin Saleh, K., Badreldin, H. A., Al Yami, M. S., Al Harbi, S., & Albekairy, A. M. (2023). Revolutionizing healthcare: The role of artificial intelligence in clinical practice. *BMC Medical Education*, 23(1), 689. DOI: 10.1186/s12909-023-04698-z PMID: 37740191

Arin, H. (2023). *AI and the Human Experience: Embracing the Age of Intelligent Machines*.

Avacharmal, R., Pamulaparthyvenkata, S., & Gudala, L. (2023). Unveiling the Pandora's Box: A Multifaceted Exploration of Ethical Considerations in Generative AI for Financial Services and Healthcare. *Hong Kong Journal of AI and Medicine*, 3(1), 84–99.

Bade, S. O., & Tomomewo, O. S. (2024). A review of governance strategies, policy measures, and regulatory framework for hydrogen energy in the United States. *International Journal of Hydrogen Energy*, 78, 1363–1381. DOI: 10.1016/j.ijhydene.2024.06.338

Baron, R., Dickenson, A. H., Calvo, M., Dib-Hajj, S. D., & Bennett, D. L. (2023). Maximizing treatment efficacy through patient stratification in neuropathic pain trials. *Nature Reviews. Neurology*, 19(1), 53–64. DOI: 10.1038/s41582-022-00741-7 PMID: 36400867

Benjamens, S., Dhunnoo, P., & Meskó, B. (2020). The state of artificial intelligence-based FDA-approved medical devices and algorithms: an online database. *NPJ digital medicine*.

Bhattamisra, S. K., Banerjee, P., Gupta, P., Mayuren, J., Patra, S., & Candasamy, M. (2023). Artificial intelligence in pharmaceutical and healthcare research. *Big Data and Cognitive Computing*, 7(1), 10. DOI: 10.3390/bdcc7010010

Blanco-Gonzalez, A., Cabezon, A., Seco-Gonzalez, A., Conde-Torres, D., Antelo-Riveiro, P., Pineiro, A., & Garcia-Fandino, R. (2023). The role of AI in drug discovery: Challenges, opportunities, and strategies. *Pharmaceuticals (Basel, Switzerland)*, 16(6), 891. DOI: 10.3390/ph16060891 PMID: 37375838

Dara, S., Dhamercherla, S., Jadav, S. S., Babu, C. M., & Ahsan, M. J. (2022). Machine learning in drug discovery: A review. *Artificial Intelligence Review*, 55(3), 1947–1999. DOI: 10.1007/s10462-021-10058-4

Desai, N., Pande, S., Gholap, A. D., Rana, D., Salave, S., & Vora, L. K. (2024). Regulatory processes involved in clinical trials and intellectual property rights around vaccine development. In *Advanced Vaccination Technologies for Infectious and Chronic Diseases* (279–309). Academic Press.DOI: 10.1016/B978-0-443-18564-9.00008-4

Díaz-Rodríguez, N., Del Ser, J., Coeckelbergh, M., de Prado, M. L., Herrera-Viedma, E., & Herrera, F. (2023). Connecting the dots in trustworthy Artificial Intelligence: From AI principles, ethics, and key requirements to responsible AI systems and regulation. *Information Fusion*, 99, 101896. DOI: 10.1016/j.inffus.2023.101896

Eskandar, K. (2023). Revolutionizing biotechnology and bioengineering: unleashing the power of innovation. *Journal of Applied Biotechnology and Bioengineering. 10*(3):81–88.

Gadade, D. D., Kulkarni, D. A., Raj, R., Patil, S. G., & Modi, A. (2024). Pushing Boundaries: The Landscape of AI-Driven Drug Discovery and Development with Insights Into Regulatory Aspects. In Khanna, A., El Barachi, M., Jain, S., Kumar, M., & Nayyar, A. (Eds.), *Artificial Intelligence and Machine Learning in Drug Design and Development* (533-561). https://doi.org/10.1002/9781394234196.ch17

Gornet, M. & Maxwell, W. (2024). The European approach to regulating AI through technical standards. *Internet Policy Review.*

Han, R., Yoon, H., Kim, G., Lee, H., & Lee, Y. (2023). Revolutionizing medicinal chemistry: the application of artificial intelligence (AI) in early drug discovery. *Pharmaceuticals, 16*(9):1259. 10.3390/ph16091259

Huang, D., Yang, M., Wen, X., Xia, S., & Yuan, B. (2024). AI-Driven Drug Discovery: Accelerating The Development Of Novel Therapeutics In Biopharmaceuticals. *Journal of Knowledge Learning and Science Technology, 3*(3), 206-224.

Janosevic, D., De Luca, T., Project, K. P. M., & Eadon, M. T. (2024). The Kidney Precision Medicine Project and Single-Cell Biology of the Injured Proximal Tubule. *The American Journal of Pathology.*

Jiménez-Luna, J., Grisoni, F., Weskamp, N., & Schneider, G. (2021). Artificial intelligence in drug discovery: Recent advances and future perspectives. *Expert Opinion on Drug Discovery*, 16(9), 949–959. DOI: 10.1080/17460441.2021.1909567 PMID: 33779453

Kumar, P., Dwivedi, Y. K., & Anand, A. (2023). Responsible artificial intelligence (AI) for value formation and market performance in healthcare: The mediating role of patient's cognitive engagement. *Information Systems Frontiers.*

Larson, D. B., Harvey, H., Rubin, D. L., Irani, N., Justin, R. T., & Langlotz, C. P. (2021). Regulatory frameworks for development and evaluation of artificial intelligence–based diagnostic imaging algorithms: Summary and recommendations. *Journal of the American College of Radiology*, 18(3), 413–424. DOI: 10.1016/j.jacr.2020.09.060 PMID: 33096088

Mak, K. K., Wong, Y. H., & Pichika, M. R. (2024). Artificial intelligence in drug discovery and development. In *Drug discovery and evaluation: safety and pharmacokinetic assays* (1461-1498). doi.org/10.1007/978-3-030-73317-9_92-1

Meskó, B. & Topol, E. J. (2023). The imperative for regulatory oversight of large language models (or generative AI) in healthcare. *NPJ digital medicine.*

Mhlanga, D. (2021). Artificial intelligence in the industry 4.0, and its impact on poverty, innovation, infrastructure development, and the sustainable development goals: Lessons from emerging economies? *Sustainability*. 10.3390/su13115788

Mirakhori, F., & Niazi, S. K. (2025). Harnessing the AI/ML in Drug and Biological Products Discovery and Development: The Regulatory Perspective. *Pharmaceuticals, 18*(1), 47. https://doi.org/10.3390/ph18010047

Nayarisseri, A., Khandelwal, R., Tanwar, P., Madhavi, M., Sharma, D., Thakur, G., & Singh, S. K. (2021). Artificial intelligence, big data and machine learning approaches in precision medicine & drug discovery. *Current Drug Targets*, 22(6), 631–655. DOI: 10.2174/18735592MTEzsMDMnz PMID: 33397265

Oladoyinbo, T. O., Olabanji, S. O., Olaniyi, O. O., Adebiyi, O. O., Okunleye, O. J., & Ismaila Alao, A. (2024). Exploring the challenges of artificial intelligence in data integrity and its influence on social dynamics. *Asian Journal of Advanced Research and Reports*, 18(2), 1–23. DOI: 10.9734/ajarr/2024/v18i2601

Osasona, F., Amoo, O. O., Atadoga, A., Abrahams, T. O., Farayola, O. A., & Ayinla, B. S. (2024). Reviewing the ethical implications of AI in decision making processes. *International Journal of Management & Entrepreneurship Research*, 6(2), 322–335. DOI: 10.51594/ijmer.v6i2.773

Ozcelik, F., Dundar, M. S., Yildirim, A. B., Henehan, G., Vicente, O., Sánchez-Alcázar, J. A., Gokce, N., Yildirim, D. T., Bingol, N. N., Karanfilska, D. P., Bertelli, M., Pojskic, L., Ercan, M., Kellermayer, M., Sahin, I. O., Greiner-Tollersrud, O. K., Tan, B., Martin, D., Marks, R., & Dundar, M. (2024). The impact and future of artificial intelligence in medical genetics and molecular medicine: An ongoing revolution. *Functional & Integrative Genomics*, 24(4), 138. DOI: 10.1007/s10142-024-01417-9 PMID: 39147901

Padmanaban, H. (2023). Navigating the intricacies of regulations: Leveraging AI/ML for Accurate Reporting. *Journal of Knowledge Learning and Science Technology, 2*(3), 401-412.

Pandey, M., Fernandez, M., Gentile, F., Isayev, O., Tropsha, A., Stern, A. C., & Cherkasov, A. (2022). The transformational role of GPU computing and deep learning in drug discovery. *Nature Machine Intelligence*, 4(3), 211–221.

Patel, V. & Shah, M. (2022). Artificial intelligence and machine learning in drug discovery and development. *Intelligent Medicine*.

Raparthi, M., Gayam, S. R., Nimmagadda, V. S. P., Sahu, M. K., Putha, S., Pattyam, S. P., & Kuna, S. S. (2022). AI assisted drug discovery: Emphasizing its role in accelerating precision medicine initiatives and improving treatment outcomes. *Human-Computer Interaction Perspectives*, 2(2), 1–10.

Rasool, S., Ali, M., Shahroz, H. M., Hussain, H. K., & Gill, A. Y. (2024). Innovations in AI-Powered Healthcare: Transforming Cancer Treatment with Innovative Methods. *BULLET: Jurnal Multidisiplin Ilmu*, 3(1), 118–128.

Schlander, M., Hernandez-Villafuerte, K., Cheng, C. Y., Mestre-Ferrandiz, J., & Baumann, M. (2021). How much does it cost to research and develop a new drug? A systematic review and assessment. *PharmacoEconomics*, 39(11), 1243–1269. DOI: 10.1007/s40273-021-01065-y PMID: 34368939

Selvaraj, C., Chandra, I., & Singh, S. K. (2021). Artificial intelligence and machine learning approaches for drug design: challenges and opportunities for the pharmaceutical industries. In *Molecular diversity*. doi.org/10.1007/s11030-021-10326-z

Suriyaamporn, P., Pamornpathomkul, B., Patrojanasophon, P., Ngawhirunpat, T., Rojanarata, T., & Opanasopit, P. (2024). The artificial intelligence-powered new era in pharmaceutical research and development: A review. *AAPS PharmSciTech*, 25(6), 188. DOI: 10.1208/s12249-024-02901-y PMID: 39147952

Uzzan, M., Bouhnik, Y., Abreu, M., Ahmad, H. A., Adsul, S., Carlier, H., Dubinsky, M., Germinaro, M., Jairath, V., Modesto, I., Mortensen, E., Narula, N., Neimark, E., Oortwijn, A., Protic, M., Rubin, D. T., Oh, Y. S., Wichary, J., Peyrin-Biroulet, L., & Reinisch, W. (2023). Declining enrolment and other challenges in IBD clinical trials: Causes and potential solutions. *Journal of Crohn's and Colitis*, 17(7), 1066–1078. DOI: 10.1093/ecco-jcc/jjad020 PMID: 36738443

Vasey, B., Nagendran, M., Campbell, B., Clifton, D. A., Collins, G. S., Denaxas, S., & McCulloch, P. (2022). Reporting guideline for the early stage clinical evaluation of decision support systems driven by artificial intelligence: DECIDE-AI. 10.1136/bmj-2022-070904

Vatansever, S., Schlessinger, A., Wacker, D., Kaniskan, H. Ü., Jin, J., Zhou, M. M., & Zhang, B. (2021). Artificial intelligence and machine learning-aided drug discovery in central nervous system diseases: State-of-the-arts and future directions. *Medicinal Research Reviews*, 41(3), 1427–1473. DOI: 10.1002/med.21764 PMID: 33295676

Yadav, S., Singh, A., Singhal, R., & Yadav, J. P. (2024). Revolutionizing drug discovery: The impact of artificial intelligence on advancements in pharmacology and the pharmaceutical industry. *Intelligent Pharmacy.*

Zeb, S., Nizamullah, F. N. U., Abbasi, N., & Fahad, M. (2024). AI in Healthcare: Revolutionizing Diagnosis and Therapy. *International Journal of Multidisciplinary Sciences and Arts*, 3(3), 118–128. DOI: 10.47709/ijmdsa.v3i3.4546

Chapter 2
AI in Clinical Trial Design and Patient Recruitment

Bancha Yingngam
https://orcid.org/0000-0001-7215-9123
Ubon Ratchathani University, Thailand

ABSTRACT

The application of artificial intelligence in the design and conduct of patient recruitment in clinical trials is targeted at addressing some of the key inefficiencies, including longer timelines and the lack of some participant characteristics. This chapter presents readers with the opportunities and advantages of using AI to make protocols more specific and execute patient recruitment more efficiently. This chapter integrates thorough discussions that explain how predictive analytics, machine learning, and other tools such as natural language processing can be used to identify participants and refine the design of trials. Moreover, this chapter contains a description of the use and results of AI implementation with the help of the provided case studies. In this way, it is possible to learn how to increase the efficiency of a trial, the number of sourced participants, and recruitment issues using AI technology. Ethical and regulatory issues are also discussed in this chapter, which provides an overview of the role and functions AI can play in the process of clinical trials.

INTRODUCTION

Artificial intelligence (AI) has substantially reshaped pharmaceutical research, claiming to be a tool for optimizing drug development and evaluation processes. By comparing traditional methods and AI-based approaches, one can determine how patient recruitment and clinical trial design have changed (Loomans et al., 2024). Before AI, some of these processes were ineffective, leading to both excessive

DOI: 10.4018/979-8-3693-6270-9.ch002

timelines and escalated costs. Furthermore, there was always a threat of under-enrollment and extensive dropout rates that could result in ineffective trials with no applicability in real-world scenarios (Williamson et al., 2024). However, AI has the potential to revolutionize this field, offering methods that will optimize these resources and time-devouring processes by creating extensive endpoints in clinical trial designs. The integration of AI ensured far better trial precision, providing comprehensive and scrupulous data analysis and complex predictive modeling. Such an approach allows AI to make automated decisions about the optimal patient candidate and then tailor clinical trial protocols regarding their specificities (Swathi & Kumar, 2024; X. Yao et al., 2024). Machine learning (ML) is used for sifting through extensive arrays of historical data obtained from previous trials to predict outcomes and suggest detailed protocols and participant candidate profiles. These implications are sure to reduce the cost and time consumption and increase the effectiveness and comprehensiveness of clinical trials (Miller et al., 2023). In this way, the period during which research and development efforts take place and the release of their respective treatments are likely to accelerate. Moreover, AI can be utilized to manage and process numerous big data arrays in real time, which will facilitate adaptive study designs. Such designs respond to various information they acquire throughout the study period, trying to ensure the scientific validity and ethical robustness of the study (Nene et al., 2024).

AI has a significant impact on the integration of both clinical trial design and patient recruitment in the process of conducting a clinical trial. In this way, the clinical trial is a process that consists of dozens of smaller tasks and meta-tasks, and even the clinical trial itself, in the final analysis, can be thought of as one large meta-task. The scheduling and length of the trial, its structure, methods, and incorporation of incentives and other factors all influence the final goal of the clinical trial. AI can help to easily and flexibly integrate the design of all these factors as applied to actual patients (Harrer et al., 2024). First, AI can be employed to analyze the data of clinical trials that have come before and use the available modern and real-world data on the possible course of such a trial given the specific conditions. This includes selecting the most precise biomarkers with the best predictive value for the tasks at hand. It also includes setting the most relevant parameters for the trial, such as the population to be invited, including and excluding patients based on their age, sex, and other, more precisely selected parameters (Ellen et al., 2024). In this way, AI has the potential to streamline and improve patient recruitment. The data that can be stored is almost unlimited, and information on tens or even hundreds of thousands of patients' conditions can be processed by AI to select the patients for a trial that will have the best prognosis. Moreover, the AI can also predict which patients are likely to reach the end of the trial (Bertsimas et al., 2024). Overall, AI accelerates the process and can make more successful clinical trials more frequent, which in turn has the potential to revolutionize the industry. The subject of clinical trials is rather complex and problematic since among the most pressing issues are inefficient trial designs and patient recruitment processes, which typically take considerable time, thus prolonging the period in which potentially life-saving treatment remains unavailable. In most cases, the use of traditional methods eventually leads to under-enrollment, high dropout rates, and unrepresentative populations of patients, which jeopardize not only the smoothness of the process but also the credibility and applicability of further trial results. In this way, not only are financial losses incurred, but innovations are also not implemented in healthcare on time. Moreover, the overall speed and safety of the process of new medical technology reaching the market are determined by the speed and success of clinical trials (Alskaf et al., 2024).

This chapter aims to present the role of AI in clinical trial design and recruitment. This chapter seeks to explain how AI technologies help address the typical issues of clinical trial design, protracted recruitment processes, and large data management. This chapter explores individual AI applications, from prediction models and ML algorithms to natural language processing (NLP), each offering an in-depth breakdown of how they improve the accuracy, efficiency, and participant diversity with which trials are conducted. Furthermore, the author explores the ethical, regulatory, and implementation challenges that face AI technologies in clinical research frameworks. Based on a synthesis of the latest literature, case studies, and expert opinions, this chapter sets out to provide readers with deep knowledge about AI possibilities today, which is not yet possible today but may be realistic for future clinical trials.

FOUNDATIONAL CONCEPTS

Basics of Clinical Trials

Clinical trials are intentionally being conducted to evaluate the safety and effectiveness of interventions designed to enhance individual health. As illustrated in Figure 1, there are four phases at which trials are usually divided. In phase I, the intervention is usually tested on a small group of people regarding its working mechanisms and the proper dosage that needs to be set. In phase II, the number of patients in the group usually increases, and the extent of the treatment effect and its side effects are usually measured. In phase III, the group is increased once more to prove whether the treatment is useful, measures to minimize and treat possible side effects, and comparisons of the treatment with those accepted by practice. In phase IV, the treatment is already on the market and is being tested for side effects on people who are part of an extended population over a more extended period (Yingngam et al., 2024).

Concerning key stakeholders and their responsibilities, pharmaceutical companies, academic researchers, healthcare providers, and regulatory agencies are the main stakeholders in relation to clinical trials, and each plays an important role. The first category often sponsors the trial and provides all the funding and necessary resources. The second component designs the experiments, conducts them, analyses the data, and makes it possible to promote the published results. The third group of stakeholders, i.e., nurses and physicians, is directly involved in treatments and controls the health and safety of patients. The last category, often represented by the Food and Drug Administration (FDA), serves as a regulatory body that maintains the highest ethical standards for trials and ensures their conduction based on sound science to keep data valid and persons safe (Yingngam & Sethabouppha, 2024).

Figure 1. Phases of clinical trials

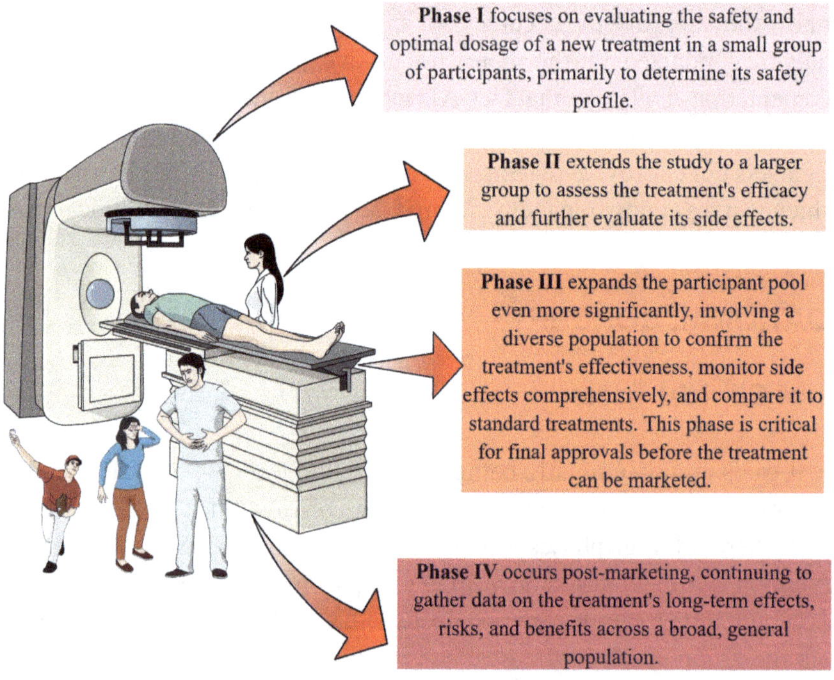

(created by the author using the licensed Mind the Graph software)

In terms of clinical trial types, randomized clinical trials (RCTs) have become the gold standard. These trials rely on a rigorous investigation of a test compound, as all results are obtained with the smallest amount of bias, and the randomization method advances disparate therapies above other variables. As confirmed by the authors, "Randomized placebo-controlled trials are the most favored trial design for controlling potential biases, as results are obtained with the minimum bias". These outcomes are accomplished by assigning both an intervention and a control therapy to research participants, eliminating any other factors. In the case of a double-blind placebo-controlled trial, experiments should guarantee that neither the patient nor the care provider is conscious of which one is used to reduce the possibility of bias (Dasarathy et al., 2024; Han et al., 2024). After considering this type of trial, it is reasonable to say that while such trials are powerful, they are also expensive, time-consuming, and have moral concerns. On the other hand, other trials offer additional flexibility. The first illustration of this is allowing patients to crossover to a control group after taking the experiment to enable relatively more minor variations within themselves, which is generally less expensive and time-consuming and can yield better information. When new tests of potentially superior compounds are acquired, it is reasonable to argue that this kind of evaluation is often inaccurate. On the other hand, patients must wash out the first medicine before beginning the test of other compounds at different times, which is a rigorous process (Lee et al., 2024). Additionally, factorial trials use multiple potential interventions for varying patients for multiple purposes, even though combined intervention use complicates the outcomes (Swendeman et al., 2024). Although each of these trials has its own set of benefits and drawbacks, it is possible to conclude that their selection is dependent on the study's objective, the ethical implications of different types of tests for patients, their prices, and their storage.

Artificial Intelligence

AI is composed of many technologies that can be used to accomplish actions, often requiring human intelligence. An AI technology called ML trains computers to learn and then uses available data to improve performance. Usually, they do not need to be programmed. Another technology called deep learning is primarily a kind of ML that uses multilayered artificial neural networks to model patterns in a large volume of data (Ryan et al., 2024). There is also another AI discipline called NLP, which is designed to enable computers to interpret human language and generate new human-like text (Alskaf et al., 2024). AI is used in the framework of clinical trials for speeding up monitoring as well as the velocity of decision-making based on various types of advanced data processing. In the majority of cases, as stated in the chapter, the main AI technologies applied in the field of clinical trials with respect to predictive modeling, automated monitoring, real-time data analysis, etc., have assisted in the prompt and timely success of phase I and phase II clinical trials. More specifically, it concerns the field of oncology and neurological disorders.

Predictive modeling is an advanced method that can suggest potential outcomes for patients or trials in general (Lou et al., 2024). In addition, automated monitoring is a technology that suggests various detection methods, such as adverse reactions and patient compliance, as well as providing suggestions based on the analysis of available patient safety data. Then, real-time data analysis allows researchers to adjust the trial protocols and enables the users of the technology to adjust the trial to new trends in emerging data (Witharana et al., 2024).

AI IN CLINICAL TRIAL DESIGN

Optimizing Protocol Design through AI

Protocol design in clinical trials, referring to detailed planning and documentation, is the first step in any research and outlines how a clinical trial will be performed. The protocol is crucial to the study because it safeguards the participants' safety and the correctness of the data that will be collected to show whether a product is effective or harmful. Thus, to ensure that this process is optimized, a clinical trial protocol presents a blueprint for the conduct of the trial, which provides guidance to stakeholders. The information on the protocol design is compiled in Figure 2, and the information is as follows:

1. Objective(s) of the Study

The objectives of a clinical trial are to identify the overall goal that the trial aims to achieve, serving as the foundation of the protocol. The objectives are characterized by guiding every element of the trial's design and to ensure that the research question is answered. The objectives include defining the purpose of the trial, such as assessing the efficacy of a new acne treatment in the target population. Another critical consideration is the bioavailability of this treatment, as this trial will seek to determine the adverse effects of acne treatment and measure the overall risk-benefit ratio. Moreover, some objectives refer to what the trial is intended to reveal, elucidating the biological or chemical applications and deficiencies. Thus, the objectives are defined according to primary and secondary objectives, where primary questions are the main objectives, the trial tries to answer, and secondary objectives reveal in more detail the surrounding effects and issues (K. Wang et al., 2024). The clearly stated objectives are necessary for the construction of the methodology, meaning selecting the correct population, performance criteria, and statistical analysis to safeguard the appropriate refinement, performance, and ability to avoid arbitrary mischief to support the ethical arguments surrounding the importance of randomness.

Figure 2. Key elements typically included in a protocol design in clinical trials

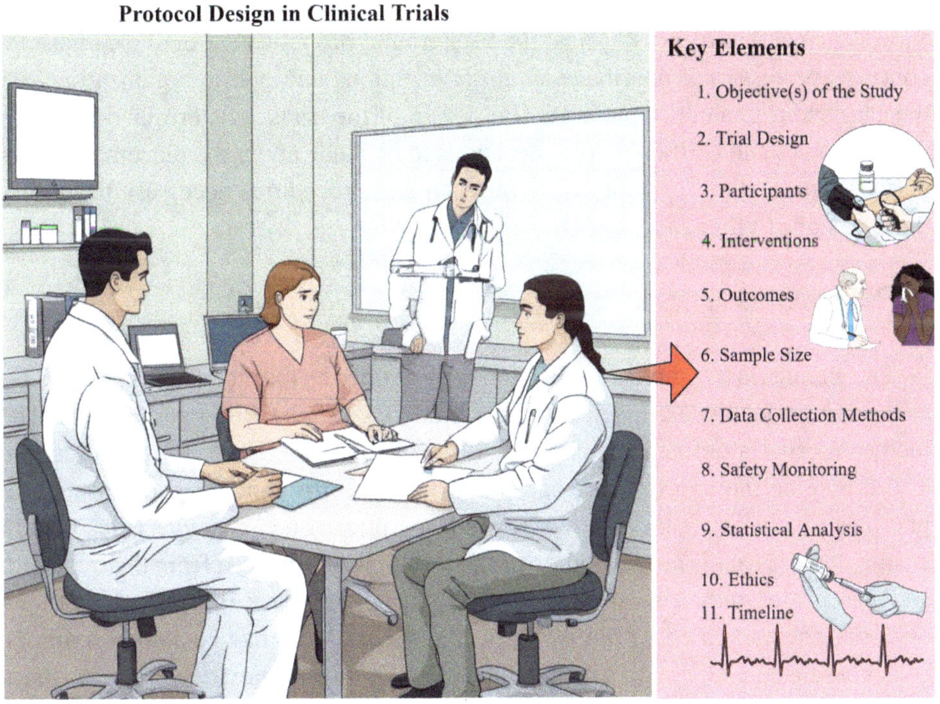

(created by the author using licensed Mind the Graph software)

2. Trial Design

The trial design of a clinical trial protocol describes the structure and methodology of a study, a critical component to ensure that the objectives of a trial will be met reliably and efficiently. The type of study is defined, such as randomized, which consists of randomly selecting study participants and assigning them to various treatment groups, which eliminates bias (L. Yao et al., 2024). In the placebo-controlled group, the effects of the new treatment were compared to the effects of a placebo, allowing one to assess the true therapeutic effects of the new treatment (Cold et al., 2024; Viraswami-Appanna et al., 2024). Open labels are used when blinding is not practical for researchers or the study participants. Both of these factors include which treatment is administered and the method and objective-specific phase of the trial. For specific purposes, phase I trials aimed to determine the safety and appropriate dosage of the new treatment through its administration to a small group of approximately 20-80 healthy volunteers or patients. Phase II studies the efficiency and safety of the libido drug for a longer period. Trials further expand the group of patients for analysis of the effects on various populations. Phase III studies are designed to verify the lethal effects of acute-step therapy on diseases as well as its effectiveness against the background of innovative therapy. Phase IV concerns professional pharmaceutical organizations and public organizations for the care and treatment of patients. The design of the trials is determined based on the objectives and further enables decisions to be made about the placement, comparison, and method of conducting the data and procedures necessary to modify these designs (Yingngam, 2024).

3. Participants

Participants in the clinical trial protocol are defined by the inclusion and exclusion criteria. Both factors are essential for the study's generalizability and validity. The inclusion criteria defined the characteristics of patients eligible for participation. These may be the approximate age range, sex, specific diagnosis, disease stage, previous treatment, or lack thereof for this condition. Such characteristics help to ensure that the trial is conducted on patients who would benefit from the treatment and answer the study's question (Shi et al., 2024). Moreover, the exclusion criterion is that the patient could not participate in the study. It may be a comorbidity, a possibly related medication used by the patient, or a secondary condition. As these exclusion criteria are likely to confuse the results, introducing them allows for maintaining the study's internal validity (Ellen et al., 2024). For example, not allowing patients with medical allergies to undergo treatment with more significant adverse effects shows that the study's goals are relevant and do not harm the participants. Thus, defining a specific type of patient prevents several ethical issues, makes the study more scientific and consistent, and increases the safety and applicability of the intervention.

4. Interventions

The interventions of a clinical trial protocol are vital because they supply all the needed information regarding the testing treatments or procedures. This is important because all being tested must be implemented in a steady and undeviating way for each of the given trial sites or trial participants. The first of the details is an intervention and always involves a certain drug, device, or procedure. It provides all of the given information on the treatment's subcomponents, such as biochemical reactions, use, and action. Furthermore, the specific dose to be given is included and, in most cases, varies not only from phase to phase but also depends on factors such as the disease and the patient's age. The intervention also includes the time and rate of consumption – how often and at what times the intervention should take place. Next is the stop duration – for how long the participant is subjected to the given intervention. In terms of duration, it can break into several hours that the intervention should be administered for, or other significantly long periods, even years. This kind of multiple definition only serves to make the subject more controlled and reliable, as it ensures that the intervention can be administered in a uniform and repetitive way, which is vital for the results to provide exact validity. It ensures that any positive or negative results are derived from the intervention and not from a different way in which it is or is not administered (Abusamaan et al., 2024).

5. Outcomes

The outcomes of a clinical trial protocol are the key aspects of what the trial will measure to determine whether the studied intervention is effective and safe. Among the types of outcomes that can be determined in such trials are primary outcomes. These outcomes are the results that the study is trying to evaluate, and commonly, they are chosen carefully with respect to their relevance to a direct effect of the intervention. They are also usually the most important changes, either clinical or statistical, expected from the treatment under study, e.g., an improvement in a disease's symptoms or a decrease in mortality rates. The choice of primary outcomes is crucial because it determines the focus of the trial, and power calculations of the trial are based on it, influencing the size and duration of the investigation (Shi et al., 2024). In contrast, secondary outcomes are additional endpoints that may provide more information about the effects of the intervention under study. They may also help clinicians better understand the primary outcomes or explore additional effects of the treatment (Williamson et al., 2024). An example of a secondary outcome may be measurements of the effects on quality of life, economic effects, or side effects of the intervention. While they are not used as the main outcomes of the trial, they can still provide important information about the intervention's effects. Both types of outcomes must be specified before the trial begins to prevent outcome switching and ensure that the trial is objective and that the results can be understood and used. Doing so is important for the overall scientific relevance of the study with all its implications, which is necessary for different stakeholders to understand the real effects of the intervention, such as regulatory bodies, healthcare providers, and, ultimately, patients.

6. Sample Size

The sample size of a clinical trial protocol is an absolute requirement to ensure the validity and long-lasting nature of the trial's outcomes. The approach requires that accurate statistical calculations be adopted in terms of consideration of effect size, the difference that is expected between the effect of the intervention and the alternative, the power of the statistics, or the probability that a check will yield a positive result if one does, adding a consideration of sample size. Greater power serves to lower the power of Type II errors or the chance that the true effect of an intervention will not be recognized in a comparison of two groups. This error is due to the sample's limitations, and an underpowered sample may lead to the trial's conclusions not being legitimated by statistics (Ellen et al., 2024). Moreover, calculating the accurate sample size and recognizing the considerable number of factors that influence it allows little probability of committing a Type I error or the existence of a difference between two otherwise largely similar populations. This error is also avoidable, as long as the sample size is accounted for in terms of the number of aspects under consideration or the range of the likely varieties, and additional testing is necessary. It also accounts for the nature of the sampling, which is likely to be problematic, with more than the powerfully associated reference population difference dropping out or being lost from the sample (Abusamaan et al., 2024). Therefore, the process ensures that a large enough sample is taken, which covers the planned sample that is likely to not be subsumed in the actual trial until the end. Altogether, this results in the calculation of a population variety estimate that covers all the predictable varieties in the sample and should be accounted for in terms of a notionally acceptable dropout or attrition rate. It also ensures that they are powered properly to reach plausible conclusions that are applicable to generalizing the results to a larger population.

7. Data Collection Methods

The section on data collection methods in the clinical trial protocol document describes the processes and tools that allow us to record the data regarding the intervention and the effects that it may cause. This section is detailed because the process of data collection directly affects the validity and reliability of trial outcomes. This ensures that the data is collected uniformly and accurately from all participants who are engaged in the trial; thus, they can properly describe and analyze these data. The specific tools and processes include a protocol that may indicate the use of medical imaging, blood sampling, scales of patient-reported outcome measures, electronic health records (EHRs), or other techniques. The timing of these data measurements is also carefully included in the section since they should be taken during the specific phases of the trial that may correspond to a particular activity of a certain intervention and a specific clinical milestone of an intervention effect. These tools and processes are usually standardized at all trial sites since they may vary across practices or due to the limited training of personnel. Furthermore, these processes allow the data to be aggregated in a statistically valid and comparable way to have an opportunity to analyze them. This section describes the procedures for training personnel and avoiding human mistakes in the process of data collection. It also explains the record-keeping rules and the responsibility for data accuracy. Proper crediting procedures are set to ensure reliability and clarify any data. These reliable and valid methods are key for a clinical trial because they determine whether the trial will produce valid and reliable outcomes (K. Wang et al., 2024).

8. Safety monitoring

Safety monitoring is designed to protect the health and general well-being of clinical trial subjects. This section outlines the procedures required for the ongoing capture and collection of safety information during the trial and defines the adverse safety effects that will trigger the termination of the trial. The independent Data Safety and Monitoring Board (DSMB) comprises people who are not involved in the trial. The DSMB is an independent advisory body of experts who possess appropriate collective qualifications and experience in clinical as well as basic science, medicine, ethics, and statistics and who are not involved in the conduct of the trial. The DSMB periodically reviews the accumulated trial data and recommends whether to continue, modify, suspend, or prematurely terminate a trial. Serious adverse events include any effects that are untoward or noxious in nature in participants, resulting in any of the following: death or life-threatening; requirement for hospitalization or prolongation of existing hospitalization; or other such criteria overall or in combination. The protocol should state the functions and specify the role of the mechanism for recording all it determines. In no case should DSMB be made aware of group-specific data or results, except where total trial data monitoring is feasible. The DSMB should not become biased in the process and should conduct its responsibilities with confidentiality and full cooperation with all partners. Adverse screening and reporting processes should be defined in the protocol. The protocol needs to describe the methods whereby direct benefit/risk comparisons will be made during the trial and after the trial. Actions, time frames, and means by which severe adverse incidents will be reported to competent national authorities and major safety events to the sponsor, investigators, and the ethical committee must be described in the protocol. The central issue of such reporting is ensuring stakeholder awareness and providing appropriate measures. Not only does correct safety feature monitoring protect patients, but it also provides relevant data that aid in identifying the features of the drug submitted to the test (Wolf et al., 2024).

9. Statistical analysis

A statistical analysis of a clinical trial protocol is a carefully designed document aimed at providing a clear definition of how the collected data will be thoroughly and systematically analyzed to answer the research questions. This document is important because it predefines the statistical methods that will be used, thus making their application objective and data interpretation fair. As a rule, there are primary and secondary analyses. The primary analysis includes tests that help answer the main objectives of a trial, such as the estimation of treatment efficacy compared with a placebo, another treatment, and more. Secondary analyses are also aimed at providing answers to some of the secondary objectives or additional hypotheses. For example, they may include tests informing on the safety or feasibility of the treatment of the attack, examination of deferred outcomes, or answers to other hypotheses regarding different subgroups of the trial population. The imputation of missing data is an important part of any statistical plan, as missing data may introduce bias to the results and inferentially affect the whole trial. As a rule, incomplete data are handled using a few imputation techniques, such as the last observation carried forward, the updated range, or others, depending on whether the missingness is systematically related to the trial's outcomes. Moreover, subgroup analyses are usually described in the statistical plan to test the difference between the effect of the intervention between some predefined subgroups, depending on age, sex, disease severity, stage, and other factors. Subgroup analyses help clarify the extent to which different factors affect the variability of treatment effects and whether the effects of the intervention are similar across different populations (Lin et al., 2024). Thus, a well-designed statistical analysis plan is a document that guarantees that the trial's findings are based on a robust, transparent, and adequate analysis, which, as a result, should be reproducible.

10. Ethics

The ethics of a clinical trial protocol are primary, describing how the protocol's execution should be guided by the highest standards of ethical practice. This should be elaborated based on concepts of respect for persons, beneficence, and justice, which form the core foundation of any ethical research involving humans. The primary way to ensure that these principles are followed is through informed consent. Such terms generally mean that all subjects should be fully aware of the nature of the trial, the risks, and the benefits thereof, including their free will and right to leave it at any time and without any consequences. The study can only be voluntary if the decision to participate is fully informed. The regulatory bodies and independent ethics committees must approve the protocol to ensure the scientific validity of the study and manage and minimize risks for the subjects and their ratio. In addition, it confirms accountability by the investigators for their actions and promises. It can also be said that the latter minimum guarantees that the study will maintain all ethical standards during its implementation (Shaw et al., 2024). It is also worth saying that strict adherence to the guidelines described is the main and last protective element for both the research subjects and the evidence and data obtained, so one can ensure its credibility and maintain honesty and trust throughout the entire study.

11. Timeline

The timeline of a clinical trial protocol is a major section that denotes the expected length and milestones of the study, thereby indicating to participants and stakeholders the pace at which the trial is proceeding. This solid timeline describes the start and end day of each phase, be it a setup, recruitment, test, or final analysis. It describes the main events, such as patient enrollment, interim analyses, and the actual times when the data will be locked in evaluation. This timeline also provides deadlines for sending interim reports to regulators and ethics committees, which is important for their own tempo of compliance and oversight. If the trial consists of several phases, the time points that separate them are indicated so that the investigators and sponsoring company can timely consider the results. In addition, each stage is thoroughly planned so that its goals do not outweigh the total aims of the trial in accordance with which the resources should be allocated. In this way, many possible delays in the study can be avoided or prevented, which facilitates interteam and intersite coordination (van Dam et al., 2024). As a result, trials that have strong timelines, alongside all other significant aspects described in the protocol, are more likely to be completed on time and within budget.

Figure 3 is a detailed flowchart of the AI-based process for clinical trial design. The focus of the presented picture is the importance of ML for improving protocol optimization and feasibility assessment. The work starts with deciding what kind of trial needs to be performed, which means that objectives and hypotheses are determined for the study. The process includes important steps, such as the collection of data from multiple sources, including not only the results of historical trials but also real-world evidence. Then, the data are prepared, and integration occurs inside an AI tool that cleanses and normalizes it. The next step is the use of ML algorithms to analyze the data and plan trial protocols, construct dose–response curves, and predict the most effective intervention schedules. For writing the protocol, a feasibility assessment is carried out, and the simulation of patient recruitment and the quantity of needed resources are performed using AI tools. Afterward, the derived findings are analyzed, and the protocol is adjusted according to the insights received and the feedback from stakeholders. The process ends with the submission of the final version of the trial protocol to the regulator authority and trial initiation. This flowchart shows how the use of AI and ML stages the process of clinical trial planning and conducting. This approach also makes decision-making more exact and personal for obtaining more effective results in medical research.

Figure 3. Flowchart depicting the AI-driven process for clinical trial design

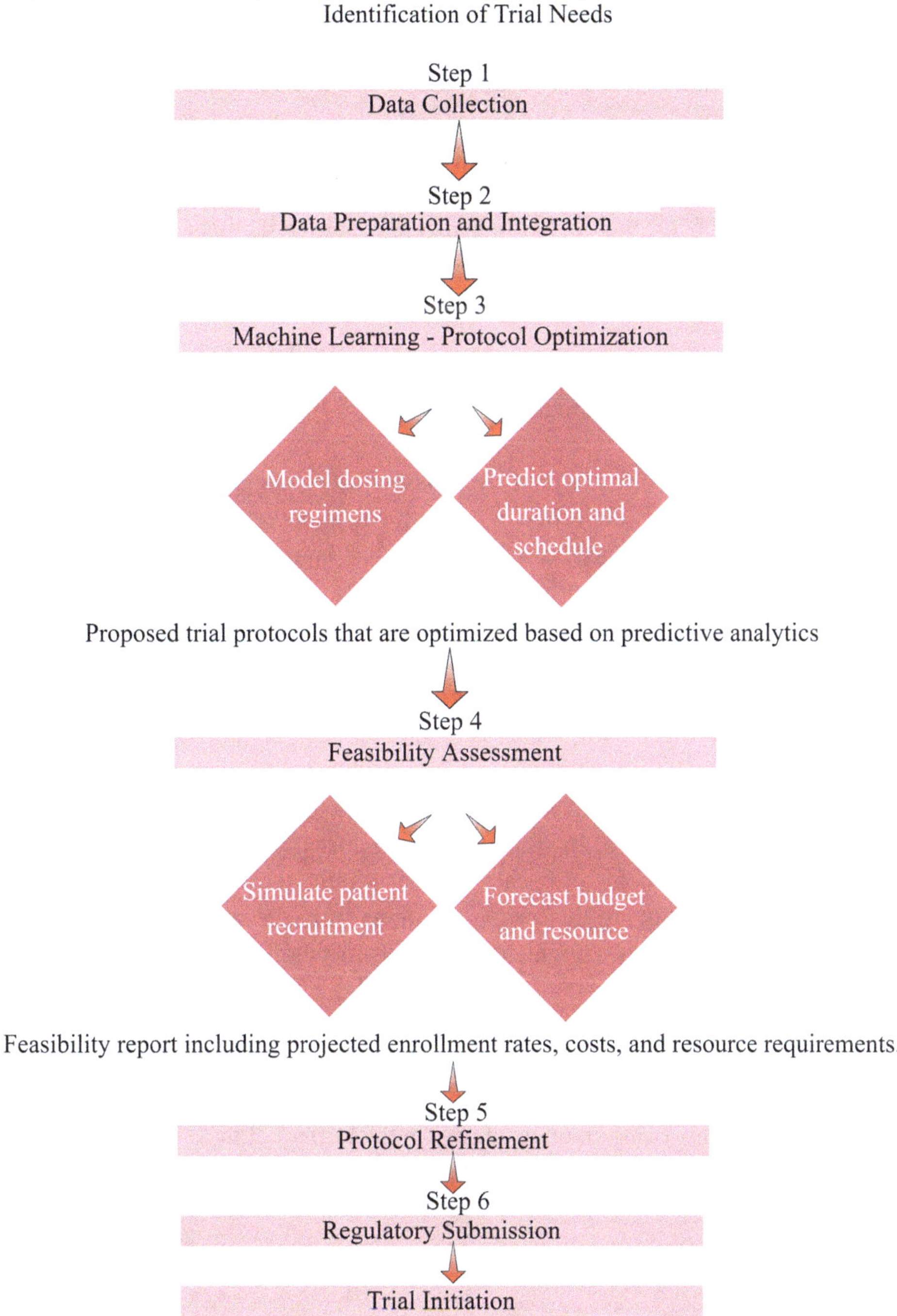

(created by the author using licensed Mind the Graph software)

One advanced field of AI, which is currently in the developing stage in terms of application, is its use to optimize protocol design in clinical trials. This development refers to the use of advanced algorithms to interpret the data associated with trials and the combination of differing types of data to forecast, develop, and optimize clinical studies. By retracing historical data that were noted as part of clinical trials, AI may be used to develop an optimal protocol for a study that is likely to yield scientifically robust results and is tailored to attain certain outcomes (Schepps et al., 2024). This transformation is anticipated to enable refinement of such elements of a protocol design as successful doses of a tested product, duration of a trial, and the wearable period following completion of the trial.

(1) Examples of AI in Protocol Design Optimization

(1.1) Dosing Optimization

AI algorithms can analyze data from past trials to suggest an optimal dosing regimen that maximizes the efficacy of the medication while minimizing the associated risk. In this case, ML is a form of AI that is used in the pharmacometric modeling of a drug and its effects across an entire population, which includes the phenotypes and various attributes of individuals who need to be considered when creating a personalized regimen, such as genetics, age, and comorbidities (Viraswami-Appanna et al., 2024). For example, ML for the optimization of dosing involves warfarin (Figure 4a), which is an oral anticoagulant used for the prevention of blood clots in veins and arteries. The medication often requires the use of a specific regimen since it has a narrow therapeutic effect and high variability in patient response. Therefore, an optimal warfarin dose is achieved when the drug is effective in preventing hematological thrombosis without causing any hemorrhage. The difficulty in achieving this primarily stems from the fact that many factors are determined by the rates at which individuals metabolize and react to the drug, regarding which existing dosing techniques are flawed, as they are often based on clinical trials and unknown trial–and–error assumptions. As a result, the frequency of side effects and the mortality rate can increase, which is where ML is used as an AI to optimize warfarin dosing (Lam et al., 2024). The way in which this works is through an analysis of vast amounts of data in the form of clinical trials and patient information to suggest the optimal dosing regimen.

Figure 4. Chemical structures of (a) warfarin and (b) temozolomide

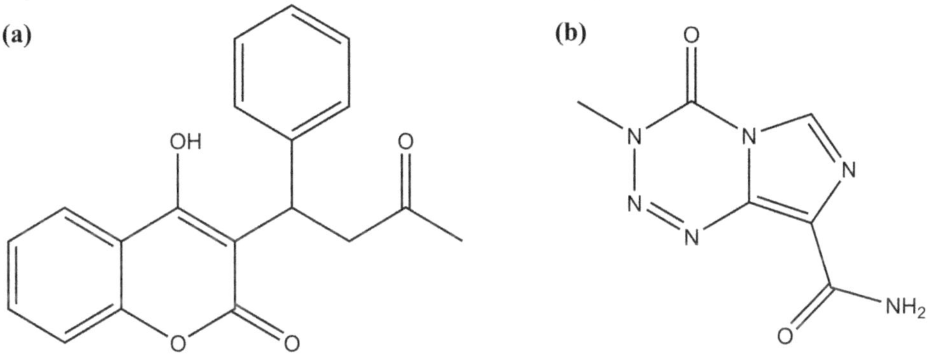

Warfarin

Temozolomide

(created by the author using ChemDraw 20.1.1)

As shown in Table 1, the AI utilizes different factors to optimize the dose of warfarin. Each of these factors is important to pharmacometrics, and the dosing for each patient-specific dataset is adjusted. In pharmacometrics, MLs are used to create various predictive models to adjust the dosage of a particular drug and its therapeutic effects on a diverse population. This type of model considers many factors, including genomics, age, comorbidities, and concurrent medications. These factors are all very important for adjusting and optimizing personal treatment. For warfarin, genetic variations in the VKORC1 and CYP2C9 genes affect how patients metabolize the drug. VKORC1 is related to the sensitivity of the internal vitamin K cycle, which is blocked by taking warfarin. The other gene, CYP2C9, affects how quickly warfarin is removed from the body. Patients with a certain form or mutation of the VKORC1 gene usually need lower doses of warfarin. VKORC1 is related to the sensitivity of the vitamin K cycle, which is inhibited by warfarin. Individuals with normal warfarin sensitivity to VKORC1 have a more limited range of rock sensitivity and therefore require a lower dose to avoid long-term anticoagulation and increased risks of bleeding (Xue et al., 2024).

For genetic variations, patients with specific CYP2C9 genotypes may require a lower dose, as warfarin is metabolized slowly. CYP2C9 is an enzyme that metabolizes warfarin. Variations in the CYP2C9 gene could slow the process of metabolism, leading to increased blood concentrations of the drug and decreased dosing. Demographic conditions, such as age, diet, and lifestyle, and other medical conditions, such as liver disease and heart failure, complicate the dosing. Older patients require lower doses of warfarin. As people age, their metabolism tends to slow, and they become more sensitive to drugs. Older people are more prone to its effects, and at the same dose, their antithrombotic effect might increase, leading to reduced dosing. Patients with liver disease or heart failure may require adjusted dosing of warfarin. These diseases affect the metabolism and sensitivity of the drug (M. Wang et al., 2024). For example, patients with liver disease may leave more warfarin unmetabolized, leading to elevated blood drug concentrations and requiring dose reduction. Diet is a major factor determining warfarin doses, as dietary intake of vitamin K can modulate warfarin dosing. Green leafy vegetables are a rich source of vitamin K that neutralizes the effect of warfarin on blood coagulation. A stable dose can therefore be modulated by a stable pattern of vitamin K intake; however, sudden changes in diet require dose modification. Lifestyle factors such as smoking might affect the metabolism of warfarin, requiring dose modification. Smoking induces liver enzymes that metabolize warfarin, and smokers are more prone to the anticoagulant actions of the drug and require a higher dose to achieve the same effect.

Table 1. Warfarin dosing optimization using AI

Factor	Impact on Dosing
Genetic variations (VKORC1)	Patients with specific VKORC1 genotypes might require lower doses due to increased sensitivity to warfarin.
Genetic variations (CYP2C9)	Patients with specific CYP2C9 genotypes might require lower doses due to slower metabolism of warfarin.
Age	Older patients often require lower doses due to decreased metabolism and increased sensitivity.
Comorbidities	Patients with liver disease or heart failure may need adjusted doses due to altered drug metabolism.
Diet	Dietary intake of vitamin K (found in green leafy vegetables) can affect warfarin dosing.
Lifestyle	Lifestyle factors such as smoking can influence warfarin metabolism, requiring dose adjustments.

In oncology, ML models are also reshaping this field by improving the accuracy and personalization of treatment strategies. For example, this technology is used to optimize the dosing schedules of temozolomide (Figure 4b), an agent applied for curing one of the most malignant forms of brain cancer called glioblastoma. This kind of cancer is challenging to treat mostly because of its heterogeneity. On the other hand, the efficacy of therapy can be significantly different among patients. Dosing regimens offered by experts tend to be rather universal and are not aimed at taking into account the individual peculiarities of a patient. ML models, however, can solve this problem by combining a variety of factors specific to a person to make the treatment more suitable for them. The methylation of the O6-methylguanine-DNA methyltransferase (MGMT) gene, which encodes the MGMT enzyme, is particularly important. By protecting cancer cells, this enzyme can stop the action of temozolomide. When an MGMT promoter is methylated, it does not work, and the impact of the drug on malignant cells is more efficient.

The factors considered for optimizing temozolomide regimens for glioblastoma therapy using ML models are shown in Table 2. Each variable specifies how the amount should change, subject to individual details. First, patients with a methylated MGMT promoter need lower dosages of temozolomide. MGMT is a DNA repair enzyme that becomes inactive when its promoter is methylated, disabling the ability to respond to potential harm from temozolomide. Consequently, cancer cells become more prone to temozolomide and are influenced by this measure, unlike those without methylation. In turn, older people also require lower doses as metabolic processes decline with age, potentially making the treatment toxic. The drug removal pathway and how well it is tolerated can fluctuate among patients, so dosing should be adjusted to circumvent harm while ensuring efficacy. Furthermore, comprehensive tumor characteristics, such as tumor dimension, site, disease stage, and patient sex, similarly impact the requisite tumor volume (Belue et al., 2024).

On the other hand, vital organs such as the liver and kidney may perform below the optimal levels due to comorbid conditions. Since organs are known to assist in drug metabolism and excretion from the body, their underperformance exposes patients to the risk of developing toxicity problems. As such, they have a direct influence on the needed adjustment. Consequently, it is crucial to consider this relationship by adjusting the dose relative to the patient's health condition. In this case, the flexibility needed for the prediction of the optimal dosing strategy is achieved by incorporating genetic alterations in the patient-derived cancer model, along with other crucial patient-specific data in the ML model. With such considerations, it would be possible to identify the optimal dosage strategy for different tumors, hence enhancing drug efficacy and reducing patient exposure to toxicity.

Mutations in specific genes of tumor cells can also affect the rate of their sensitivity to temozolomide; hence, adjustments are needed to optimize dosing. These genes are involved in DNA repair mechanisms in tumors. In this event, the ML model should be adjusted to incorporate these deviations, thereby predicting the expected dosing regimen in reference to such revelation. Such inclusion would inform the initial and follow-up adjustments needed in a patient who has shown resistance to the treatment. Similarly, dosing may be informed by the patient's sensitivity to the previously used therapy. Such information may assist in optimizing ML model predictions by considering adjusted regimens that will be nuanced accordingly (Xie et al., 2024).

The use of ML in customizing dosing regimens demonstrates the ability of this technology to work with complicated, multidimensional data that would otherwise not be processed effectively with traditional methods. To create such models, a large dataset that can account for genetic profiles, the clinical history of the patient, imaging results, and much more is used to create personalized treatment plans. ML works with this information to analyze correlations and patterns within this dataset, identifying various combinations of key factors that make the positive effect of the therapy most likely. Thus, the precision of the operation is not only improved by making the drug more effective but also safer, as over- and underdosing the patient becomes less likely. Therefore, patients receive a dosing regimen that is specifically developed for their biological and clinical profile, which heralds the beginning of truly individualized oncology. With increasing progress being made in the de-pressurizing of more features predicting the effect of therapy, the use of ML can become the basis of a new generation of methods focused on predictive analytics and personalized medicine in the care of cancer patients. This shift will potentially improve the outcome of some oncology patients with a dismal prognosis, such as those with glioblastoma.

Table 2. Optimizing the dose of temozolomide using AI

Factor	Impact on Dosing
MGMT promoter methylation status	Patients with methylated MGMT promoter may require lower doses due to increased sensitivity to temozolomide.
Patient age	Older patients may require adjusted doses due to decreased metabolism and increased sensitivity.
Tumor characteristics	Detailed tumor characteristics (size, location, grade) can influence the required dose to maximize efficacy.
Genetic mutations	Specific genetic mutations in tumor cells can affect drug sensitivity and require dose adjustments.
Previous treatment responses	Responses to previous treatments can inform the adjustments needed in current dosing regimens.
Comorbidities	Comorbid conditions like liver or kidney dysfunction may necessitate dose modifications to avoid toxicity.

(1.2) Predictive Modeling for Treatment Duration

Predictive modeling is an advanced AI application that substantially transforms the strategic planning of clinical trials. It allows the prediction of the optimal duration of a particular treatment based on aggregated data on patient responses associated with previous studies. With the help of this AI feature, researchers can customize a treatment period to make it optimal and aimed at achieving the most robust therapeutic results possible within the shortest period feasible (Khaligh et al., 2024). For example, concerning the state of oncology, AI has already been applied to determine the optimal duration of chemotherapy for particular types of cancer.

One of the applications of AI was to determine the optimal period of treatment for glioblastoma patients treated with temozolomide. The following aggregated data on patient response were collected: the decrease in the size of the tumors over time and the tolerance of the patients to the drug. The use of temozolomide as a drug for glioblastoma treatment can also be optimized by AI, which, concerning the case, considers the responses to the drug associated with a series of other factors. Such AI models process multidimensional data that cannot be simply analyzed analytically. They showed that some of the patients had drastically decreased tumors and were not able to tolerate the full treatment; as a result, the dose of temozolomide needed to be changed. However, some patients may need a longer treatment period before a significant effect is observed. AI can learn to predict such a response after the diagnosis of the first side effect. As a result of such an approach, patients receive only treatments suitable for them.

In the same way that AI and ML have helped in identifying novel compounds for treating infections and cancer, these technologies have transformed how the management of chronic wholly owned disease is practiced. An illustrative example is methotrexate, a mainstay of treatment for rheumatoid arthritis (Coskun et al., 2024). Decisions on the course of methotrexate development have had to rely on cookbook recommendations that provide rough guidelines for the duration of treatment. AI and ML allow developers to use large trial datasets and those from real-life clinical use to predict the amount of time needed to achieve therapy in this case, to be disease-free after the end of a given treatment, or to find the minimum amount of time such carriers need to reach the same degree of therapeutic effect. An astonishing number of variables, such as patient age, sex, weight, ethnic plasticity of the disease, and genotype, can be measured in greater detail. AI can use this number and many thousand patients, and by identifying patterns of correlation, how to predict the behavior of individuals over time can be determined. Thus, some patients will be seen reaching remission grades faster than others, and some will be seen ceasing therapy and remain in remission grades, while others will be seen to need longer durations to register the same value. This can lead to different recommended durations based on certain biomarker characteristics. Thus, in some cases, the treatment may be discontinued because of the risk of side effects, and in other cases, because the patient shows poor improvement. The net effect is the prevention of both overtreatment and undertreatment. These patients will not be subject to the potential liver toxicity and bone marrow depression consequences of taking the medication for a long period. They are also subject to the potential loss of their joints. In other words, the company also increases the safety of clinical trials by reducing the time patients are exposed to potentially ineffective and potentially harmful treatments.

(1.3) Dynamic Publications Supporting AI in Protocol Design

A dynamic follow-up schedule utilizing AI tools is a major achievement in clinical trial management. It enables precision and efficiency in how studies monitor participants. AI-driven systems are capable of analyzing a range of data from baseline participant characteristics to ongoing clinical responses and emerging risk factors and adjusting follow-up schedules for each individual. Such a personalized schedule ensures that each participant is monitored appropriately to their actual needs (Bindra & Jain, 2024). For example, in a clinical trial of a new cardiovascular drug, an AI system may be used to analyze the blood pressure, cholesterol, and genetic biomarkers of each individual in the study, identifying whose risk of adverse events is greater. For individuals who may be at greater risk, follow-up treatments might be scheduled more frequently. For those whose risk is lower, the drug performs well, and the actual treatment causes no severe side effects; hospital visits and model tests can be scheduled more infrequently. In this way, the use of an AI tool ensures that no extra hospital time and no extra tests are administered to participants who do not benefit from them, which saves resources. It also ensures that no participant is exposed to less than necessary monitoring, as those at higher risk are examined and followed as closely as necessary, which ensures a higher level of safety. Beyond patient safety, dynamic scheduling also ensures efficient data collection, which constitutes the primary aim of clinical trials. Clinically relevant data can only be collected at enough time points and with enough precision. By using a dynamic follow-up schedule, which utilizes AI tools to determine when follow-up is unnecessary and when new data collection points are needed, the study ensures high-quality data. This enables more efficient trials where potential problems with new drugs can be identified early, as the system intervenes with more frequent, less frequent, or more closely scheduled follow-up times. Furthermore, the use of AI tools ensures that no extra resources are wasted, which increases the feasibility of larger or longer trials. Tribulations are expensive in terms of human resources, as much of the workload is based on extra work for professionals. There is also pressure caused by the constant scheduling of equipment and administration time. Dynamic scheduling can alleviate the pressure caused by both reducing the total costs of studies and increasing the feasibility of larger or longer trials.

AI-Driven Predictive Modeling for Trial Feasibility

AI-driven predictive modeling can predict whether clinical trials will prove practical prior to commencing. Such predictive algorithms assess diverse variables involving anticipated patient recruitment rates, projected costs of potential interventions, and geographic contexts to anticipate feasibility. This aids organizations in deciding where to dedicate resources and by what means. Predictive algorithms may also reduce the number of patients likely to enroll and withdraw from evaluations. By relying on these prognoses, trial coordinators can subsequently calibrate recruitment tactics or target populations to guarantee an adequate number and diversity of participants (Yingngam et al., 2024).

Table 3 presents a summary of the demonstration of AI technologies, such as predictive analytics, NLP, or ML, used for clinical trial design, detailing what they are used for and how, and detailing specific examples. Predictive analytics enable the creation of statistical models that can predict the likelihood of future event occurrence, such as the rate of patient recruitment in a clinical trial, the likelihood of adverse events, or the best dosing schedule for particular patients. This is crucial for planning and risk management throughout the trial. NLP helps process large scales of unstructured text data, such as processing electronic health records and extracting patient characteristics based on which they were eligible for the trial or reviewing literature by condensing and identifying appropriate data within published articles as relevant. It is also used to interpret patient feedback for improving their experience participating in or dropping out of the trial. ML helps identify data patterns and refine trial or trial protocol planning based on past trials, such as optimizing dosing based on past patient treatment impacts or diagnosing and treatment response assessment through automated picture analysis. It may also be used to monitor how a trial is going and for corrective action if the measurement of certain data, for example, shows a significant negative impact. All these technologies play a significant role in making trials faster, more efficient, adaptable, and better aligned with modern medical needs and possibilities. At the same time, they also shorten the time by which innovative treatments are developed, tested, and approved under high safety standards and are delivered to the market.

Table 3. Summary of key AI technologies in clinical trial design

AI Technology	Function	Examples
Predictive analytics	Utilizes statistical models and historical data to predict future outcomes.	**- Patient Recruitment** Predicting patient enrollment rates by analyzing demographic and health data from past trials to optimize recruitment strategies **- Adverse Event Forecasting** Using historical trial data to model and predict the likelihood of specific adverse events allows for proactive risk management. **- Dosing Optimization** Estimating the most effective dosing schedules by analyzing outcomes from previous studies, considering variables such as age, weight, and genetic markers.
Natural language processing (NLP)	Processes and interprets large volumes of unstructured text data.	**- Eligibility Screening** Automating the extraction of patient information from EHRs to quickly identify individuals who meet specific trial criteria. **- Literature Review** Streamlining the review of scientific literature to extract pertinent data such as drug interactions and previous trial results, aiding in protocol development. **- Patient Feedback Analysis** Analyzing open-ended responses in patient surveys or online forums to gauge participant satisfaction and concerns regarding the trial experience.
Machine learning	Analyzes data patterns to automate and improve decision-making processes.	**- Trial Protocol Refinement** Learning from data on previous trial outcomes to refine trial protocols, improving efficacy and safety measures. **- Image Analysis** Using advanced image recognition and analysis for diagnostic purposes, such as identifying tumor responses in oncology trials. **- Real-Time Monitoring** Implementing real-time data analysis to adjust trial parameters dynamically based on incoming patient data, enhancing adaptive trial designs.

Enhancing the Trial Efficiency with AI Algorithms

AI algorithms can substantially enhance the productivity of clinical trials. First, they can perform a variety of routine tasks that require little cognitive input. Such tasks also tend to leave room for error, meaning that humans should direct their attention elsewhere. At the same time, these programs can interpret data in real time. This information can be used to dynamically adjust the protocols used by researchers, for example, changes in dosage (Patel et al., 2024). AI relies on the earliest data produced by a clinical trial to make adjustments. This is known as the adaptive nature of such programs. The main benefit of their use is that they substantially increase the probability of completion and can significantly reduce the cost and time of clinical studies.

PATIENT RECRUITMENT WITH AI

Key Aspects of Patient Recruitment

Patient recruitment is a crucial stage in clinical trial conduction and is dedicated to finding and involving participants in meeting a set of requirements in medical research studies. Since the number of suitable participants depends on the success and reliability of the clinical trial, effective recruitment provides an opportunity to achieve scientific goals and obtain statistically valuable results that can be generalized. The key aspects of patient recruitment are presented in Figure 5.

(1) Eligibility Criteria

Before developing effective patient recruitment, it is necessary to design inclusion and exclusion criteria that are created to explain specifically and explicitly who is eligible for participation in a clinical trial. For this purpose, researchers must decide on specific aspects, such as age, sex, personal characteristics, previous health status, stage of the disease, or other individual parameters. In addition, researchers need to specify who is not included in this examination (K. Wang et al., 2024). For instance, a clinical trial for a new medication approach for reducing the threat of postmenopausal acquired osteoporosis might include women who are more than 50 years old with a postmenopausal diagnosis of osteoporosis. Simultaneously, excluding women with recent fractures and those who currently use any kind of treatment for improving their bone density is important for preventing the development of potential side effects caused by the combination of drugs. In addition, excluding women in such categories increases the scientific validity of the work by decreasing the level of the sample's heterogeneity.

Figure 5. Key aspects of patient recruitment in clinical trials

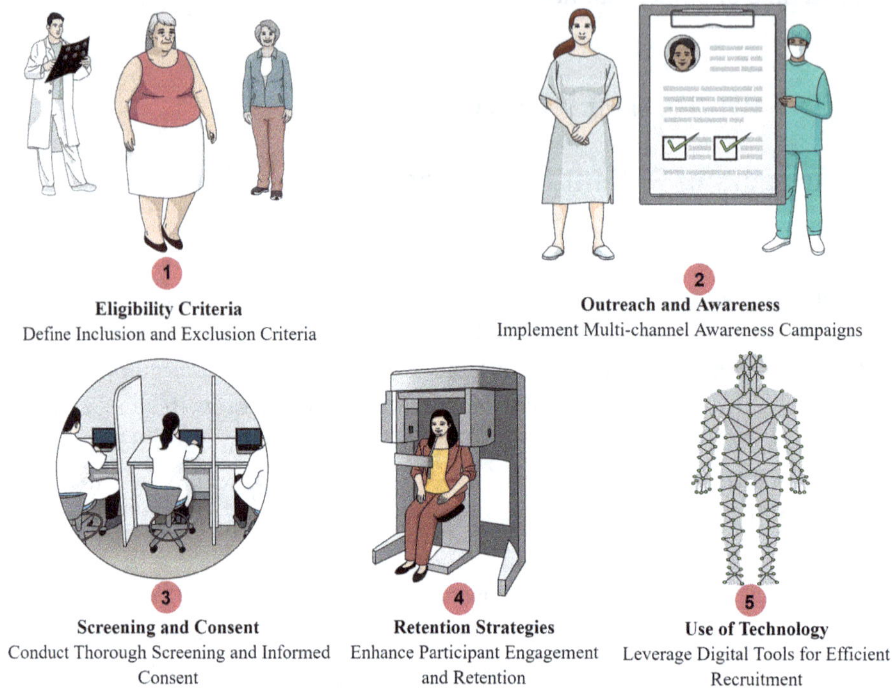

(created by the author using licensed Mind the Graph software)

(2) Outreach and Awareness

Efficient strategies of outreach and awareness represent one of the key essentials of patient recruitment success in clinical trials. These often comprise a combination of solutions. For more traditional advertising, advertising through radio and newspapers reaches a diverse range of individuals. Social media platforms provide an opportunity for targeted advertising and engagement within specific communities, attracting those who correspond to specific demographic conditions. In addition, cooperation with patient advocacy groups is another strategy aimed at reaching people directly affected by these conditions. At the same time, healthcare providers play a crucial role in the process. Patients who met the inclusion criteria for the trial and were potential beneficiaries were referred to the providers for the research (Abusamaan et al., 2024). For example, in the case of a new type of insulin therapy, the diabetes clinic may inform patients directly and hence have relatively quick access to the extremely relevant and, at the same time, likely to be interested in the population. This not only requires the maximum result regarding the trial's visibility but also works in reaching the diverse range of individuals who may be outside the particular reach of a single type of communication.

(3) Screening and Consent

Screening and consent are essential ethical aspects of new treatments or medical procedure trials. Before the beginning of any clinical trial, potential participants should pass a rigorous screening to determine if they fit the predefined criteria. Once the patients are acknowledged as eligible, they are provided with a careful consent process, which helps them to give their consent to become participants. During the process, the possible participants receive and acknowledge the detailed information regarding the trial, such as the purposes, scope, methods, drugs, and outcomes. The information should be provided as clearly as possible; as a result, consent may be provided in several formats at once or in a specific language if the assumptions are that not all possible participants have a high education or may have vision problems (Wolf et al., 2024). For instance, in my practice setting, the consent process implied documentation regarding the clinical trial of a new Alzheimer's disease drug, and the participants were provided with an explanation about the scope and side effects of the drug and required hospital visits, the monthly treatment duration, analysis visits, etc. Thus, the consent process ensured that the participant understood the meaning and conditions of the research and provided the information to be decided upon by the patient alone.

(4) Retention Strategies

If participants agree to participate in a clinical trial, the next step should be to retain them within the stipulated period. The dropout rate in multiple types of trials can be significantly high; hence, there is a need for retention strategies to increase the likelihood of participants completing the study (Chandra et al., 2024). Examples of strategies include the provision of constant communication updates such as through emails. Follow-ups should be organized when most convenient for the participants, and side effects should be managed to ensure that participants are as comfortable as possible. For long-term clinical trials on rheumatoid arthritis, monthly newsletters update participants on the progress of the trials. Participants also received their appointment dates at the clinic for the next month. In addition, the constant availability of the hotline can help participants feel supported and appreciate the value of the clinical trial.

(5) Use of Technology

The trend of technology entering various spheres of human life has also affected clinical trials. Currently, technological advancements have been frequently made in the process of patient recruitment since such strategies appear to be highly efficient. The use of digital tools allows researchers to facilitate the identification of potential participants and expand the scope of their research (Nashwan & Hani, 2023). For example, EHRs are used to scan data at no time and distinguish people whose health characteristics correspond to the criteria defined for a particular study. In this way, the first phases of recruitment become much swifter. In addition, it is possible to create advertisements that will target those groups of the population that are more likely to have a specific health problem using such systems as Google or Facebook and employ AI-driven algorithms to achieve the greatest effectiveness. Thus, a smart algorithm can analyze EHR data, detect severe patients who have experienced several asthma attacks in the recent past but who have not found an appropriate remedy, and invite them to participate in a study testing a new medication for asthma.

AI in Patient Recruitment

Challenges in Traditional Patient Recruitment

The traditional methods of patient recruitment in clinical trials usually face challenges, such as low enrollment and high dropout rates, as well as failures to address diverse target populations effectively. The process is often time-consuming and associated with considerable costs that are dependent on manual labor aimed at identifying and engaging the right patients. In addition, the conventional approaches struggle with precise and targeted matching of the patients who meet the necessary inclusion criteria to the patients included in the trial. As a result of such inefficiencies and the absence of accuracy, the trial outcomes can lose their quality and be hardly applicable to broader populations (Askin et al., 2023).

AI Solutions for Patient Identification and Recruitment

One of the primary obstacles in conducting clinical trials and health studies is finding suitable volunteers and ensuring that they are actively engaged throughout the research. Automated intelligence solutions offer entrancing solutions by using data analytics because AI systems can run through various patient databases in the field of health care and, as such, pinpoint the exact patient who is tailoring the characteristics of a clinical trial. It will then be helpful to predict and monitor such patients throughout the research. In addition, the same AI system can be used to send these patients automated follow-up messages and reminders as a way of remarking them on their scheduled visits.

Ethical Considerations and Patient Privacy

The use of AI in enhancing the efficiency of patient recruitment is feasible. However, the use of AI raises some ethical issues. One of the most crucial problems associated with the use of AI is patient privacy and consent. In this regard, there is a considerable risk of violating the sensitive personal and medical information of patients, and proper data protection and data usage policies are essential. In addition, AI may carry a risk of constant learning based on the existing data and, as a result, subject matter and its potentially biased selection of patients. In this regard, strict control and critical selection of data for teaching AI are needed to prevent biased and equal use of AI in the corresponding domain.

Improving Patient Diversity with AI

The Importance of Diversity in Clinical Trials

Diversity in the aspect of clinical trials is one of the crucial concepts. It determines whether a certain medical intervention is safe and efficient in regard to different races, ethnicities, ages, and genders. In the past, some groups of people did not participate in the research. Unfortunately, this led to so-called "gaps" in the outcomes and interventions. Thus, by enhancing diversity, people will be able to obtain a full overview of what is working and what is not in a broader spectrum of the population.

AI Approaches to Address Underrepresentation

Some AI technologies are able to analyze user demographic data and inform administrators of which groups they are underperforming to suggest ways to reach a broader number of people. Additionally, using the same technology, it is possible to track the activity of those users who can potentially participate in clinical trials. Moreover, some AI systems can adjust their recruitment language or methods to be more appropriate for different cultural backgrounds and languages to improve participation.

Strategies for Broadening the Eligibility Criteria Using AI

AI provides an opportunity and tools for refining and broadening the eligibility criteria without compromising the scientific validity of a clinical trial. By making predictions based on vast amounts of data collected from patients' histories, AI models can identify broader patterns and underpin correlations, allowing more extensive groups of participants. Moreover, the use of AI to refine the parameters of a trial can not only make it more diverse but also more applicable to different groups of patients.

To provide readers with a detailed description of how AI is used for patient recruitment in clinical trials, the author describes all the necessary steps in Figure 6. The recruitment of such patients is one of the essential parts of clinical trial design; however, it can become an obstacle mainly because of its time- and resource-consuming nature. The importance of recruitment is even more significant in regard to rare diseases, and although traditional methods of recruitment can still be employed, they are usually associated with obstacles and approximately 50% of delays in clinical trials and thousands of dollars wasted. At the same time, a systematic and AI-based approach to development is effective, as it usually allows for identifying the necessary participants and the most suitable conditions and engaging these people as necessary. Data collection is the first step, and there is no shortage of sources for such training: historical clinical data for respiratory disease trials, electronic health records in hospitals, and real-world data from patient registries and insurance claims. Then, these data are collected, and the first step is to ensure that the data are diverse and sufficiently large. After that, an ML model is developed, and this model is validated on a test set, in contrast to the training set. However, practical recruitment is the second problem with model-type recruitment. This model was also developed based on the more or less universal inclusion and exclusion criteria for the trials, which were compared with the obtained data to identify potential participants. Then, the data from multiple sources are integrated into a centralized database, with an emphasis on the data quality ensured by inadequate standardization and data cleaning processes. The surgical concern is ensuring that only one category of data and the most valuable data from the same source must be used, as real-world data can also sometimes be less useful because of biases. The AI candidate search also proposes the possibility of employing other machines, for example, a phone or a tablet app. This ranked list is then inspected by coordinators and other employees who should validate the list by contacting the best candidates by phone. This includes the use of automated communication systems, ensures that all potential participants are contacted, and includes all important information up to their high level. At the same time, another AI also maintains the real-time monitoring of this group of potential participants to prevent any repetitions or being ignored as necessary. Special algorithms for such systems can be used simultaneously to identify factors that would allow a more personal approach, taking differences between people into account. At the same time, the large variety of data available allows the AI to also inspect some data. The third step is the long-term retention of participants, as the engagement crisis intensifies; AI is now also from them to be employed for personal engagement. Finally, these recruitment methods also allow for real-time monitoring, and the site-wide strategies employed here reduce costs and allow more participants who are as close as possible to receiving a fill-and-dosage by the end of the published monitor.

Figure 6. Examples of the use of AI for patient recruitment in clinical trials

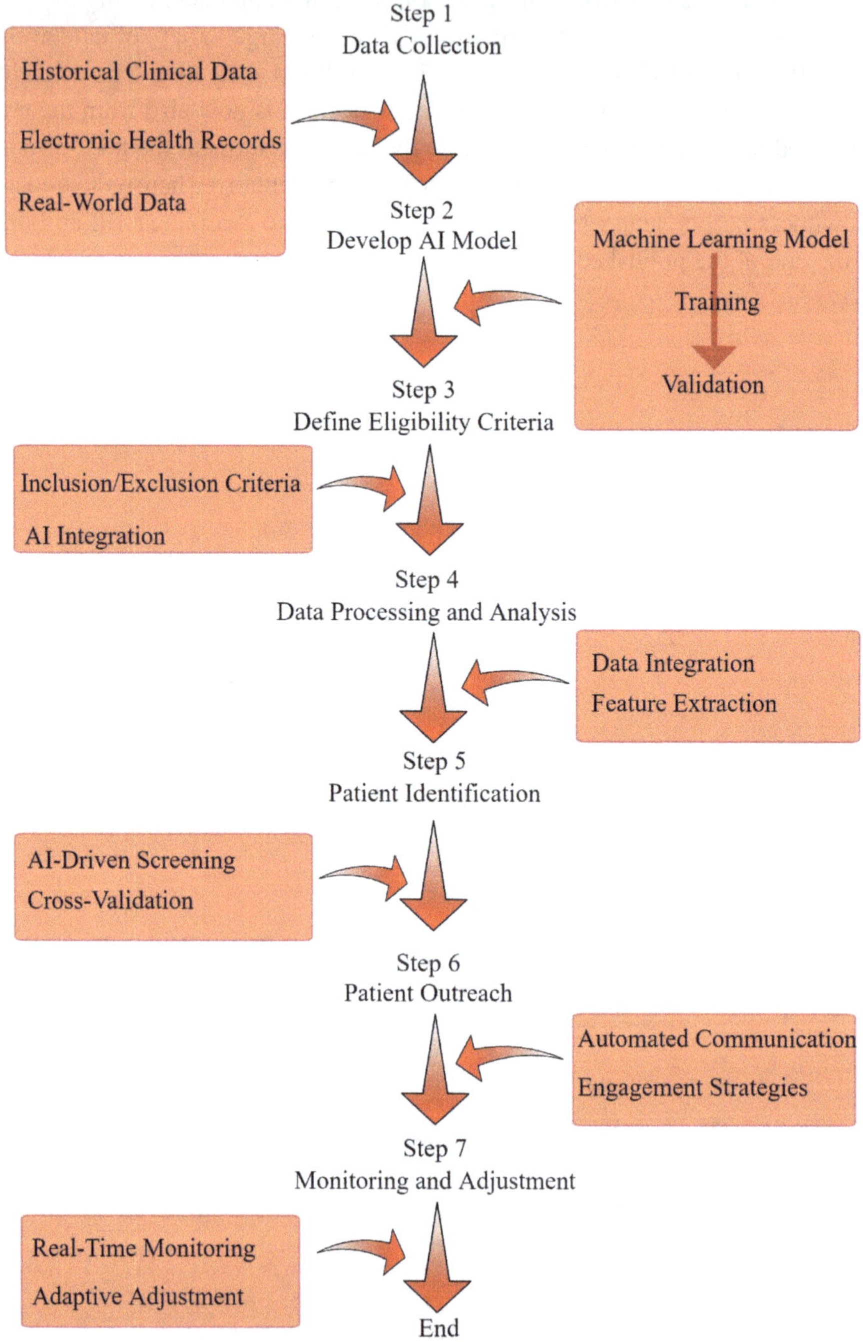

(created by the author using licensed Mind the Graph software)

In addition, Table 4 summarizes a wide selection of recently published journal articles from both the PubMed and Scopus databases, gathered up until July 2024, that focus intensively on integrating AI into clinical trial processes. These articles were pinpointed using the following search query: ("Clinical Trials" AND "Artificial Intelligence"). This table offers a high-level view of current AI applications in clinical trial design and patient recruitment, highlighting five pivotal studies. AI for age-related macular degeneration trials significantly enhanced patient recruitment by identifying more eligible candidates with greater precision than traditional approaches, achieving positive predictive values as high as 63% and 86% when combined with electronic health records (Williamson et al., 2024). AI also plays a vital role in advancing health equity in trials by leveraging participant flow charts to monitor demographic shifts and ensure that representative sampling stays are consistent (Ellen et al., 2024). In another example, an AI-based system for matching lung cancer patients to clinical studies demonstrated 91.6% accuracy, high sensitivity (83.3%), and specificity (93.8%), greatly reducing the time spent screening (Alexander et al., 2020). Automated eligibility screening for pediatric oncology trials enhanced the efficiency of matching and demonstrated high specificity (95.5%) as well as a negative predictive value of 100% (Ni et al., 2015). In addition, NLP and ML applications effectively assessed trial eligibility for HIV patients, achieving F2 scores ranging from 77% to 91% for various classifications (Zhang et al., 2013).

Table 4. Overview of recent AI applications in clinical trial design and patient recruitment

Main Topics	Examples of AI Applications	Main Findings for Observational Studies	References
AI in macular degeneration trial recruitment	AI for recruiting patients with geographic atrophy for macular degeneration trials	AI shortlisted more eligible patients with higher precision (positive predictive value: 63%) than traditional methods. The combined AI-electronic health record approach improved positive predictive value to 86%. AI adjusts to different trial criteria, aiding feasibility.	Williamson et al. (2024)
AI for health equity in trials	Participant flow diagrams for ensuring health equity in AI clinical trials	AI can help identify and mitigate selection biases in clinical trials by using detailed participant flow diagrams to track demographic shifts and ensure representative sampling.	Ellen et al. (2024)
AI-based clinical trial matching system	Evaluation of AI system for matching lung cancer patients to clinical trials	The AI system demonstrated 91.6% accuracy for overall eligibility assessment, with high sensitivity (83.3%) and specificity (93.8%). It significantly reduced the time required for patient screening.	Alexander et al. (2020)
Automated eligibility screening	Automated clinical trial eligibility prescreening for pediatric oncology patients	The system increased efficiency in trial-patient matching, improved precision (36%) and recall (100%) and demonstrated high specificity (95.5%) and negative predictive value (100%).	Ni et al. (2015)
Natural language processing (NLP) and machine learning (ML) for trial eligibility	Application of NLP and ML in evaluating clinical trial eligibility for human immunodeficiency virus patients	Achieved F2 scores ranging from 77% to 91% for different eligibility classifications, demonstrating effective use of AI in processing and matching eligibility criteria from unstructured data.	Zhang et al. (2013)

CHALLENGES

Technical, Ethical, and Regulatory Hurdles in Applying AI to Clinical Trials

While AI in clinical trials shows promise, it comes with many technical, ethical, and regulatory challenges that need to be resolved before full leverage can truly commence. Nevertheless, AI is fundamentally data-driven, and there are significant requirements regarding the storage of large datasets, which can be a major hurdle, especially for small research entities. The second challenge is the need for continuous training and validation of AI systems to ensure accuracy and reliability, which means an ongoing operational strain point. Using AI also raises interesting ethical issues regarding the consent involved in sharing patient data. More broadly, researchers and companies using AI in clinical trials should maintain transparency among trial participants on how ML fits into the picture and how their data are being used or processed. There is also an ethical risk that AI will maintain or possibly intensify access-related disparities found in health care if not properly channeled. There are also substantial regulatory hurdles, as existing laws and guidance might not completely cover elements of how AI is used in clinical studies. As AI continues to evolve at a breakneck pace, regulators still lag, which makes for an uncertain but very jumbled landscape in which organizations that perform international multisite trials need to navigate to stay compliant (Romagnoli et al., 2024).

Data Privacy, Bias, and Equity

One of the top concerns with AI clinical trials is data privacy. As with any type of sensitive health data, it should be well protected and in compliance with the applicable regulations (such as the GDPR in Europe or the HIPAA in the United States). The cornerstone of trust and ethical integrity in clinical trials is ensuring that the data generated by patients remain secure while being used only as agreed upon between patients. Bias in AI models is another issue of concern. The results of such studies may be less useful for underrepresented groups because AI systems are trained on nondiverse data (Kamel, 2024). Therefore, the inclusion of all patient populations must be reflected in training datasets so that AI algorithms can produce fair health outcomes. It is not just that data may incorrectly capture our experiences; this extends to getting access to AI-enabled trials equitably. A major concern is that these highly advanced technologies do not perpetuate or exacerbate existing healthcare inequalities but ameliorate them. Those include things such as making trials available to a diverse population—not just those who can afford it or live near the location of the trial. This necessitates an equal level of ongoing technological innovation, ethical vigilance, and regulatory processes that are all in sync with one another to develop a well-rounded approach to AI use within the context of clinical trials such that we can ensure the greatest prescribed benefits while also minimizing risks (Romagnoli et al., 2024).

Table 5 illustrates a broad range of challenges, as well as AI-based solutions for streamlining the application of AI to clinical trial processes in terms of related technical, ethical, and regulatory considerations. AI analytics platforms with ML and NLP capabilities help overcome technical challenges such as data integration complexity arising from diverse sources (e.g., genomic, clinical) to facilitate automated data cleaning/integration into comprehensive analyses. Technical challenges include addressing algorithmic biases, as well as recognizing variability among algorithms (which can be overcome by using existing ensemble methods) and ensuring that AI applications generalize to broad populations. Currently, ethical concerns such as patient privacy are being handled with cutting-edge encryption and dynamic access controls reinforced by AI to stay ahead of future threats while protecting the sanctity of data. Interactive, AI-driven consent platforms demystify what it means for an AI system to be at work in a trial, help make sense of the murky issues surrounding informed consent in trials with AI support and inform participants about how an algorithm works (to improve understanding and compliance). Using AI-enabled systems to monitor and adapt to global regulatory changes while maintaining continuous compliance in the face of rapidly evolving standards is one aspect of this topic. Second, the absence of uniform standards in AI application evaluation is addressed by designing so-called standardization protocols for AI that enable consistent testing and validation across trials. The solution in Table X works to address a distinct set of problems while making any clinical trials that include AI technologies more robust, transparent, and efficient.

Table 5. Challenges and solutions in AI implementation for clinical trials

Challenge Category	Challenge Description	AI-Driven Solution	Solution Description
Technical	Data Complexity and Integration: The challenge of managing, integrating, and interpreting diverse, voluminous, and complex data types from multiple sources such as genomic, clinical, and wearable device data.	Advanced Data Analytics Platforms with Machine Learning Capabilities: Utilize sophisticated AI tools equipped with machine learning and natural language processing to handle, integrate, and analyze large and complex datasets efficiently.	These platforms automate the processes of data cleaning, normalization, and integration, ensuring that data from different sources can be combined to provide a holistic view of trial outcomes. They also employ advanced analytics to derive actionable insights from integrated data.
Technical	Algorithm Bias and Variability: AI algorithms can inadvertently develop biases based on training data, leading to skewed or unfair trial results, and variability in algorithm performance across different populations.	Bias Detection and Mitigation Algorithms: Implement robust AI systems designed to identify, quantify, and correct biases within datasets and algorithm outputs. Utilize ensemble methods to reduce variability and improve generalizability.	Regular audits, updates, and the use of diverse training datasets ensure that AI algorithms remain unbiased and effective across various demographic groups, maintaining the integrity and applicability of trial results.
Ethical	Patient Privacy and Data Security: Safeguarding the privacy and security of sensitive patient data used in AI models against breaches and unauthorized access.	Advanced Encryption Techniques and Dynamic Access Controls: Deploy AI-enhanced cybersecurity measures including state-of-the-art encryption and dynamic access controls that adapt to evolving threats.	AI-driven security systems continuously monitor data access and usage, automatically adjusting security protocols based on real-time threat analysis to protect patient data throughout the trial process.
Ethical	Informed Consent Complexity: Enhancing the informed consent process to adequately cover AI-specific considerations, ensuring that participants are fully aware of how AI will be used in the study and the implications for their data.	Interactive AI-Powered Consent Platforms: Develop interactive, AI-driven tools that use simple, clear language to explain the roles of AI in trials, potentially augmented by virtual or augmented reality to improve understanding.	These platforms provide tailored, engaging, and comprehensive explanations of AI functionalities and data usage policies, helping participants make well-informed decisions about their involvement.
Regulatory	Keeping Up with Rapid Regulatory Changes: Navigating the rapidly evolving regulatory landscape regarding AI applications in clinical trials, which may differ significantly across jurisdictions.	AI-Enabled Regulatory Tracking and Compliance Systems: Leverage AI to monitor regulatory changes globally and automatically update trial protocols and documentation to ensure compliance.	These AI systems are designed to scan and interpret vast amounts of regulatory data, providing real-time updates and recommendations for maintaining compliance with local and international standards.

Table 6 shows the predicted effects of AI in the future of clinical trials according to the author's assessment and information from the literature. Currently, AI is used in rather simple actions in clinical trials, i.e., patient acquisition, data analysis, and monitoring. Once it is implemented in the future, it will affect the entire range of actions occurring during a trial, integrating real-time data and increasing the complexity of decision-making. It will employ new types of models, allowing for flexibility and autonomy in running trials and patient activities. As a result, the way trials are controlled will be adjusted. Currently, laws and regulations do not have time to react to the implications of AI for a variety of uses. The future, however, will create an entirely encompassing approach that will be particularly designed to legislate the ethical implications of AI. For example, such laws may focus on how the trials are run, how the data are handled and shared, how patient identities are protected, and how the AI decision is being audited. The entire process of trial design will also change. According to the current state, it starts with a fixed paradigm hinged on an adaptive design able to change in real-time according to the outcomes of AI data collection. The whole collection will also adapt depending on how the data is used. The positive effects of the trial today can only be calculated several years after its end. The future will likely be able to predict positive actions before individuals become known. It is also important to mention the predicted effects on the patient's care. The ultimate decisions will be personalized according to the AI's real-time analysis of the patient's data. Naturally, it will be beneficial for the health of patients and for the general safety of treatments.

Table 6. Predictions for the future impact of AI on clinical trial processes

Area of Impact	Current State	Predicted Future State	Impact Description
Advancements in technology	AI is primarily used for patient recruitment, data analysis, and monitoring.	Integration of AI across all trial aspects, including real-time data integration, complex decision-making, and patient management.	AI will evolve to include more sophisticated models like deep learning and reinforcement learning, which will automate and optimize even more complex aspects of clinical trials, such as real-time patient monitoring and adaptive dosing. These technologies will enhance the precision of trials and enable more dynamic responses to data as it is collected.
Regulatory adaptations	Existing regulations are adapting slowly, with basic frameworks focusing on data security and ethical AI use.	Development of advanced regulatory frameworks specifically designed to govern comprehensive AI applications in clinical trials, including ethical AI use, data sharing, and patient privacy.	Regulatory bodies will increasingly focus on creating standards and guidelines that address the specific challenges posed by AI, including how AI decisions are made and audited. This will ensure that AI applications are both safe and effective while maintaining high ethical standards, particularly concerning patient consent and data handling.
Shifts in trial design paradigms	Trials are typically designed with fixed protocols and predetermined endpoints.	Shift toward fully adaptive trial designs facilitated by AI, where protocols and endpoints can evolve based on ongoing data analysis.	The use of AI will lead to a significant shift in how clinical trials are designed and conducted. With AI's capability to analyze data on the fly, trial protocols will become more adaptive, allowing for modifications based on real-time insights. This could include adjusting treatment dosages, changing study endpoints, and even reallocating resources dynamically, making trials more responsive to individual patient needs and potentially leading to quicker, more decisive trial outcomes.

continued on following page

Table 6. Continued

Area of Impact	Current State	Predicted Future State	Impact Description
Enhancement in data utilization	Data utilization is currently linear, primarily retrospective analysis of trial data.	Predictive and prescriptive analytics will dominate, utilizing both historical and real-time data for forward-looking insights and decision-making.	Future AI applications will not only analyze existing data but will also predict future trends and outcomes, enabling prescriptive actions that guide ongoing clinical trial processes. This proactive use of data will minimize risks and enhance the efficiency of trials by predicting potential issues and opportunities for intervention before they arise.
Personalization of Patient Care	Patient care in trials is somewhat standardized, with little customization based on individual data.	Personalized trial experiences and treatment plans based on AI-driven analysis of patient-specific data.	As AI technologies gain the ability to process and learn from vast amounts of individual patient data, clinical trials will increasingly be able to offer personalized care paths. This will adjust treatments and monitoring to the individual's response, enhancing patient safety, treatment efficacy, and overall trial effectiveness.

CONCLUSION AND FUTURE SCOPE

This chapter explores the impact of AI on clinical trial design and patient recruitment. The author has shown that AI, especially with the help of ML, deep learning, and NLP models, provides benefits for various trials. AI has helped in optimizing trial protocol design and allowed the use of efficient methods of patient recruitment. Predictive modeling with the help of various available information has streamlined feasibility assessments that add to the effectiveness of trials. Although concerns still exist, especially concerning the issue of ensuring patient privacy and managing data security, the benefits of AI adoption are a continuation. The challenges of patient diversity and the adaptability of clinical trials have also been addressed. AI makes it possible to increase the speed and efficiency of clinical trials, and its further adoption can make the whole process more effective. In the future, more trials will be more effectively designed, with adequate progress tracking and data safety ensured. This will undoubtedly benefit the thousands of patients involved in trials and the hundreds of scientists carrying out trials.

In conclusion, it is essential to pay attention to trends and research areas that are likely to shape the future of AI in clinical trials. The next focus can be on the further adoption of real-world data and real-world evidence, as they will make the trials even more predictive, and their results will be more representative of actual patients. The use of federated learning models will also become more popular, as they will allow the use of data in a decentralized manner that ensures that the data is not stolen. Ethical decisions in the context of data use must be considered to prevent the use of data in the wrong way. AI ethics and governance will improve with the help of the latest tools and algorithms that eliminate biases and promote equal health outcomes. AI will also contribute to the better use of other technologies, such as blockchain and IoT devices. Finally, future research is likely to develop algorithms capable of dealing with even the most complex data and trials. These technologies will not only refine many of the current practices in biomedical research but also fundamentally change the paradigms of future research practice in the field of digital medicine.

REFERENCES

Abusamaan, M. S., Ballreich, J., Dobs, A., Kane, B., Maruthur, N., McGready, J., Riekert, K., Wanigatunga, A. A., Alderfer, M., Alver, D., Lalani, B., Ringham, B., Vandi, F., Zade, D., & Mathioudakis, N. N. (2024). Effectiveness of artificial intelligence vs. human coaching in diabetes prevention: A study protocol for a randomized controlled trial. *Trials*, 25(1), 325. DOI: 10.1186/s13063-024-08177-8 PMID: 38755706

Alexander, M., Solomon, B., Ball, D. L., Sheerin, M., Dankwa-Mullan, I., Preininger, A. M., Jackson, G. P., & Herath, D. M. (2020). Evaluation of an artificial intelligence clinical trial matching system in Australian lung cancer patients. *JAMIA Open*, 3(2), 209–215. DOI: 10.1093/jamiaopen/ooaa002 PMID: 32734161

Alskaf, E., Frey, S. M., Scannell, C. M., Suinesiaputra, A., Vilic, D., Dinu, V., Masci, P. G., Perera, D., Young, A., & Chiribiri, A. (2024). Machine learning outcome prediction using stress perfusion cardiac magnetic resonance reports and natural language processing of electronic health records. *Informatics in Medicine Unlocked*, 44, 101418. DOI: 10.1016/j.imu.2023.101418 PMID: 38173908

Askin, S., Burkhalter, D., Calado, G., & El Dakrouni, S. (2023). Artificial Intelligence Applied to clinical trials: Opportunities and challenges. *Health and Technology*, 13(2), 203–213. DOI: 10.1007/s12553-023-00738-2 PMID: 36923325

Belue, M. J., Harmon, S. A., Chappidi, S., Zhuge, Y., Tasci, E., Jagasia, S., Joyce, T., Camphausen, K., Turkbey, B., & Krauze, A. V. (2024). Diagnosing progression in glioblastoma—Tackling a neuro-oncology problem using artificial-intelligence-derived volumetric change over time on magnetic resonance imaging to examine progression-free survival in glioblastoma. *Diagnostics (Basel)*, 14(13), 1374. DOI: 10.3390/diagnostics14131374 PMID: 39001264

Bertsimas, D., Antonios Margonis, G., Sujichantararat, S., Koulouras, A., Ma, Y., Antonescu, C. R., & Singer, S. (2024). Interpretable artificial intelligence to optimize use of imatinib after resection in patients with localized gastrointestinal stromal tumors: An observational cohort study. *The Lancet. Oncology*. DOI: 10.1016/S1470-2045(24)00259-6 PMID: 38976997

Bindra, S., & Jain, R. (2024). Artificial intelligence in medical science: A review. *Irish Journal of Medical Science*, 193(3), 1419–1429. DOI: 10.1007/s11845-023-03570-9 PMID: 37952245

Chandra, S., Prakash, P. K. S., Samanta, S., & Chilukuri, S. (2024). ClinicalGAN: Powering patient monitoring in clinical trials with patient digital twins. *Scientific Reports*, 14(1), 12236. DOI: 10.1038/s41598-024-62567-1 PMID: 38806536

Cold, K. M., Xie, S., Nielsen, A. O., Clementsen, P. F., & Konge, L. (2024). Artificial intelligence improves novices' bronchoscopy performance: A Randomized controlled trial in a simulated setting. *Chest*, 165(2), 405–413. DOI: 10.1016/j.chest.2023.08.015 PMID: 37619664

Coskun, B. N., Yagiz, B., Ocakoglu, G., Dalkilic, E., & Pehlivan, Y. (2024). Assessing the accuracy and completeness of artificial intelligence language models in providing information on methotrexate use. *Rheumatology International*, 44(3), 509–515. DOI: 10.1007/s00296-023-05473-5 PMID: 37747564

Dasarathy, S., Tu, W., Bellar, A., Welch, N., Kettler, C., Tang, Q., Liangpunsakul, S., Gawrieh, S., Radaeva, S., & Mitchell, M. (2024). Development and evaluation of objective trial performance metrics for multisite clinical studies: Experience from the AlcHep Network. *Contemporary Clinical Trials*, 138, 107437. DOI: 10.1016/j.cct.2024.107437 PMID: 38215876

Ellen, J. G., Matos, J., Viola, M., Gallifant, J., Quion, J., Anthony Celi, L., & Abu Hussein, N. S. (2024). Participant flow diagrams for health equity in AI. *Journal of Biomedical Informatics*, 152, 104631. DOI: 10.1016/j.jbi.2024.104631 PMID: 38548006

Han, R., Acosta, J. N., Shakeri, Z., Ioannidis, J. P. A., Topol, E. J., & Rajpurkar, P. (2024). Randomized controlled trials evaluating artificial intelligence in clinical practice: A scoping review. *The Lancet. Digital Health*, 6(5), e367–e373. DOI: 10.1016/S2589-7500(24)00047-5 PMID: 38670745

Harrer, S., Menard, J., Rivers, M., Green, D. V. S., Karpiak, J., Jeliazkov, J. R., & Sternke, M. C. (2024). Artificial intelligence drives the digital transformation of pharma. In Krittanawong, C. (Ed.), *Artificial Intelligence in Clinical Practice* (pp. 345–372). Academic Press., DOI: 10.1016/B978-0-443-15688-5.00049-8

Kamel, I. (2024). Artificial intelligence in medicine. *Journal of Medical Artificial Intelligence*, 7, 4. DOI: 10.21037/jmai-24-12

Khalighi, S., Reddy, K., Midya, A., Pandav, K. B., Madabhushi, A., & Abedalthagafi, M. (2024). Artificial intelligence in neuro-oncology: advances and challenges in brain tumor diagnosis, prognosis, and precision treatment. *npj Precision Oncology, 8*(1), 80. DOI: 10.1038/s41698-024-00575-0

Lam, B. D., Dodge, L. E., Zerbey, S., Robertson, W., Rosovsky, R. P., Lake, L., Datta, S., Elavakanar, P., Adamski, A., Reyes, N., Abe, K., Vlachos, I. S., Zwicker, J. I., & Patell, R. (2024). The potential use of artificial intelligence for venous thromboembolism prophylaxis and management: Clinician and healthcare informatician perspectives. *Scientific Reports*, 14(1), 12010. DOI: 10.1038/s41598-024-62535-9 PMID: 38796561

Lee, M. C. M., Parker, C. H., Liu, L. W. C., Farahvash, A., & Jeyalingam, T. (2024). Impact of study design on adenoma detection in the evaluation of artificial intelligence–aided colonoscopy: A systematic review and meta-analysis. *Gastrointestinal Endoscopy*, 99(5), 676–687.e616. DOI: 10.1016/j.gie.2024.01.021 PMID: 38272274

Lin, C., Liu, W.-T., Chang, C.-H., Lee, C.-C., Hsing, S.-C., Fang, W.-H., . . . Cheng, C.-C. (2024). Artificial intelligence–powered rapid identification of ST-elevation myocardial infarction via electrocardiogram (ARISE)—A pragmatic randomized controlled trial. *NEJM AI, 1*(7), DOI: 10.1056/AIoa2400190

Loomans, B. A. C., Mendes, F. M., Vinayahalingam, S., Xi, T., Opdam, N. J. M., Kreulen, C. M., Pereira-Cenci, T., & Cenci, M. S. (2024). Challenges in conducting clinical research in primary care dentistry. *Journal of Dentistry*, 144, 104958. DOI: 10.1016/j.jdent.2024.104958 PMID: 38522408

Lou, N., Cui, X., Lin, X., Gao, R., Xu, C., Qiao, N., Jiang, J., Wang, L., Wang, W., Wang, S., Shen, W., Zheng, X., & Han, X. (2024). Development and validation of a deep learning-based model to predict response and survival of T790M mutant non-small cell lung cancer patients in early clinical phase trials using electronic medical record and pharmacokinetic data. *Translational Lung Cancer Research*, 13(4), 706–720. DOI: 10.21037/tlcr-23-737 PMID: 38736496

Miller, M. I., Shih, L. C., & Kolachalama, V. B. (2023). Machine learning in clinical trials: A primer with applications to neurology. *Neurotherapeutics; the Journal of the American Society for Experimental NeuroTherapeutics*, 20(4), 1066–1080. DOI: 10.1007/s13311-023-01384-2 PMID: 37249836

Nashwan, A. J., & Hani, S. B. (2023). Transforming cancer clinical trials: The integral role of artificial intelligence in electronic health records for efficient patient recruitment. *Contemporary Clinical Trials Communications, 36*, 101223, 101223. DOI: 10.1016/j.conctc.2023.101223

Nene, L., Flepisi, B. T., Brand, S. J., Basson, C., & Balmith, M. (2024). Evolution of drug development and regulatory affairs: The demonstrated power of artificial intelligence. *Clinical Therapeutics*. DOI: 10.1016/j.clinthera.2024.05.012 PMID: 38981791

Ni, Y., Wright, J., Perentesis, J., Lingren, T., Deleger, L., Kaiser, M., Solti, I. (2015). Increasing the efficiency of trial-patient matching: Automated clinical trial eligibility prescreening for pediatric oncology patients clinical decision-making, knowledge support systems, and theory. *BMC Medical Informatics and Decision Making, 15*(1), 28, 28. DOI: 10.1186/s12911-015-0149-3

Patel, S. J., Yousuf, S., Padala, J. V., Reddy, S., Saraf, P., Nooh, A., Fernandez Gutierrez, L. M. A., Abdirahman, A. H., Tanveer, R., & Rai, M. (2024). Advancements in artificial intelligence for precision diagnosis and treatment of myocardial infarction: A comprehensive review of clinical trials and randomized controlled trials. *Cureus*, 16(5), e60119. DOI: 10.7759/cureus.60119 PMID: 38864061

Romagnoli, A., Ferrara, F., Langella, R., & Zovi, A. (2024). Healthcare systems and artificial intelligence: Focus on challenges and the international regulatory framework. *Pharmaceutical Research*, 41(4), 721–730. DOI: 10.1007/s11095-024-03685-3 PMID: 38443632

Ryan, D. K., Maclean, R. H., Balston, A., Scourfield, A., Shah, A. D., & Ross, J. (2024). Artificial intelligence and machine learning for clinical pharmacology. *British Journal of Clinical Pharmacology*, 90(3), 629–639. DOI: 10.1111/bcp.15930 PMID: 37845024

Schepps, M. A., Wong, W. K., Austin, M., & Anisimov, V. (2024). Optimizing patient recruitment in global clinical trials using nature-inspired metaheuristics. *Statistics in Biopharmaceutical Research*, 1–15. DOI: 10.1080/19466315.2024.2308882

Shaw, J., Ali, J., Atuire, C. A., Cheah, P. Y., Español, A. G., Gichoya, J. W., Hunt, A., Jjingo, D., Littler, K., Paolotti, D., & Vayena, E. (2024). Research ethics and artificial intelligence for global health: Perspectives from the global forum on bioethics in research. *BMC Medical Ethics*, 25(1), 46. DOI: 10.1186/s12910-024-01044-w PMID: 38637857

Shi, Z., Hu, B., Lu, M., Chen, Z., Zhang, M., Yu, Y., Zhou, C., Zhong, J., Wu, B., Zhang, X., Wei, Y., & Zhang, L. J.China Aneurysm. (2024). Assessing the impact of an artificial intelligence-based model for intracranial aneurysm detection in CT angiography on patient diagnosis and outcomes (IDEAL Study)—A protocol for a multicenter, double-blinded randomized controlled trial. *Trials*, 25(1), 358. DOI: 10.1186/s13063-024-08184-9 PMID: 38835091

Swathi, N. L., & Kumar, A. (2024). Advanced technologies in clinical research and drug development. In Kumar, R., Joshi, A., Sharan, H., Peng, S., & Dudhagara, C. (Eds.), *The Ethical Frontier of AI and Data Analysis* (pp. 1–17). IGI Global., DOI: 10.4018/979-8-3693-2964-1.ch001

Swendeman, D., Rotheram-Borus, M. J., Arnold, E. M., Fernández, M. I., Comulada, W. S., Lee, S.-J., Ocasio, M. A., Ishimoto, K., Gertsch, W., Duan, N., Reback, C. J., Murphy, D. A., Lewis, K. A., Abdalian, S. E., Bolan, R., Bryson, Y., Cortado, R., Flynn, R., Kerin, T., & Weiss, R. E. (2024). Optimal strategies to improve uptake of and adherence to HIV prevention among young people at risk for HIV acquisition in the USA (ATN 149): A randomized, controlled, factorial trial. *The Lancet. Digital Health*, 6(3), e187–e200. DOI: 10.1016/S2589-7500(23)00252-2 PMID: 38395539

van Dam, P. M. E. L., van Doorn, W. P. T. M., van Gils, F., Sevenich, L., Lambriks, L., Meex, S. J. R., Cals, J. W. L., & Stassen, P. M. (2024). Machine learning for risk stratification in the emergency department (MARS-ED) study protocol for a randomized controlled pilot trial on the implementation of a prediction model based on machine learning technology predicting 31-day mortality in the emergency department. *Scandinavian Journal of Trauma, Resuscitation and Emergency Medicine*, 32(1), 5. DOI: 10.1186/s13049-024-01177-2 PMID: 38263188

Viraswami-Appanna, K., Buenconsejo, J., Baidoo, C., Chan, I., Li, D., Micsinai-Balan, M., Tiwari, R., Yang, L., & Sethuraman, V. (2024). Accelerating drug development at Bristol Myers Squibb through innovation. *Drug Discovery Today*, 29(5), 103952. DOI: 10.1016/j.drudis.2024.103952 PMID: 38508230

Wang, K., Cui, H., Zhu, Y., Hu, X., Hong, C., Guo, Y., An, L., Zhang, Q., & Liu, L. (2024). Evaluation of an artificial intelligence-based clinical trial matching system in Chinese patients with hepatocellular carcinoma: A retrospective study. *BMC Cancer*, 24(1), 246. DOI: 10.1186/s12885-024-11959-7 PMID: 38388861

Wang, M., Qian, Y., Yang, Y., Chen, H., & Rao, W.-F. (2024). Improved stacking ensemble learning based on feature selection to accurately predict warfarin dose. *Frontiers in Cardiovascular Medicine*, 10, 1320938. DOI: 10.3389/fcvm.2023.1320938 PMID: 38312950

Williamson, D. J., Struyven, R. R., Antaki, F., Chia, M. A., Wagner, S. K., Jhingan, M., Wu, Z., Guymer, R., Skene, S. S., Tammuz, N., Thomson, B., Chopra, R., & Keane, P. A. (2024). Artificial intelligence to facilitate clinical trial recruitment in age-related macular degeneration. *Ophthalmology Science*, (6), 100566. DOI: 10.1016/j.xops.2024.100566 PMID: 39139546

Witharana, P., Chang, L., Maier, R., Ogundimu, E., Wilkinson, C., Athanasiou, T., & Akowuah, E. (2024). Feasibility study of rehabilitation for cardiac patients aided by an artificial intelligence web-based programme: A randomized controlled trial (RECAP trial)—a study protocol. *BMJ Open*, 14(4), e079404. DOI: 10.1136/bmjopen-2023-079404 PMID: 38688664

Wolf, R. M., Channa, R., Liu, T. Y. A., Zehra, A., Bromberger, L., Patel, D., Ananthakrishnan, A., Brown, E. A., Prichett, L., Lehmann, H. P., & Abramoff, M. D. (2024). Autonomous artificial intelligence increases screening and follow-up for diabetic retinopathy in youth: The ACCESS randomized control trial. *Nature Communications*, 15(1), 421. DOI: 10.1038/s41467-023-44676-z PMID: 38212308

Xie, X., Luo, C., Wu, S., Qiao, W., Deng, W., Jin, L., Lu, J., Bu, L., Duffau, H., Zhang, J., & Yao, Y. (2024). Recursive partitioning analysis for survival stratification and early imaging prediction of molecular biomarker in glioma patients. *BMC Cancer*, 24(1), 818. DOI: 10.1186/s12885-024-12542-w PMID: 38982347

Xue, L., Singla, R. K., He, S., Arrasate, S., González-Díaz, H., Miao, L., & Shen, B. (2024). Warfarin–A natural anticoagulant: A review of research trends for precision medication. *Phytomedicine*, 128, 155479. DOI: 10.1016/j.phymed.2024.155479 PMID: 38493714

Yao, L., Li, X., Wu, Z., Wang, J., Luo, C., Chen, B., Luo, R., Zhang, L., Zhang, C., Tan, X., Lu, Z., Zhu, C., Huang, Y., Tan, T., Liu, Z., Li, Y., Li, S., & Yu, H. (2024). Effect of artificial intelligence on novice-performed colonoscopy: A multicenter randomized controlled tandem study. *Gastrointestinal Endoscopy*, 99(1), 91–99.e99. DOI: 10.1016/j.gie.2023.07.044 PMID: 37536635

Yao, X., Attia, Z. I., Behnken, E. M., Hart, M. S., Inselman, S. A., Weber, K. C., Li, F., Stricker, N. H., Stricker, J. L., Friedman, P. A., & Noseworthy, P. A. (2024). Realtime Diagnosis from Electrocardiogram Artificial Intelligence-Guided Screening for Atrial Fibrillation with Long Follow-Up (REGAL): Rationale and design of a pragmatic, decentralized, randomized controlled trial. *American Heart Journal*, 267, 62–69. DOI: 10.1016/j.ahj.2023.10.005 PMID: 37913853

Yingngam, B. (2024). Machine Learning Applications for Drug Repurposing. In *Artificial Intelligence and Machine Learning in Drug Design and Development* (pp. 251–294). Wiley-Scrivener., DOI: 10.1002/9781394234196.ch9

Yingngam, B., Navabhatra, A., & Sillapapibool, P. (2024). AI-Driven Decision-Making Applications in Pharmaceutical Sciences. In Nguyen, T. V. T., & Vo, N. T. M. (Eds.), *Using Traditional Design Methods to Enhance AI-Driven Decision Making* (pp. 1–63). IGI Global., DOI: 10.4018/979-8-3693-0639-0.ch001

Yingngam, B., & Sethabouppha, B. (2024). Advanced AI applications for drug discovery. In *Advances in Computational Intelligence for the Healthcare Industry 4.0* (pp. 42–86). IGI Global., DOI: 10.4018/979-8-3693-2333-5.ch003

Zhang, M., Del Fiol, G., Grout, R. W., Jonnalagadda, S., Medlin, R.Jr, Mishra, R., & Fiszman, M. (2013). Automatic identification of comparative effectiveness research from medline citations to support clinicians' treatment information needs. *Studies in Health Technology and Informatics*, 192, 846–850. PMID: 23920677

Chapter 3
Real-World Evidence and AI in Healthcare Analytics

Nur Ozturk
Istanbul Medipol University, Turkey

ABSTRACT

This chapter discusses the transformational role of artificial intelligence (AI) across real-world evidence (RWE) analysis throughout health care. It shows how AI (through Machine learning and Natural language processing) is powerful enough to help deal with voluminous, heterogeneous amounts of semantic-rich healthcare data; full-text records coming from clinical notes. Most notably, AI applications such as predictive models, risk stratification and pattern analysis, or adverse event detection (ADE) are reviewed to underscore how new technologies could enable improved data accuracy along with meaningful information extraction in patient care personalization. Importantly, this complete review highlights the promise of AI to modernize health analytics in a truly meaningful sense and achieve better clinical results.

INTRODUCTION

Nowadays, real-world evidence (RWE) has been essentially synonymous with healthcare analytics and represents a critical component of the story needed to shed light on how well medical interventions work in either practice or only publishable data. RWE is broadly understood as clinical information on the utilization and potential benefits or risks of a medical product derived from Real-World Data (RWD). Patient-generated data distributed by the National Institutes of Health (NIH), such as from wearables, stored in electronic health records (EHRs), retrieved in patient registries, or even through insurance claims are especially loaded with informa-

DOI: 10.4018/979-8-3693-6270-9.ch003

tion that can be crowd-sourced into a dataset for AI but also to arrive at verifiable evidence-based conclusions. RWE synthesis provides a broader understanding of the real-world clinical effectiveness and safety of medical interventions used in unselected patient populations outside controlled randomized clinical trials (RCTs) environments.

Artificial intelligence (AI) has the potential to transform large-scale real-world evidence from a new opportunity into an automatic tool for radical changes in research and pharmaceutical delivery. Such vast and complex datasets that make up RWD are impossible to handle by human beings, but AI with technology like machine learning (ML) or natural language processing (NLP), provides high-end tools for the management of these large datasets present in the healthcare industry. Such technologies help to extract actionable patterns and understanding, which could improve evidence-based decision-making in healthcare (Bhatt, 2019). Various dimensions of healthcare analytics, ranging from drug safety monitoring and personalized medicine to patient journey analysis and comparative effectiveness research have the potential to be reinvented by marrying AI with RWE.

The explosive growth of RWD provides a big opportunity along with challenges. The primary challenges in working with and analyzing RWD rose by the four V's of big data—volume, velocity, variety, and veracity (Geldof et al. 2019). EHRs generate vast amounts of data, and adequate computational power is needed to store the information for analysis. Insurance claims also can add up at high volume, along with patient registries (groupings based on similar health conditions). The rate at which this data is being churned out requires real-time or near-real-time analysis to deliver the insights in a timely manner. Different types of data (e.g. structured, numeric patient demographics; unstructured free-text clinical notes) require specific approaches to process integration and analysis. Also, RWD often lacks veracity primarily because it arises from incomplete or inconsistent data (Batko & Ślęzak, 2022).

Several AI technologies, especially ML and NLP provide solutions for the aforementioned problems by facilitating intelligent use of RWE in healthcare analytics. MacKay et al., (2021) mention ML algorithms are able to analyze a large amount of data through their learning capability which facilitates detecting patterns, predicting clinical outcomes, and stratifying patients with risk profiles. These algorithms can then be trained on RWD to build prognostic models that guide clinical decisions and direct resources For example, clustering and association rule mining methods can be used to discover the hidden patterns from RWD which is beneficial for detecting patient subgroups that have some common characteristics or exposure of similarities towards treatments (Peng et al., 2021). These insights can be used to develop individual treatment plans that lead to better patient outcomes, and more efficient use of healthcare resources.

NLP, a vital AI technology, is ideal for interpreting unstructured data such as clinical notes and medical reports. NLP techniques can be used to collect necessary information from these texts and process them in a structured format for analysis. The NLP approach therefore becomes very useful for recognizing adverse drug events (ADE), researching treatment patterns, and insight from feedback or social media to support the curation of patient experience rather than clinical data (Nawab et al., 2020; Murphy et al., 2023). Automation of medical record data extraction and coding using NLP minimizes manual workload, improves the level of precision in available healthcare analytics, and assures uniformity.

Several use cases illustrate AI applications in healthcare analytics powered by RWE. For example, AI in pharmacovigilance; ADE detection, and drug safety surveillance are significantly improved by AI-driven systems, both playing a crucial role within the framework of pharmacovigilance. NLP has been reported to be useful in automating the extraction of ADEs from unstructured data mediums like EHR and medical case reports by enhancing the productivity and accuracy of pharmacovigilance activities (Gurulingappa et al., 2012; Warrer et al., 2012). Likewise, AI has helped standardize and capture unstructured clinical information from EHRs, and NLP systems can provide structured data for a variety of clinical and research applications (Kreimeyer et al., 2017).

These AI approaches have even been successfully used to validate drug repurposing signals with EHR data. For example, Xu et al. (2015) utilized automated informatics to verify the signal for metformin in reducing cancer mortality, demonstrating validation of AI could identify novel therapeutic indications for extant drugs. These apps highlight the potential of AI to revolutionize how RWE can be applied toward better healthcare impacts.

While the future vision is exciting, incorporating AI and RWE into healthcare analytics does present its fair share of difficulties. Data quality & standardization, AI model validation improvements, and ethics/privacy questions are critical and seem to be ignored. Alongside the absence of common benchmarks, heterogeneous reporting within this space also presents a challenge for assessing AI-based systems in clinical deployment (Choudhury & Asan 2020). In addition, the protection of patient information and ethical considerations around the use of AI in health care is also really important for ensuring trust and adoption of these technologies.

Focus of the Chapter

The chapter attempts to clarify the vital position of AI in enabling the use of RWE for improving healthcare analytics. This chapter has a twofold objective - first, to offer an overarching exploration of the ways in which AI technologies and especially ML & NLP are revolutionizing primary care as well as patient/disease-specific medical research on one hand, and secondly, to further show how machine-learning algorithms permit simultaneous discovery and outcomes translation. AI can analyze RWD from multiple sources like EHRs, patient registries, insurance claims, and real-world data generated by patients through wearable devices to gather actionable insights that may inform evidence-based decision-making.

The chapter discusses the multifaceted challenges of RWE analysis due to the complexity, quantity, and diversity of all types of secondary data. It also demonstrates how AI solutions are a great way to deal with these problems, as they provide advanced analytics that can analyze huge amounts of data, find patterns, and predict clinical results shine in the field for detecting conditions and promoting individualized treatment. The emphasis is on showcasing the practical uses of AI in real-world healthcare settings such as prognostic modeling, risk stratification, ADE identification, and medication repurposing.

The chapter demonstrates the real-world impact of AI on medication safety surveillance, standardizing unstructured clinical information, and increasing overall healthcare delivery quality through thorough case studies and research findings. It also covers the ethical and privacy concerns that arise when integrating AI into healthcare analytics, highlighting the importance of strong data governance structures and model validation methods.

THE ROLE OF AI IN ANALYZING RWE

Challenges in RWE Analysis

Volume, Velocity, Variety, and Veracity of Data

The analysis of RWE is dependent on the appropriate management and interpretation of RWD, which is highly complicated. The four main dimensions of RWE analysis are volume, velocity, variety, and data validity. The healthcare industry has a high amount of data, which it generates in copious amounts every single day. These sources include EHR. This data explosion is driven by a variety of sources, including EHRs, insurance claims, patient registries, genetics, wearable devices, and social media. For example, EHRs contribute to a vast repository of data recording regarding patient histories at the most granular level across all associated treatment regimens, lab results received, and clinically documented care. The healthcare industry produces about 2.5 quintillion bytes of data daily (Jee & Kim, 2013; Raghupathi & Raghupathi, 2014). Such volume creates complexity regarding their storage, management, and analysis. There is a need to switch over to newer, big data technologies and architectures because traditional storage and processing infrastructures cannot easily cater to such huge datasets in many instances.

Velocity represents the speed at which data is created and processed. In the healthcare sector, data is continuously created at high velocity. The processing of real-time data streams can be beneficial for EHRs, monitoring devices, and other digital health technologies to make them offer insights that matter. Continuous glucose monitors and wearable fitness trackers provide raw information streams that new insights need to live in real-time but also need hardware capable of performing sensors at a high speed - all the vital signs calculated lag behind (Murdoch & Detsky, 2013). The need for real-time or near-real-time analysis also complicates the integration and use of RWD, requiring that operational data management have strong elements involving both robust data pipelines as well as essentially an infrastructure associated with somewhat resembling real-time analytics.

RWD is extremely complex because it includes a wide variety of data types and formats. This variety of data represents structured data (numeric lab results, coded diagnoses, etc.); semi-structured data (HL7 messages and XML files) as well as unstructured free-text clinical notes (containing numerical values, medical images, or genomics). Each type of data has different properties, and integration demands certain research approaches for all purposes. While structured data is easier to work with, it doesn't necessarily capture the entirety of patient information. Alternatively, the unstructured data (like physician's notes or imaging studies) can be more clinically meaningful but will typically require advanced post-processing techniques like NLP and image analysis to extract meaning from them (Gandomi & Haider, 2015). RWE has substantial challenges in integrating these disparate data sources into a cohesive dataset that can be efficiently evaluated.

In the era of RWD, veracity is a real problem as data quality varies. Data collected outside of research settings will be filled with inconsistencies, inaccuracies, and biases. EHRs, for instance, may be incomplete or incorrect because of human error in data entry combined with differences among clinical documentation practices and levels of detail recorded by individual healthcare providers (Cabitza et al. 2018). Moreover, patient-reported outcomes or wearable device data could contain bias due to self-reporting or inaccuracy. RWD's validity is ensured by rigorous data cleaning, validation, and harmonization procedures that discover and repair mistakes, and fill in missing information, along with standardized data formats.

Structured vs. Unstructured Data

One of the most difficult aspects of studying RWE is distinguishing between organized and unstructured data. Each category brings distinct obstacles and opportunities for investigation. Structured data is the information that lies within predefined fields, tables, and so on, e.g. databases, spreadsheets, or coded segments located in EHRs. Structured healthcare data might include patient demographics, laboratory test results, billing codes, and medication lists. However, the real benefit of structured data is that one can easily read and interpret it with traditional data processing tools. Structured data are easily queried, summarized, and analyzed to generate descriptive statistics (e.g. counts of patients with different diagnoses), predictive modeling (e.g. algorithms for predicting readmission risk), or other forms of clinical and operational analysis.

Structured data, however, has its own set of constraints as well. Not only does structured data lack the specificity and nuance we get with unstructured data. For example, a structured database might show that an individual has been diagnosed with diabetes but not the symptoms experienced by one; lifestyle factors, or why the doctor decided to prescribe certain treatments. This limitation can result in inaccurate assessments of patient health and outcomes (Murphy et al. 2007).

Unstructured data is information that does not adhere to a model or set structure. Unstructured data within the medical field is extensive, and it comprises clinical notes, discharge summaries, imaging reports, pathology slides, genetic sequences, and even audio and video recordings. This data is rich in clinical context, and it provides detailed narratives of patient disease progression, treatment, and response information absent from structured data. The main issue with unstructured data is its linearity and the problem of identifying relevant information. This raw form of data is just too much for the traditional methods to handle, and so this demands more advanced techniques like NLP or Deep Learning capabilities and many others such as image recognition technologies. For example, NLP can parse clinical notes or reports to pull out symptom mentions and a diagnosis and response to treatment over time by taking free text information many times in the flow of analysis (Kreimeyer et al., 2017).

Comprehensive RWE analysis requires structured and unstructured data to be integrated into an end-to-end software analytics framework. This allows researchers and clinicians to capture the benefits of both data types; quantitative reliability stemming from structured data, combined with qualitative depth gained through unstructured clinical notes. This integration can improve the accuracy and depth of clinical findings, enabling more nuanced and effective healthcare decision-making.

Data Completeness and Accuracy

Ensuring data completeness and correctness is critical to the validity and reliability of RWE analyses. Inadequate or inaccurate data might result in skewed results, incorrect conclusions, and eventually, poor patient care and research outcomes.

Data completeness measures how accurately all required data points are captured and provided for analysis. This completeness can be compromised by gaps in data entry, variability of clinical documentation practices, and inherent limitations associated with certain types of data sources within the realm of RWD. For example, EHRs may have incomplete patient records due to patients receiving care from multiple providers whose (often paper-based) records are not fully integrated; they could also arise from discrepancies in the documentation of clinical encounters (Weiskopf & Weng, 2013).

Limited data complicates RWE analysis. Missing values can distort statistical analyses, lower the performance of prediction models, and undermine their ability to generalize. Some strategies to overcome missing data are through the techniques of imputation that estimate what the value would be based on other information available in a dataset, and by using multiple data sources as potential avenues for filling gaps. Nevertheless, none of these approaches are accurate; if not properly used they could potentially add more bias to the prediction (Little & Rubin, 2020).

Data accuracy applies to the reliability and accuracy of data entries. Errors in manual data input, incorrect coding, and differences between collection methods are just a few of the ways that inaccurate data can come within the system. For instance, coding errors in a diagnosis or medication dose can cause serious mistakes in clinical research and patient care decisions (Marino et al., 2021).

Data accuracy calls for a rigorous approach to data validation and cleansing. The process of validating is used to verify the accuracy with which data has been recorded against legitimate sources or rules. Cleaning operations are designed to detect and correct mistakes, standardize data formats, and assure consistency among datasets. In RWE analysis, for example, these methods are even more important as the accuracy of findings depends on data quality.

Additionally, the heterogeneity of sources of RWD introduces challenges in accurate data quality. Healthcare providers themselves use different terminologies, codes, and data entry procedures which may not be consistent. Standardization of data using shared terminology and ontology (e.g., SNOMED, ICD-10) is necessary to improve the precision of data as well as for meaningful comparisons across datasets (Xu et al., 2016).

Ongoing data completeness and accuracy are a challenge for RWD and need continuous efforts across levels to address. Healthcare providers need to adopt comprehensive data governance models inclusive of clear-cut defined standards, clean audit trails, and processes for continuous quality management. Such frameworks need to include the representation of stakeholders from all levels in the ecosystem - clinicians, data scientists, and IT professionals alike- for an end-to-end sound approach to managing data quality.

In addition, technology has a huge part to play in overcoming these challenges. A variety of specialized tools are available for the automated capture of data like interfaces into EHRs that ease up manual entry and reduce human errors, hence increasing completeness and accuracy. It is more likely that an AI-driven data validation and cleaning tool will bring into play complicated algorithms for identifying errors, filling missing value slots (imputation), standardizing data formats, etc. For example, they can be trained to detect anomalies in data entries and signal potential errors (Nassif et al., 2021).

AI Solutions to RWE Challenges

Machine Learning (ML)

ML is a subset of artificial intelligence that focuses on the development and use of algorithms. ML has become a formidable weapon in overcoming some of the limitations faced with real-world evidence analysis; specifically, those related to variety, velocity, volume, and variety of data.

One of the most important uses of ML in RWE analysis is handling the enormous volume and velocity of data produced in medical facilities. Traditional data processing techniques do not measure up in handling the large-scale, real-world datasets that underlie RWD. Unlike humans, which are slow and prone to errors while processing a large amount of data at once, ML algorithms, especially those designed for big data applications, can do this fast and accurately enough. Parallel computation along with distributed computing allows for effective management of huge datasets, resulting in rapid interpretation and analysis (Dean & Ghemawat, 2008).

As an example, one of the most common applications for ML is predictive modelling which uses historical data to forecast future outcomes. This ability is critical for spotting changing health patterns, predicting disease outbreaks, and guiding public health actions. For instance, ML algorithms like random forests or support vector machines can analyze complex datasets spang across millions of records to produce accurate predictive insights (Obermeyer & Emanuel 2016).

RWD is complex, both formatted and unformatted data, which makes it difficult to analyze. ML algorithms are effective in working with heterogeneous data. Feature engineering techniques can turn raw data into a format amenable to analysis by extracting meaningful features from both structured and unstructured data. Deep learning replicas, notably CNNs, and RNNs, have shown extraordinary performance in analyzing unstructured information, like medical photos as well as medical records (Shickel et al., 2018).

Also, ensemble learning methods aggregate multiple ML models, which can increase the reliability and accuracy of analysis by capturing the benefits of several unique algorithms. For example, ensembles of decision trees with logistic regression models can perform better predictions in the presence of heterogeneous data sources leading to a clearer view, which defines health outcomes for patients (Breiman, 2001).

Verification of RWD is essential to guarantee the reliability and quality of RWE analysis. ML algorithms are used to find and fix errors, inconsistencies, and biases in the data. With data processing, anomaly detection algorithms are able to highlight outliers as well as doubtful entries. It is easy and saves time when performing data cleaning and validation. For example, some data mining techniques discover clusters and principal components in the data that can serve as a sort of unsupervised pre-processing step, highlighting potential trouble spots (Chandola et al., 2009).

In addition, ML algorithms may be designed to detect and repair data entry mistakes. Natural language processing (NLP) approaches, as detailed in the next part, may be used to analyze as well as standardize clinical writing, therefore reducing variation and improving data accuracy. These skills are critical for maintaining good quality data and making sure RWE-derived insights are accurate and useful.

Natural Language Processing (NLP)

NLP is an area of AI that studies how computers interact with human language. In the setting of RWE, NLP is critical for analyzing and extracting unstructured information from various textual sources, including discharge summaries, clinical notes as well as patient detailed results.

A considerable amount of RWD, unstructured data has intrinsic clinical information that is not formalized into structured data fields. NLP techniques allow this information to be gleaned from text, providing a transformation of free text into well-structured data that can then be subjected to quantitative analysis. For instance, named entity recognition (NER) algorithms scan clinical text for entities such as drugs of interest, diseases, and symptoms to enable identification or extraction into electronic structured resources where disease concept highlighter would extract the relevant details from all available sources, facilitating studies capturing the clinical details; if at least one can be identified (Wei et al., 2013).

An additional NLP application, sentiment analysis can also be used to determine treatment satisfaction and outcomes directly from patient-reported data. Analyzing patient feedback could offer insight into the sentiment and context behind it, allowing both researchers and healthcare providers to view the data as humans would, which can lead to improved care quality (Gohil et al., 2018).

Integration and standardization of different data sources are also supported by NLP. Clinical text often contains spoken terms, synonyms, and abbreviations which can create problems during the integration of data generally use different standardized terminology. These variations can be normalized using NLP algorithms, which map the terms to medical standard vocabularies like SNOMED CT (Systematized Nomenclature of Medicine Clinical Terms), or ICD-10. Standardization is important to keep the data consistent and comparable (Liu et al., 2019).

Additionally, NLP can also support harmonization of multi-source data where clinical narratives and the structured fields. These changes can yield data completeness and accuracy gains by using NLP techniques to assign codes in EHRs (e.g., from symptoms and diagnoses listed in clinical notes) that fuel automated adverse event detection. This ensures all necessary patient information is collected side-by-side, and as such easier to coordinate a full RWE analysis across the data stack (Brom et al., 2020).

Through NLP, the structured data that can be acquired from raw text is used to improve predictions and decision-making. Predictive models perform best when informed by relevant details from clinical notes and more unstructured text sources. For instance, NLP-enhanced predictive models that capitalize on the rich clinical context present in unstructured data have demonstrated accuracy improvements for disease progression predictions, patient readmissions, and treatment responses (Miotto et al., 2018).

In addition, NLP can support clinical decision-making by analyzing real-time documentation. For instance, clinical decision support systems (CDSS) use NLP to parse through detailed information about patients in the form of clinical notes and profile prescription patterns or missed diagnoses so that healthcare providers can detect potentially dangerous scenarios via alerts to higher patient safety as well as care quality (Jung et al., 2013).

The deployment of NLP in RWE analysis is, however, not without hindrances despite its promise. A major issue is clinical language and documentation practices differ widely. Variations in the nomenclature, abbreviations, and documentation style of healthcare providers can make NLP processing significantly challenging. In addition, advanced NLP models based on deep learning for large corpora of clinical text are under development to handle various languages (Yin et al., 2016).

One such problem is the requirement of huge, annotated datasets for training and validating NLP models. Clinical text annotation is a time-consuming procedure that requires the proficiency of domain experts, consequently restricting large-scale training data availability. Efforts to develop systematized as well as publicly available medical text databases are critical for improving NLP skills in healthcare (Murphy et al., 2007).

Machine Learning Applications in RWE Analysis

Prognostic Models for Clinical Outcomes

ML has greatly facilitated the development of prognostic models for clinical outcomes enabling more accurate predictions on patient trajectories than traditional statistical methods. Prognostic models are invaluable for predicting the course of a disease, choosing treatment strategies, and managing patients. Doing so ML allows the discovery of patterns and relationships in the data that are not easily accessible via traditional analytics due to the use of large quantities of RWD.

Researchers found that ML included in prognostic models significantly improved the accuracy of these models. Classic models like Cox proportional hazards and logistic regression rely on fixed relationships between variables. In contrast to linear regression, ML, such as decision trees, random forests (RFs), gradient boosting machines (GBMs), and neural networks can be used in a non-linear fashion which helps them fully capture complex nonlinear interactions within the data leading to increased accuracy and robustness of predictions (Obermeyer & Emanuel 2016).

In cancer patients, ML models have been used to predict the risk of disease recurrence. Kourou et al. (2015) found that ML methods such as support vector machines and neural networks surpassed standard statistical models for cancer prediction. Using these algorithms, the team analyzed clinical, genetic, and demographic data simultaneously to identify intricate patterns in a manner that could more effectively guide treatment decisions and follow-up strategies.

ML has the property of being able to work with high-dimensional data, i.e. datasets where there are a vast number of predictors available for use in creating predictions. Data such as genomic data with its thousands of variables are not well suited for traditional statistical methods due to the complexity and number of predictors. ML techniques, especially regularized regression methods such as LASSO (Least Absolute Shrinkage and Selection Operator) and Ridge regression, can handle large datasets by selecting and regularizing variables, avoiding overfitting, and improving model generalizability (Tibshirani, 1996).

ML models consistently outperform in combining data from different proprietary and open-source providers for improved accuracy. One example is the fact that by comparing EHR data with imaging and genomic information, one can gain a full view of a patient's state of health. Convolutional neural networks (CNNs) have recently shown promise in examining medical image data such as MRIs and CT scans, a frontline use-case being their successful combination with clinicopathologic information to prognosticate outcomes like tumor recurrence or therapeutic response (Esteva et al., 2017).

Risk Stratification and Personalized Medicine

Risk stratification and personalized medicine are game-changing areas in healthcare where ML aids to analyze RWD. It is being leveraged for categorizing patients according to their risk profile, as well as treatment individualization. In the context of care and public health, this strengthens disease control while directing attention (and limited resources) to those most at risk.

Risk stratification involves divvying up patients into groups with different risks of the worst health outcomes. Through processing large amounts of data, ML algorithms can capture fine subtle risk factors and interactions that traditional methods do not. ML models may stratify individuals with chronic illnesses such as diabetes or cardiovascular disorders, predicting the probability of consequences like stroke or myocardial infarction (Miotto et al., 2018).

In a study, Rajkomar et al. (2018) designed an ML model on EHR records for predicting patient mortality, readmission, and prolonged length of stay. This model was built for many different things, including laboratory results and vital signs with medication info demographics, etc. The ability to predict is very high compared to other scoring systems. Such models help healthcare professionals detect high-risk patients early on, allowing for prompt treatments and perhaps lowering negative consequences.

Personalized medicine seeks to personalize medical therapy to the unique features of each patient. ML is perfect for this kind of problem because it can interpret multidimensional data (genetic, environmental, and lifestyle) which means its potential value in personalized medicine is massive. ML models can recommend individualized courses of treatment that are tailored to the convoluted profile of every patient and optimize response without adding any excess disease burden.

Pharmacogenomics is one of the essential applications in personalized medicine where ML plays a critical role as it helps us to understand how genes affect the response and metabolism of drugs. For instance, ML algorithms can mine the volumes of genomic data to determine how a patient is expected to respond at an individual level before designing solutions for cure and care providing both accurate treatment selections from the widest spectrum of available drugs yet ensuring inimical selected drug elimination. For example, ML has been successfully used to predict warfarin dosing based on genetic variants that impact drug metabolism (Johnson & Cavallari, 2013).

ML also helps in improving treatment plans by constantly learning from new patient data. Adaptive treatment strategies, which update the given therapy based on individual responses, have been developed as a subset of ML reinforcement learning. Such as in oncology, where reinforcement learning algorithms can be used to determine optimal chemotherapy dosing schedules that are both effective and less toxic overall improving patient outcomes (Liu et al., 2019).

In the meantime, predictive models with ML can help to find patients for clinical trials who might benefit from experimental treatment. ML can use this information to match the criteria of who would likely be positively responding to patients, and analyze patient data for evaluation-related purposes, allowing clinical trials to expedite their process along with increasing chances of success (Ryan et al., 2014).

Although potentially beneficial, several obstacles hinder the utilization of ML in risk stratification and personalized medicine. These present significant challenges such as data quality and completeness, model interpretability, and clinician understanding present some major challenges. Understanding ML models by clinicians is important in building clinician trust and acceptability for uptake (Caruana et al., 2015).

Future research should work on developing powerful but also explainable ML models and deal with the ethical questions around personalized medicine. The key will be to protect patient privacy and secure the databases. Furthermore, a multidisciplinary collaboration among data scientists, physicians, and policymakers will be required to transform machine-learning discoveries into actual health advantages (Topol, 2019).

Pattern Analysis in RWD

Patterns are the most significant part of raw healthcare data that transforms into informative insights and thus is a critical point. This is articulated in combing through massive datasets to tease out trends, correlations, and anomalies that instruct the practice of clinical care, and health policy decision-making at a macro level and lay the framework for personalized patient care. The conjunction of ML algorithms has greatly improved the analytical possibilities to analyze patterns and unveil all kinds of sophisticated relationships that classical methods might be missing out.

Pattern analysis utilizes a number of different ML techniques, each with its own strengths. K-means and hierarchical clustering are among the popular grouping methods where all similar patients are published into a cluster to make it easier for disease sub-typing or patient stratification (Gao et al., 2023) For example, these methods have been employed to find patient subgroups with similar responses to treatment in oncology which improve understanding of treatment response and tailored therapies.

An equally important technique is association rule learning, which reveals associations or relationships among variables in large data sets. The Apriori algorithm and FP-Growth methods are used to find out frequent itemsets and in turn the association rules. These have been used in pharmacovigilance to detect possible drug interactions and adverse effects via analyzing patterns within patient records of prescribed medications (Borgelt 2005).

Pattern analysis via ML has several applications within healthcare. One such example is the use of ML technology to predict hospital re-admissions. ML may be used in a targeted manner, assessing patterns of patient data such as specific demographics but also comorbidities and previous hospitalizations to identify "high-risk" readmitted patients. Such patients will be able to benefit from focused interventions that have been found successful at decreasing readmission rates (Shameer et al. 2017).

In chronic disease care, pattern analysis assists professionals in tracking the progress of the patient's condition and also helps determine how effective different treatment modalities are in mitigating that particular issue. In diabetes management, ML models process patient glucose levels and compliance to medication or lifestyle factors revealed patterns which in turn would seem a complication such as cardiovascular disease therefore determine the most appropriate course of action (Miotto et al., 2018).

Despite its promise, pattern analysis in RWD has several hurdles. Healthcare data is heterogeneous in nature (structured-e.g., laboratory results, unstructured- e.g. - clinical notes), and even the analysis adds complexity to this process. There is also the issue of data ethics/data governance where it works to ensure that measurement and informational ecosystems operate correctly. Another problem is ensuring data quality and completeness since missing or erroneous data can have a major influence on the validity of detected patterns (Murphy et al., 2007).

Furthermore, there is ongoing worry about the interpretability of ML models. Although complicated models like deep neural networks are extremely accurate, their black-box nature renders it difficult to grasp the underlying patterns they find. This dearth of transparency may impede clinical uptake and confidence in ML-driven insights (Caruana et al., 2015).

ANALYZING UNSTRUCTURED DATA WITH DEEP LEARNING

Unstructured data, like clinical notes, medical photographs, and patient narratives, make up a large component of healthcare information. DL (a subset of ML) has enabled groundbreaking progress in the analysis of unstructured data by offering sophisticated techniques to draw valuable conclusions from large and high-dimensional sets of structured or multidimensional sources.

One of the most important applications in DL for analyzing unstructured textual data is NLP in healthcare, because clinical notes, discharge summaries, and patient stories comprise information otherwise missing in the structured data sheets. NLP techniques, particularly deep learning-based NLP models like Recurrent Neural

Networks (RNNs) and transformers have shown promise in extracting and understanding such information from free text (Ahmed et al., 2023).

DL-based NLP models are able to distinguish between what is a medical condition vs. treatment or an outcome of patient care. A study by Miotto et al. (2018) employed DL to interpret EHRs for the prediction of disease phenotypes, highlighting NLP's ability to convert free text into valuable data.

Similarly, DL has had substantial effects on the domain of medical image analysis as well. CNNs are very useful for medical image processing such as X-rays, MRIs, and CT scans. Such models can pick up patterns and anomalies with a high degree of accuracy, often better than human capabilities in tasks such as tumor detection or classification (Esteva et al., 2017). CNNs have also been used in the analysis of retinal images for early detection of diabetic retinopathy. These models are trained on vast datasets of annotated images (data points) and can detect even the smallest anomalies in the retina indicating disease progression which allows early intervention measures to save lives (Gulshan et al., 2016)

Although DL has shown great potential for processing unstructured data there are some challenges to allow these networks to be capable of analyzing such type of information. A major challenge, however, is that DL approaches require large labeled data sets to be able to train the models well. Creating and labeling these datasets can be expensive both labor and effort-wise. Furthermore, DL models perform as a black box and are not interpretable by clinicians, thus clinicians may be skeptical about the results given which challenges mold trust issues (Samek et al., 2017).

In addition, employing DL models in clinical workflows necessitates attention to usability and regulatory compliance. However, it is critical that these models yield clinically useful and implementable recommendations for real-world effectiveness in the practice of medicine (Topol, 2019).

Future works need to develop more interpretable DL models and methods for unsupervised learning (use cases with no labeled data) which can exploit unlabelled data and provide valuable information. Moreover, partnerships among data scientists, clinicians, and policymakers are needed to overcome both the ethical and logistical issues faced in deploying DL within healthcare (Liu et al., 2019).

Natural Language Processing Applications in RWE Analysis

Extracting Information From Clinical Notes and Reports

NLP is a revolutionary technology in the context of RWE analysis, which helps extract actionable information from unstructured text data like clinical notes, reports, or patient Narratives. The advent of NLP in healthcare has enabled harnessing a vast amount of textual data produced at clinics and helped expedite decision-making as well as patient care.

Clinical notes and reports are repositories of patient data in the form of medical history, diagnoses, treatment plans, or outcomes. However, their unstructured nature is a challenge for the extraction and analysis of data. Utilization of NLP techniques, especially the one based on DL models such as transformers and RNNs has provided significant insight in overcoming these challenges.

One can train NLP models that identify and extract medical entities (concepts) as well as relationships between these concepts from clinical text. For example, named entity recognition (NER) algorithms recognize the mentions of diseases, medications, and procedures in clinical notes thus transforming free text into structured data that permits systematic analysis (Jiang et al., 2011). These data are used to establish detailed patient profiles and monitor changes in disease state over time; essential when evaluating therapies that target specific gene defects.

In addition, NLP provides potentially efficient tools like summarization and information retrieval to optimize clinical workflows. Techniques for automated summarization are used which can condense the necessary information in a long text (in particular clinical documents) into short texts giving healthcare providers useful and concise summaries of content. This function can particularly be useful in dealing with patient records and rapid clinical decisions (Liu et al., 2019).

Extracting patient traits from EHRs is one example of an excellent NLP application. NLP models can analyze clinical notes to pick out patterns that represent certain phenotypes, which may help in identifying groups of patients for research or even personalized medicine interventions (Tenenbaum, 2016). This increases the ability to identify phenotypes more accurately and also allows for large-scale epidemiological studies.

Another major NLP application for data extraction from clinical notes is medication extraction. Medication regimens are complex, with multiple drugs often for different durations and doses. NLP algorithms, including deep learning-based sequence tagging models enabling the extraction of granular medication information from unstructured clinical text, provide a novel form of data that has not been previously available for complete analysis around prescribing patterns and adherence (Yang & Kar, 2023).

Moreover, NLP enables the extraction of more chronological information from clinical notes (e.g. timing of symptom onset, progression, and treatment). In essence, one of the critical aspects of disease progression and intervention effectiveness over time is temporal information. Temporal relation extraction models exploit RNNs/transformers to adequately learn temporal information in a structured way (Hossain et al., 2023).

Also, NLP has been used on other formats of unstructured text data such as radiology reports and pathology reports. Radiology reports contain a wealth of information about imaging findings that is essential for diagnosis and treatment planning. These reports can be reconstructed by NLP models to uncover data including lesion size, location, and characteristics needed for longitudinal disease progression tracking (Kahn et al., 2013). Furthermore, pathology reports provide useful information regarding tissue samples, such as histological results and molecular markers. This information was extracted and standardized using NLP approaches, making it easier to integrate with other clinical data for full analysis (Sezgin et al., 2022).

Identifying Adverse Events and Treatment Patterns

The ability to identify ADEs as well as treatment patterns is another important application of NLP. In healthcare ADEs are a major problem, and have an impact on patient morbidity and escalating the cost of treatment. In standard identification methods such as voluntary reporting systems by medical professionals or consumers to regulatory agencies, delayed or under-reporting has been the common experience. NLP takes a proactive approach to ADE detection by simply mining clinical narratives for mentions, which catches many more and much sooner (Murphy et al., 2023).

NLP algorithms may look at clinical notes, discharge summaries, and other types of unstructured text for mentions of adverse reactions, negative effects, and treatment failures. Specifically, literature has demonstrated that high-precision and recall ADEs are more likely to be identified than other forms of ADEs using DL models such as CNN and long short-term memory (LSTM) networks for parsing clinical text (Fan et al., 2020). Additionally, these models also use contextual information to tell adversities attributed directly to treatment from those arising otherwise.

In addition to detecting ADEs, NLP allows for the investigation of treatment trends across many patient groups. NLP models can extract and aggregate data regarding prescribed drugs, dosing, and duration of use to detect normal treatment regimens as well as deviations in practice (Hripcsak & Albers, 2015). This information is vitally important to determine how efficacious treatments are in the real world and for pinpointing areas of improvement.

Another use case for NLP is pharmacovigilance, in which patient records are scanned on an ongoing basis to identify potential safety signals early. NLP systems have also been integrated into EHRs to monitor patient data in real-time, and identify potential safety issues for follow-up (Hossain et al., 2023). It improves the scope for proactive intervention which results in better monitoring and improving patient safety.

Moreover, NLP can help with healthcare policy by mapping treatment patterns. Through analyzing vast databases of clinical text, researchers can gain knowledge about the relative efficacy of various therapies, compliance with clinical guidelines, and variances in care provision. The insights from this can inform evidence-based changes in clinical practice and healthcare policy (Hong et al. 2016).

Conventional NLP is used in oncology to determine whether patients diagnosed with cancer are treated according to clinical guidelines, involving extraction of relevant information from pathology reports and clinical notes. Such evaluation is useful for assessment of the use of different types of therapy modalities like surgery, chemotherapy, and radiation therapy along with their results. NLP models have, for instance, been used to automatically identify patients receiving off-label treatments and assess the impact of those treatments on patient survival (Sheikhalishahi et al., 2019).

NLP has also made substantial advances in the investigation of chronic illnesses. NLP can discover stent details as recorded in unstructured clinical text or adherence and treatment patterns for patients with diseases like diabetes, hypertension, and chronic obstructive pulmonary disease (COPD). This can then be used to generate interventions targeting adherence and favorable treatment outcomes (Dhillon & Singh, 2018).

A more sophisticated application of NLP has been used to parse surgical notes and post-operative reports in order to create a structured analysis of outcomes from surgery. Surgical methods, complications, and the time for recovery are given in this analysis. As an example, NLP models have been employed to help identify who is at high risk for post-operative complications so early interventions may be placed as necessary which could ultimately result in improved surgical outcomes (Ghassemi et al., 2019).

Capturing Patient Sentiments and Experiences

Sentiment Analysis is a subfield of NLP that deals with identifying and classifying opinions in text data. Sentiment analysis can be used in healthcare to evaluate patient sentiment around care. A related approach is sentiment analysis where emotions and opinions are parsed from patient narratives as three types of subjectivity, positive, negative, or neutral. Support Vector Machines (SVM), Naïve Bayes, and deep learning models such as RNN and Transformer-based models like BERT have been shown to be effective in this area (Pang et al., 2002; Devlin et al., 2018).

A study by Greaves et al. (2013) also applied sentiment analysis to over 6412 online comments on patient comments on the NHS website and found meaningful trends related to patient satisfaction or the need for improvement. Similarly, another research used Twitter data to track public attitudes regarding the COVID-19 pandemic, offering real-time input on public health initiatives (Lamsal, 2020).

In addition to sentiment classification, more advanced NLP techniques like topic modeling and thematic analysis are used to find common themes in patient narratives. Topic modeling techniques such as Latent Dirichlet Allocation (LDA) and Non-Negative Matrix Factorization (NMF) have been widely used to mine the dominant topics from large text corpora (Blei et al., 2003; Lee & Seung, 1999). For example, in one study by Wallace et al. (2014) researchers reported using LDA to analyze patients, they extracted some of the main themes in terms of doctor-patient communications, treatment effectiveness, and waiting time.

Integrating sentiment data with clinical results can give a more complete picture of patient health and treatment success. Moreover, study results suggest that patient attitudes are an important correlate to clinical outcomes like treatment satisfaction overall and medication adherence (Choudhury & Asan, 2020). By combining sentiment analysis results with EHRs, researchers can identify intricate correlations between patient experiences and clinical indicators, driving individualized treatment methods.

Automating Medical Data Coding and Classification

NLP algorithms can be employed to assign standardized codes ICD-10 (International Classification of Diseases, 10th Revision) and CPT (Current Procedural Terminology) codes automatically based on clinical documentation. Several methods, such as Named Entity Recognition (NER), and rule-based systems with ML models have achieved success in this context (Friedman et al. 2004). Early applications of NLP, such as the MedLEE system, were able to automate tasking for report-based clinical information extraction and coding (Friedman et al. 2004).

Recent advances in deep learning have improved automated coding skills. CNN and Transformer architectures have achieved a high accuracy on medical text classification tasks. Recent research by Shi et al. (2015) demonstrated that CNNs were highly effective when applied to ICD-10 code assignment, and represented state-of-the-art performance in large-scale EHR datasets.

Automated coding and categorization increase data quality as well as interoperability. Standardized coding enables better communication of information between diverse healthcare systems, and allows for consistent documentation. Standardization is important for studies utilizing large-scale RWE, as it allows the data from different sources to be combined in an analysis (Hripcsak et al., 2015).

In addition to the above-mentioned benefits, real-time clinical decision support (CDS) is one of the most important advantages of automated medical data coding. Combining NLP-based coding systems with CDS tools enables healthcare practitioners to get timely warnings and suggestions based on the most recent clinical guidelines along with patient-specific data. An NLP-driven CDS system, for example, can automatically detect possible drug interactions or recommended diagnostic tests which will improve clinical decision-making (Wang et al., 2018).

Use Cases of AI in RWE-based Healthcare Analytics

Adverse Drug Event (ADE) Detection and Drug Safety Surveillance

ADEs are unanticipated and undesirable outcomes of pharmaceutical usage. Identifying and monitoring adverse drug events is critical for patient safety and successful pharmacovigilance. Traditional methods of detecting ADEs frequently depend on spontaneous reporting systems, which are subject to underreporting and delays. AI provides significant capabilities for improving ADE detection and drug safety surveillance through automated evaluation of massive volumes of real-world data.

Case Studies and Research Findings

One well-known use of AI in ADE identification is the analysis of clinical notes and patient narratives in EHRs using natural language processing. NLP algorithms can extract useful information about medication responses, symptoms, and outcomes that may not be represented in structured data fields. Wang et al. (2018) demonstrated a high-throughput NLP-based system able to deliver more accurate identification of ADEs and superior performance when compared with traditional methods in identifying them from clinical notes.

Using massive datasets containing information from patient demographics to medical histories as well as laboratory results, ML algorithms can pick out patterns and risk factors linked with ADEs. Denck et al. (2023) provided a summary of the systematic review using EHR data; which includes a predictive model for early identification and prediction of adverse drug reactions using electronic health record data.

Also, post-market drug safety can be monitored using AI-driven surveillance systems. These systems perform ongoing analysis of data from a wide range of sources such as social media, forums, and patient reviews to identify new safety trends. For example, Freifeld et al. (2014) used an NLP-based technique to evaluate information from Twitter for early identification of medication safety concerns, indicating the social media possibilities as a supplemental source of information for pharmacovigilance.

AI has been used in the FDA's Sentinel Initiative to monitor the safety of products under regulation by this agency. By reviewing the EHR and claims data of millions of patients, AI algorithms can identify safety issues far more quickly and with greater accuracy than conventional approaches. Moreover, this work also depicts the large-scale pharmacovigilance potential of AI as a tool to improve drug safety monitoring (Platt et al., 2012)

Besides, machine learning using AI such as deep study has been used in SRS (spontaneous reporting system) databases. For example, Mohsen et al. (2021) used a deep learning model to predict ADEs from the FDA Adverse Event Reporting System (FAERS). The model outperformed conventional statistical approaches in detecting uncommon and severe ADEs, highlighting AI's potential for improving the accuracy and specificity of ADE identification.

Standardization and Capture of Unstructured Clinical Information

Unstructured healthcare data, like free-text clinical notes, can be difficult to integrate and analyze. AI technologies, notably NLP, help to standardize and gather unstructured clinical information, translating it into structured, usable data.

NLP Systems for Structuring Clinical Data

NLP systems can automatically recognize clinical concepts from free text and encode the recognition, for instance, mapping to standardized terminologies like ICD-10, and SNOMED CT. This step improves data interoperability and makes it easier to gather clinical evidence.

The most famous example is cTAKES, an open-source NLP system aiming at extracting structured information from clinical text (Savova et al., 2010). cTAKES is heavily used in the research and clinical arenas as a tool for processing EHRs to extract diagnoses, procedures medications, and other types of clinical entities.

The Mayo Clinic uses cTAKES to actually extract data from pathology reports as a way to reduce human error and increase the efficiency of getting this information in a computable format. It is an entirely closed system, which has been integrated into the EHR of a clinic in order to improve clinical decision and research support (Savova et al., 2010). For example, the Veterans Health Administration (VHA) has employed NLP tools to create standardized clinical documents that enhance health data quality and enable ease of use for both research and patient care (Murphy et al. 1999).

Case Studies and Research Findings

The success of NLP systems at structuring clinical data has been demonstrated in a number of studies. Murff et al. (2011) accomplished high sensitivity and specificity when using an NLP-based approach to identify postoperative complications from narrative surgical notes. Additionally, Meystre et al. (2008) used NLP to detect instances of pneumonia in EHRs, highlighting NLP's potential for disease monitoring and epidemiological studies.

AI technologies for structured data extraction enabled patient-reported outcome (PRO) capture enhancements. Using all the unstructured data in patient surveys, NLP algorithms can analyze them and map this to standard metrics indicating the state of patient's experiences with treatment. This feature is particularly advantageous for PROs because of their critical contribution to validating the real-world effectiveness of interventions as demonstrated through large-scale RWE studies.

For example, Sim et al. (2023) employed natural language processing to assess patient-reported outcomes (PROs) from social media platforms, revealing important themes associated with patient satisfaction and adverse occurrences. This strategy has provided an in-the-moment perspective on patient experience, helping healthcare providers respond to issues more rapidly and improve the quality of care.

In addition to this, NLP has been used for normalizing and extracting information from radiology reports. A study by Mozayan et al. (2021) applied an NLP system to tapping structured data from radiology reports that have demonstrated benefits in diagnostic correctness and research proficiency on imaging outcomes. This application demonstrates the applicability of NLP across multiple clinical domains to structure unstructured data.

Drug Repurposing and Validation

A popular strategy to accelerate drug development and save costs is to repurpose existing drugs, i.e., identify new therapeutic uses for already approved but off-patent medications. Various AI technologies, notably ML and NLP, have proven capable of recognizing repurposing opportunities by virtue of the analysis of RWE.

EHR-based Drug Repurposing Signals

EHRs are full of longitudinal patient data that includes treatment histories, and diagnoses details. ML algorithms applied to EHR data can reveal new therapeutic indications and associations of existing drugs. For example, research by Xu et al. (2014) used machine learning to evaluate EHR data and identify possible repurposing candidates for Alzheimer's disease, emphasizing the significance of RWE in drug development.

Utilizing NLP techniques to extract information from unstructured text sources (e.g. scientific literature and clinical trial reports) can enhance drug repurposing efforts. NLP allows the extraction of all three aspects critical in validating repurposing hypotheses - drug-disease associations, molecular mechanisms, and clinical outcomes. A study by Wang et al. (2022) also used NLP for the rapid curation of potential repurposing candidates in COVID-19 using biomedical literature, underlining how quickly this technology can be applied to newly emerging health crises.

Moreover, these AI-enabled methods can incorporate a wide range of data sources from EHRs to omics data and patient registries for the discovery of new drug repositioning opportunities. The combination of a multitude of data types increases the resilience to use de-validation signals and support hypothesis validation by cross-referencing across various evidence streams.

Case Studies and Research Findings

Many noteworthy case studies demonstrate the promise of AI-powered medication repurposing. A classic example is the repurposing of sildenafil (Viagra) for the treatment of pulmonary arterial hypertension (PAH). Sildenafil, initially created for the treatment of erectile dysfunction was adapted to PAH due to its effect on pulmonary blood pressure. Backed initially by retrospective data mining of clinical records, this repurposing is no exception (Grinnan et al., 2019).

Repurposing of metformin, a commonly used antidiabetic drug for cancer treatment is one other such example. Subsequent analysis with algorithms for EHR data, as well as literature exploration using AI platforms, highlights potential anticancer features of metformin due to established clinical trials evaluating its effects (Lal et al., 2022).

AI has been playing a big role in the infectious disease space for identifying potential candidates available for repurposing in case of COVID-19. A study by Beck et al. (2020) screened existing drugs for potential activity against SARS-CoV-2 using deep learning. The model flagged certain drugs such as atazanavir and remdesivir, which were later validated in COVID-19 clinical trials.

In addition, AI methods have been applied to drug repositioning for neurological diseases. For example, Aliper et al. (2016) created an ML model that examined transcriptome data to identify medications with potential neuroprotective benefits, leading to the discovery of novel indications for numerous pharmaceuticals. This strategy demonstrates AI's potential to accelerate the identification of innovative medicines for difficult ailments.

Challenges and Future Directions

Addressing Data Quality and Standardization

One of the main hurdles to consistent analysis is that data quality and standardization differ. RWE typically takes the form of disparate EHRs and claims databases, patient-reported data; for example, hypertension may be only reported in some, reflecting heterogeneous or incomplete capture. Finally, unreliable and reproducible AI models, inconsistent coding practices among professionals as well as the absence of data or format differences can hamper reliability (Benchimol et al., 2015).

One possible way to overcome this is by creating standardized data formats and ontologies that enforce the homogeneity between independent datasets. Efforts such as the Observational Medical Outcomes Partnership (OMOP), and Common Data Model (CDM) strive to standardize heterogeneous RWD sources, which in turn permits more rigorous and reliable analyses across data sets; within what they refer to as a data network, especially with respect to patient cohorts' identification and confounder adjustment using an increasing repertoire of source codes spread among large diverse structured clinical databases (Hripcsak et al., 2015). In turn, implementing stricter data quality assessment procedures can improve the reliability of RWE studies as well.

Improving AI Model Validation and Benchmarking

The verification and evaluation of models in healthcare are important for validating the model's performance and capabilities. Validations currently happen using historical data that may not be modeled accurately for real-world clinical environments. There is a requirement for large-scale, real-time clinical validation studies to test the performance of such AI models in practice (Luo et al., 2016).

In addition to different AI models being compared, standardized benchmarking frameworks and performance metrics have also been developed. These frameworks need to take several considerations into account, such as data diversity and clinical relevance alongside model interpretability. Joint initiatives such as the Health AI Partnership seek to set these standards and drive open science for a more transparent, reproducible future in AI research (Topol, 2019).

Enhancing AI Adoption in Real-world Clinical Settings

AI is not widely used in clinical settings due to several barriers, such as resistance to change and distrust in AI systems, on top of requiring large infrastructure investments. Clinicians and health systems can be leery of adopting AI-powered recommendations over concerns for reliability, liability, or the fearsome disruption to present workflows (Nguyen et al., 2014).

To encourage AI adoption, it is critical to prioritize user-focused design and include doctors in the invention process. Ensure that AI solutions are intuitive, clear, and easily incorporated into healthcare workflows to improve usage as well as adoption. Furthermore, educating and training healthcare workers about the advantages and limits of AI can increase confidence and trust in these advancements.

Ethical and Privacy Considerations

There are also serious ethical and privacy concerns related to the use of AI in RWE analytics. Vulnerability to sensitive data and so much personal health information necessary for the AI models are at risk in terms of security, privacy, and potential misuse. Adherence to data protection requirements like the General Data Protection Regulation (GDPR) is critical for protecting healthcare data (Hafen, 2019).

In addition, it is critical that guidelines and ethical frameworks for AI in healthcare are developed to address bias, transparency, and accountability issues. For example, unrepresentative training data in AI models can introduce bias leading to healthcare outcomes being affected by disparity. Ethical frameworks should incorporate fairness, inclusivity, and patient-centeredness in AI development place (Obermeyer & Emanuel, 2016).

Future Directions

Solving these problems together in a cross-disciplinary fashion is the way forward for AI-enhanced RWE analytics. Quality assessment, standardization, and data integration will become more advanced making RWE studies much more robust. Further development of validation and benchmarking standards is essential to provide reliability in AI models. Designing with users in clinical environments and engaging clinicians early will be critical to the practical impact of AI.

CONCLUSION

The role of AI in RWE analysis may henceforth further bring healthcare within the purview with its complete automation providing a more targeted and efficient medical intervention. This chapter has discussed the power of AI in improving RWE and its possible game-changing capabilities to address modern healthcare issues.

The issue began with a primer on RWE, and its significance in the context of modern healthcare was well established while AI surfaced as an enabling technology for reinforcing capabilities if combined properly. Inherent difficulties associated with the quest for meaningful methods in RWE analysis to reconcile data heterogeneity, volume, and increasingly unstructured formats are tractable via AI methodologies; notably ML and NLP. These advances in methodology can help healthcare analytics unlock new findings from large, embodied datasets, which more traditional approaches cannot provide.

In this chapter applications of AI in RWE were explored. Framework for developing personalized medicine, risk stratification, and prognostic models can become easy with the help of AI. ML models can predict patient outcomes from the prognosis of patients who may benefit from a particular therapy whereas NLP techniques extract useful information from unstructured clinical notes or EHR. Applications like detecting ADE and safety surveillance, as well as for repurposing old drugs from RWE analysis owing to AI are real-world applications of ML and AI that can change the care course.

While the future of AI for RWE analytics is bright, the promise will only be realized by overcoming several hurdles. Maintaining the quality and standardization of data is important for ensuring good AI models. These data will be generated and shared for the operation, but it is important to find such datasets and link them across multiple biorepositories if possible. Furthermore, improving the validation as well as benchmarking of AI models using standard structures in future research would ensure their durability and usefulness in practical clinical situations.

The application of AI in healthcare requires a good user experience, design, seamless integration into clinical workflows, and professional engagement. However, defeating the inherent resistance to change and establishing trust in AI systems are two important steps required before it can happen on a large scale. However, these advances cannot occur at the expense of ethical and privacy concerns for patients whose data has been collected, or indeed on whether all this effort is going to improve healthcare results equitably.

In summary, the blending of AI with RWE analytics is a monumental step forward for pharmaceutical research and healthcare delivery. More accurate, faster, and individualized medical interventions can derive from AI-generated mechanisms that analyze extensive amounts of real-world data. Also, advances in AI technologies, the next horizon of which is already on the doorstep, will only make health informatics more powerful and capable of delivering innovations that support RWE analysis for better patient care and for achieving advances in medical precision.

Cooperation among academics, doctors, politicians, and engineers will be critical for solving the problems and reaping the advantages of AI in healthcare. By collaborating to build strict standards, practical solutions, and ethical frameworks; the healthcare sector may fully leverage AI in RWE analysis. This collaborative endeavor will set the path for an era in which AI will improve health results, help with better medications, and finally, a more effective as well as amenable healthcare structure.

REFERENCES

Ahmed, S. F., Bin, S., Hassan, M., Rozbu, M. R., Ishtiak, T., Rafa, N., Mofijur, M., Ali, A. B. M. S., & Gandomi, A. H. (2023). Deep learning modelling techniques: Current progress, applications, advantages, and challenges. *Artificial Intelligence Review*, 56(11), 13521–13617. Advance online publication. DOI: 10.1007/s10462-023-10466-8

Aliper, A., Plis, S., Artemov, A., Ulloa, A., Mamoshina, P., & Zhavoronkov, A. (2016). Deep Learning Applications for Predicting Pharmacological Properties of Drugs and Drug Repurposing Using Transcriptomic Data. *Molecular Pharmaceutics*, 13(7), 2524–2530. DOI: 10.1021/acs.molpharmaceut.6b00248 PMID: 27200455

Batko, K., & Ślęzak, A. (2022). The Use of Big Data Analytics in Healthcare. *Journal of Big Data*, 9(1), 3. Advance online publication. DOI: 10.1186/s40537-021-00553-4 PMID: 35013701

Beck, B. R., Shin, B., Choi, Y., Park, S., & Kang, K. (2020). Predicting commercially available antiviral drugs that may act on the novel coronavirus (SARS-CoV-2) through a drug-target interaction deep learning model. *Computational and Structural Biotechnology Journal*, 18, 784–790. DOI: 10.1016/j.csbj.2020.03.025 PMID: 32280433

Benchimol, E. I., Smeeth, L., Guttmann, A., Harron, K., Moher, D., Petersen, I., Sørensen, H. T., von Elm, E., & Langan, S. M. (2015). The REporting of studies Conducted using Observational Routinely-collected health Data (RECORD) Statement. *PLoS Medicine*, 12(10), e1001885. DOI: 10.1371/journal.pmed.1001885 PMID: 26440803

Bhatt, A. (2019). Conducting real-world evidence studies in India. *Perspectives in Clinical Research*, 10(2), 51. DOI: 10.4103/picr.PICR_8_19 PMID: 31008069

Blei, D., Ng, A., & Jordan, M. (2003). Latent Dirichlet Allocation. *Journal of Machine Learning Research*, 3, 993–1022. https://www.jmlr.org/papers/volume3/blei03a/blei03a.pdf

Borgelt, C. (2005). An implementation of the FP-growth algorithm. *Proceedings of the 1st International Workshop on Open Source Data Mining Frequent Pattern Mining Implementations - OSDM '05*. DOI: 10.1145/1133905.1133907

Breiman, L. (2001). Random Forests. *Machine Learning*, 45(1), 5–32. DOI: 10.1023/A:1010933404324

Brom, H., Brooks Carthon, J. M., Ikeaba, U., & Chittams, J. (2020). Leveraging Electronic Health Records and Machine Learning to Tailor Nursing Care for Patients at High Risk for Readmissions. *Journal of Nursing Care Quality*, 35(1), 27–33. DOI: 10.1097/NCQ.0000000000000412 PMID: 31136529

Cabitza, F., Locoro, A., & Banfi, G. (2018). Machine Learning in Orthopedics: A Literature Review. *Frontiers in Bioengineering and Biotechnology*, 6, 75. Advance online publication. DOI: 10.3389/fbioe.2018.00075 PMID: 29998104

Caruana, R., Lou, Y., Gehrke, J., Koch, P., Sturm, M., & Elhadad, N. (2015). Intelligible Models for HealthCare. *Proceedings of the 21th ACM SIGKDD International Conference on Knowledge Discovery and Data Mining - KDD '15*. DOI: 10.1145/2783258.2788613

Chandola, V., Banerjee, A., & Kumar, V. (2009). Anomaly Detection: A Survey. *ACM Computing Surveys*, 41(3), 1–58. DOI: 10.1145/1541880.1541882

Choudhury, A., & Asan, O. (2020). Role of Artificial Intelligence in Patient Safety Outcomes: Systematic Literature Review. *JMIR Medical Informatics*, 8(7), e18599. DOI: 10.2196/18599 PMID: 32706688

Dean, J., & Ghemawat, S. (2008). MapReduce: Simplified data processing on large clusters. *Communications of the ACM*, 51(1), 107–113. DOI: 10.1145/1327452.1327492

Denck, J., Ozkirimli, E., & Wang, K. (2023). Machine-learning-based adverse drug event prediction from observational health data: A review. *Drug Discovery Today*, 28(9), 103715. DOI: 10.1016/j.drudis.2023.103715 PMID: 37467879

Devlin, J., Chang, M.-W., Lee, K., & Toutanova, K. (2018, October 11). *BERT: Pre-training of Deep Bidirectional Transformers for Language Understanding*. ArXiv.org. https://arxiv.org/abs/1810.04805

Dhillon, A., & Singh, A. (2018). Biology and Today's World Machine Learning in Healthcare Data Analysis: A Survey. *Journal of Biology and Today's World*, 8(2), 1–10. DOI: 10.15412/J.JBTW.01070206

Esteva, A., Kuprel, B., Novoa, R. A., Ko, J., Swetter, S. M., Blau, H. M., & Thrun, S. (2017). Dermatologist-level classification of skin cancer with deep neural networks. *Nature*, 542(7639), 115–118. DOI: 10.1038/nature21056 PMID: 28117445

Fan, B., Fan, W., Smith, C., & Garner, H. (2020). Adverse drug event detection and extraction from open data: A deep learning approach. *Information Processing & Management*, 57(1), 102131. DOI: 10.1016/j.ipm.2019.102131

Freifeld, C. C., Brownstein, J. S., Menone, C. M., Bao, W., Filice, R., Kass-Hout, T., & Dasgupta, N. (2014). Digital Drug Safety Surveillance: Monitoring Pharmaceutical Products in Twitter. *Drug Safety*, 37(5), 343–350. DOI: 10.1007/s40264-014-0155-x PMID: 24777653

Friedman, C., Shagina, L., Lussier, Y., & Hripcsak, G. (2004). Automated Encoding of Clinical Documents Based on Natural Language Processing. *Journal of the American Medical Informatics Association : JAMIA*, 11(5), 392–402. DOI: 10.1197/jamia.M1552 PMID: 15187068

Gandomi, A., & Haider, M. (2015). Beyond the Hype: Big Data Concepts, Methods, and Analytics. *International Journal of Information Management*, 35(2), 137–144. DOI: 10.1016/j.ijinfomgt.2014.10.007

Gao, C. X., Dwyer, D., Zhu, Y., Smith, C. L., Du, L., Filia, K. M., Bayer, J., Menssink, J. M., Wang, T., Bergmeir, C., Wood, S., & Cotton, S. M. (2023). An overview of clustering methods with guidelines for application in mental health research. *Psychiatry Research*, 327, 115265. DOI: 10.1016/j.psychres.2023.115265 PMID: 37348404

Geldof, T., Huys, I., & Van Dyck, W. (2019). Real-World Evidence Gathering in Oncology: The Need for a Biomedical Big Data Insight-Providing Federated Network. *Frontiers in Medicine*, 6, 43. Advance online publication. DOI: 10.3389/fmed.2019.00043 PMID: 30906740

Ghassemi, M., Naumann, T., Schulam, P., Beam, A. L., Chen, I. Y., & Ranganath, R. (2019, December 5). *A Review of Challenges and Opportunities in Machine Learning for Health*. ArXiv.org. https://doi.org//arXiv.1806.00388DOI: 10.48550

Gohil, S., Vuik, S., & Darzi, A. (2018). Sentiment Analysis of Health Care Tweets: Review of the Methods Used. *JMIR Public Health and Surveillance*, 4(2), e43. DOI: 10.2196/publichealth.5789 PMID: 29685871

Greaves, F., Ramirez-Cano, D., Millett, C., Darzi, A., & Donaldson, L. (2013). Use of Sentiment Analysis for Capturing Patient Experience From Free-Text Comments Posted Online. *Journal of Medical Internet Research*, 15(11), e239. DOI: 10.2196/jmir.2721 PMID: 24184993

Grinnan, D., Trankle, C., Andruska, A., Bloom, B., & Spiekerkoetter, E. (2019). Drug repositioning in pulmonary arterial hypertension: Challenges and opportunities. *Pulmonary Circulation*, 9(1), 1–18. Advance online publication. DOI: 10.1177/2045894019832226 PMID: 30729869

Gulshan, V., Peng, L., Coram, M., Stumpe, M. C., Wu, D., Narayanaswamy, A., Venugopalan, S., Widner, K., Madams, T., Cuadros, J., Kim, R., Raman, R., Nelson, P. C., Mega, J. L., & Webster, D. R. (2016). Development and Validation of a Deep Learning Algorithm for Detection of Diabetic Retinopathy in Retinal Fundus Photographs. *Journal of the American Medical Association*, 316(22), 2402. DOI: 10.1001/jama.2016.17216 PMID: 27898976

Gurulingappa, H., Rajput, A. M., Roberts, A., Fluck, J., Hofmann-Apitius, M., & Toldo, L. (2012). Development of a benchmark corpus to support the automatic extraction of drug-related adverse effects from medical case reports. *Journal of Biomedical Informatics*, 45(5), 885–892. DOI: 10.1016/j.jbi.2012.04.008 PMID: 22554702

Hafen, E., Kossmann, D., & Brand, A. (2014). Health data cooperatives - citizen empowerment. *Methods of Information in Medicine*, 53(2), 82–86. DOI: 10.3414/ME13-02-0051 PMID: 24514946

Hong, N., Li, D., Yu, Y., Xiu, Q., Liu, H., & Jiang, G. (2016). A computational framework for converting textual clinical diagnostic criteria into the quality data model. *Journal of Biomedical Informatics*, 63, 11–21. DOI: 10.1016/j.jbi.2016.07.016 PMID: 27444185

Hossain, E., Rana, R., Higgins, N., Soar, J., Barua, P. D., Pisani, A. R., & Turner, K. (2023). Use of ai/ml-enabled state-of-the-art method in electronic medical records: A systematic review. *Computers in Biology and Medicine*, 155, 106649. DOI: 10.1016/j.compbiomed.2023.106649 PMID: 36805219

Hripcsak, G., & Albers, D. J. (2012). Next-generation phenotyping of electronic health records. *Journal of the American Medical Informatics Association : JAMIA*, 20(1), 117–121. DOI: 10.1136/amiajnl-2012-001145 PMID: 22955496

Hripcsak, G., Duke, J. D., Shah, N. H., Reich, C. G., Huser, V., Schuemie, M. J., Suchard, M. A., Park, R. W., Wong, I. C. K., Rijnbeek, P. R., van der Lei, J., Pratt, N., Norén, G. N., Li, Y.-C., Stang, P. E., Madigan, D., & Ryan, P. B. (2015). Observational Health Data Sciences and Informatics (OHDSI): Opportunities for Observational Researchers. *Studies in Health Technology and Informatics*, 216, 574–578. https://pubmed.ncbi.nlm.nih.gov/26262116/. DOI: 10.3233/978-1-61499-564-7-574 PMID: 26262116

Jee, K., & Kim, G.-H. (2013). Potentiality of Big Data in the Medical Sector: Focus on How to Reshape the Healthcare System. *Healthcare Informatics Research*, 19(2), 79. DOI: 10.4258/hir.2013.19.2.79 PMID: 23882412

Jiang, M., Chen, Y., Liu, M., Rosenbloom, S. T., Mani, S., Denny, J. C., & Xu, H. (2011). A study of machine-learning-based approaches to extract clinical entities and their assertions from discharge summaries. *Journal of the American Medical Informatics Association : JAMIA*, 18(5), 601–606. DOI: 10.1136/amiajnl-2011-000163 PMID: 21508414

Johnson, J. A., & Cavallari, L. H. (2013). Pharmacogenetics and Cardiovascular Disease—Implications for Personalized Medicine. *Pharmacological Reviews*, 65(3), 987–1009. DOI: 10.1124/pr.112.007252 PMID: 23686351

Jung, K., LePendu, P., & Shah, N. (2013). Automated Detection of Systematic Off-label Drug Use in Free Text of Electronic Medical Records. *AMIA Joint Summits on Translational Science Proceedings AMIA Summit on Translational Science*, 2013, 94–98. https://www.ncbi.nlm.nih.gov/pmc/articles/PMC3814472/ PMID: 24303308

Kahn, C. E.Jr, Heilbrun, M. E., & Applegate, K. E. (2013). From Guidelines to Practice: How Reporting Templates Promote the Use of Radiology Practice Guidelines. *Journal of the American College of Radiology*, 10(4), 268–273. DOI: 10.1016/j.jacr.2012.09.025 PMID: 23332496

Kourou, K., Exarchos, T. P., Exarchos, K. P., Karamouzis, M. V., & Fotiadis, D. I. (2015). Machine learning applications in cancer prognosis and prediction. *Computational and Structural Biotechnology Journal*, 13(13), 8–17. DOI: 10.1016/j.csbj.2014.11.005 PMID: 25750696

Kreimeyer, K., Foster, M., Pandey, A., Arya, N., Halford, G., Jones, S. F., Forshee, R., Walderhaug, M., & Botsis, T. (2017). Natural language processing systems for capturing and standardizing unstructured clinical information: A systematic review. *Journal of Biomedical Informatics*, 73, 14–29. DOI: 10.1016/j.jbi.2017.07.012 PMID: 28729030

Lal, J. C., Mao, C., Zhou, Y., Gore-Panter, S. R., Rennison, J. H., Lovano, B. S., Castel, L., Shin, J., Gillinov, A. M., Smith, J. D., Barnard, J., Wagoner, D. R. V., Luo, Y., Cheng, F., & Chung, M. K. (2022). Transcriptomics-based network medicine approach identifies metformin as a repurposable drug for atrial fibrillation. *Cell Reports Medicine*, 3(10), 100749. Advance online publication. DOI: 10.1016/j.xcrm.2022.100749 PMID: 36223777

Lamsal, R. (2020). Design and analysis of a large-scale COVID-19 tweets dataset. *Applied Intelligence*. Advance online publication. DOI: 10.1007/s10489-020-02029-z PMID: 34764561

Lee, D. D., & Seung, H. S. (1999). Learning the parts of objects by non-negative matrix factorization. *Nature*, 401(6755), 788–791. DOI: 10.1038/44565 PMID: 10548103

Little, R. J. A., & Rubin, D. B. (2020). *Statistical analysis with missing data* (3rd ed.). John Wiley & Sons, Inc.

Liu, Y., Chen, P.-H. C., Krause, J., & Peng, L. (2019). How to Read Articles That Use Machine Learning: Users' Guides to the Medical Literature. *Journal of the American Medical Association*, 322(18), 1806–1816. DOI: 10.1001/jama.2019.16489 PMID: 31714992

Luo, J., Wu, M., Gopukumar, D., & Zhao, Y. (2016). Big Data Application in Biomedical Research and Health Care: A Literature Review. *Biomedical Informatics Insights, 8. Biomedical Informatics Insights*, S31559, BII.S31559. Advance online publication. DOI: 10.4137/BII.S31559 PMID: 26843812

MacKay, E. J., Stubna, M. D., Chivers, C., Draugelis, M. E., Hanson, W. J., Desai, N. D., & Groeneveld, P. W. (2021). Application of machine learning approaches to administrative claims data to predict clinical outcomes in medical and surgical patient populations. *PLoS One*, 16(6), e0252585. DOI: 10.1371/journal.pone.0252585 PMID: 34081720

Marino, M., Lucas, J., Latour, E., & Heintzman, J. D. (2021). Missing data in primary care research: Importance, implications and approaches. *Family Practice*, 38(2), 199–202. DOI: 10.1093/fampra/cmaa134 PMID: 33480404

Meystre, S. M., Savova, G. K., Kipper-Schuler, K. C., & Hurdle, J. F. (2008). Extracting information from textual documents in the electronic health record: A review of recent research. *Yearbook of Medical Informatics*, •••, 128–144. https://pubmed.ncbi.nlm.nih.gov/18660887/ PMID: 18660887

Miotto, R., Wang, F., Wang, S., Jiang, X., & Dudley, J. T. (2018). Deep Learning for healthcare: Review, Opportunities and Challenges. *Briefings in Bioinformatics*, 19(6), 1236–1246. DOI: 10.1093/bib/bbx044 PMID: 28481991

Mohsen, A., Tripathi, L. P., & Mizuguchi, K. (2021). Deep Learning Prediction of Adverse Drug Reactions in Drug Discovery Using Open TG–GATEs and FAERS Databases. *Frontiers in Drug Discovery*, 1, 768792. Advance online publication. DOI: 10.3389/fddsv.2021.768792

Mozayan, A., Fabbri, A. R., Maneevese, M., Tocino, I., & Chheang, S. (2021). Practical Guide to Natural Language Processing for Radiology. *Radiographics*, 41(5), 1446–1453. DOI: 10.1148/rg.2021200113 PMID: 34469212

Murdoch, T. B., & Detsky, A. S. (2013). The Inevitable Application of Big Data to Health Care. *Journal of the American Medical Association*, 309(13), 1351. DOI: 10.1001/jama.2013.393 PMID: 23549579

Murff, H. J., FitzHenry, F., Matheny, M. E., Gentry, N., Kotter, K. L., Crimin, K., Dittus, R. S., Rosen, A. K., Elkin, P. L., Brown, S. H., & Speroff, T. (2011). Automated Identification of Postoperative Complications Within an Electronic Medical Record Using Natural Language Processing. *Journal of the American Medical Association*, 306(8). Advance online publication. DOI: 10.1001/jama.2011.1204 PMID: 21862746

Murphy, R. M., Klopotowska, J. E., de Keizer, N. F., Jager, K. J., Leopold, J. H., Dongelmans, D. A., Abu-Hanna, A., & Schut, M. C. (2023). Adverse drug event detection using natural language processing: A scoping review of supervised learning methods. *PLoS One*, 18(1), e0279842. DOI: 10.1371/journal.pone.0279842 PMID: 36595517

Murphy, S. N., Mendis, M., Hackett, K., Kuttan, R., Pan, W., Phillips, L. C., Gainer, V., Berkowicz, D., Glaser, J. P., Kohane, I., & Chueh, H. C. (2007). Architecture of the Open-source Clinical Research Chart from Informatics for Integrating Biology and the Bedside. *AMIA ... Annual Symposium Proceedings - AMIA Symposium. AMIA Symposium*, 2007, 548–552. https://www.ncbi.nlm.nih.gov/pmc/articles/PMC2655844/ PMID: 18693896

Murphy, S. N., Morgan, M. M., Barnett, G. O., & Chueh, H. C. (1999). Optimizing healthcare research data warehouse design through past COSTAR query analysis. *Proceedings. AMIA Symposium*, 892–896. https://pubmed.ncbi.nlm.nih.gov/10566489/

Nassif, A. B., Talib, M. A., Nasir, Q., & Dakalbab, F. M. (2021). Machine Learning for Anomaly Detection: A Systematic Review. *IEEE Access : Practical Innovations, Open Solutions*, 9, 78658–78700. DOI: 10.1109/ACCESS.2021.3083060

Nawab, K., Ramsey, G., & Schreiber, R. (2020). Natural Language Processing to Extract Meaningful Information from Patient Experience Feedback. *Applied Clinical Informatics*, 11(02), 242–252. DOI: 10.1055/s-0040-1708049 PMID: 32236917

Nguyen, L., Bellucci, E., & Nguyen, L. T. (2014). Electronic health records implementation: An evaluation of information system impact and contingency factors. *International Journal of Medical Informatics*, 83(11), 779–796. DOI: 10.1016/j.ijmedinf.2014.06.011 PMID: 25085286

Obermeyer, Z., & Emanuel, E. J. (2016). Predicting the Future — Big Data, Machine Learning, and Clinical Medicine. *The New England Journal of Medicine*, 375(13), 1216–1219. DOI: 10.1056/NEJMp1606181 PMID: 27682033

Pang, B., Lee, L., & Vaithyanathan, S. (2002). Thumbs up? Sentiment Classification using Machine Learning Techniques. *Proceedings of the ACL-02 Conference on Empirical Methods in Natural Language Processing - EMNLP '02, 10*. DOI: 10.3115/1118693.1118704

Peng, J., Jury, E. C., Dönnes, P., & Ciurtin, C. (2021). Machine Learning Techniques for Personalised Medicine Approaches in Immune-Mediated Chronic Inflammatory Diseases: Applications and Challenges. *Frontiers in Pharmacology*, 12(1), 720694. Advance online publication. DOI: 10.3389/fphar.2021.720694 PMID: 34658859

Platt, R., Carnahan, R. M., Brown, J. S., Chrischilles, E., Curtis, L. H., Hennessy, S., Nelson, J. C., Racoosin, J. A., Robb, M., Schneeweiss, S., Toh, S., & Weiner, M. G. (2012). The U.S. Food and Drug Administration's Mini-Sentinel program: Status and direction. *Pharmacoepidemiology and Drug Safety*, 21(S1), 1–8. DOI: 10.1002/pds.2343 PMID: 22262586

Raghupathi, W., & Raghupathi, V. (2014). Big data analytics in healthcare: Promise and potential. *Health Information Science and Systems*, 2(1), 1–10. DOI: 10.1186/2047-2501-2-3 PMID: 25825667

Rajkomar, A., Oren, E., Chen, K., Dai, A. M., Hajaj, N., Hardt, M., Liu, P. J., Liu, X., Marcus, J., Sun, M., Sundberg, P., Yee, H., Zhang, K., Zhang, Y., Flores, G., Duggan, G. E., Irvine, J., Le, Q., Litsch, K., & Dean, J. (2018). Scalable and accurate deep learning with electronic health records. *NPJ Digital Medicine*, 1(1), 18. Advance online publication. DOI: 10.1038/s41746-018-0029-1 PMID: 31304302

Ryan, P., Zhang, Y., Liu, F., Gao, J., Bigger, J. T., Hripcsak, G., Weng, C., & Li, Y. (2014). A Distribution-based Method for Assessing The Differences between Clinical Trial Target Populations and Patient Populations in Electronic Health Records. *Applied Clinical Informatics*, 05(02), 463–479. DOI: 10.4338/ACI-2013-12-RA-0105 PMID: 25024761

Samek, W., Wiegand, T., & Müller, K.-R. (2017, August 28). *Explainable Artificial Intelligence: Understanding, Visualizing and Interpreting Deep Learning Models*. ArXiv.org. https://doi.org//arXiv.1708.08296DOI: 10.48550

Savova, G. K., Masanz, J. J., Ogren, P. V., Zheng, J., Sohn, S., Kipper-Schuler, K. C., & Chute, C. G. (2010). Mayo clinical Text Analysis and Knowledge Extraction System (cTAKES): Architecture, component evaluation and applications. *Journal of the American Medical Informatics Association : JAMIA*, 17(5), 507–513. DOI: 10.1136/jamia.2009.001560 PMID: 20819853

Sezgin, E., Hussain, S.-A., Rust, S., & Huang, Y. (2022). Extracting Medical Information from Free-text and Unstructured Patient-Generated Health Data using Natural Language Processing Methods: A Feasibility Study with Real-world Data (Preprint). *JMIR Formative Research*. Advance online publication. DOI: 10.2196/43014 PMID: 36881467

Shameer, K., Johnson, K. W., Glicksberg, B. S., Dudley, J. T., & Sengupta, P. P. (2018). Machine learning in cardiovascular medicine: Are we there yet? *Heart (British Cardiac Society)*, 104(14), 1156–1164. DOI: 10.1136/heartjnl-2017-311198 PMID: 29352006

Sheikhalishahi, S., Miotto, R., Dudley, J. T., Lavelli, A., Rinaldi, F., & Osmani, V. (2019). Natural Language Processing of Clinical Notes on Chronic Diseases: Systematic Review. *JMIR Medical Informatics*, 7(2), e12239. DOI: 10.2196/12239 PMID: 31066697

Shi, X., Chen, Z., Wang, H., Yeung, D. Y., Wong, W. K., & Woo, W. C. (2015). Convolutional LSTM network: A machine learning approach for precipitation nowcasting. *Advances in Neural Information Processing Systems, 28*. https://dl.acm.org/doi/10.5555/2969239.2969329

Shickel, B., Tighe, P. J., Bihorac, A., & Rashidi, P. (2018). Deep EHR: A Survey of Recent Advances in Deep Learning Techniques for Electronic Health Record (EHR) Analysis. *IEEE Journal of Biomedical and Health Informatics*, 22(5), 1589–1604. DOI: 10.1109/JBHI.2017.2767063 PMID: 29989977

Sim, J., Huang, X., Horan, M. R., Stewart, C. M., Robison, L. L., Hudson, M. M., Baker, J. N., & Huang, I.-C. (2023). Natural language processing with machine learning methods to analyze unstructured patient-reported outcomes derived from electronic health records: A systematic review. *Artificial Intelligence in Medicine*, 146, 102701–102701. DOI: 10.1016/j.artmed.2023.102701 PMID: 38042599

Tenenbaum, J. D. (2016). Translational Bioinformatics: Past, Present, and Future. *Genomics, Proteomics & Bioinformatics*, 14(1), 31–41. DOI: 10.1016/j.gpb.2016.01.003 PMID: 26876718

Tibshirani, R. (1996). Regression Shrinkage and Selection Via the Lasso. *Journal of the Royal Statistical Society. Series B, Statistical Methodology*, 58(1), 267–288. DOI: 10.1111/j.2517-6161.1996.tb02080.x

Topol, E. J. (2019). High-performance medicine: The convergence of human and artificial intelligence. *Nature Medicine*, 25(1), 44–56. https://www.nature.com/articles/s41591-018-0300-7. DOI: 10.1038/s41591-018-0300-7 PMID: 30617339

Wallace, B. C., Paul, M. J., Sarkar, U., Trikalinos, T. A., & Dredze, M. (2014). A large-scale quantitative analysis of latent factors and sentiment in online doctor reviews. *Journal of the American Medical Informatics Association : JAMIA*, 21(6), 1098–1103. DOI: 10.1136/amiajnl-2014-002711 PMID: 24918109

Wang, L., Jiang, L., Pan, D., Wang, Q., Yin, Z., Kang, Z., Tian, H., Geng, X., Shao, J., Pan, W., Yin, J., Fang, L., Wang, Y., Zhang, W., Li, Z., Zheng, J., Hu, W., Pan, Y., Yu, D., & Xu, H. (2022). Novel approach by natural language processing for COVID-19 knowledge discovery. *Biomedical Journal*, 45(3), 472–481. Advance online publication. DOI: 10.1016/j.bj.2022.03.011 PMID: 35367669

Wang, Y., Kung, L., & Byrd, T. A. (2018). Big data analytics: Understanding its capabilities and potential benefits for healthcare organizations. *Technological Forecasting and Social Change*, 126(1), 3–13. DOI: 10.1016/j.techfore.2015.12.019

Wang, Y., Wang, L., Rastegar-Mojarad, M., Moon, S., Shen, F., Afzal, N., Liu, S., Zeng, Y., Mehrabi, S., Sohn, S., & Liu, H. (2018). Clinical information extraction applications: A literature review. *Journal of Biomedical Informatics*, 77, 34–49. DOI: 10.1016/j.jbi.2017.11.011 PMID: 29162496

Warrer, P., Hansen, E. H., Juhl-Jensen, L., & Aagaard, L. (2012). Using text-mining techniques in electronic patient records to identify ADRs from medicine use. *British Journal of Clinical Pharmacology*, 73(5), 674–684. DOI: 10.1111/j.1365-2125.2011.04153.x PMID: 22122057

Wei, W. Q., Cronin, R. M., Xu, H., Lasko, T. A., Bastarache, L., & Denny, J. C. (2013). Development and evaluation of an ensemble resource linking medications to their indications. *Journal of the American Medical Informatics Association : JAMIA*, 20(5), 954–961. DOI: 10.1136/amiajnl-2012-001431 PMID: 23576672

Weiskopf, N. G., & Weng, C. (2013). Methods and dimensions of electronic health record data quality assessment: Enabling reuse for clinical research. *Journal of the American Medical Informatics Association : JAMIA*, 20(1), 144–151. DOI: 10.1136/amiajnl-2011-000681 PMID: 22733976

Xu, H., Aldrich, M. C., Chen, Q., Liu, H., Peterson, N. B., Dai, Q., Levy, M., Shah, A., Han, X., Ruan, X., Jiang, M., Li, Y., Julien, J. S., Warner, J., Friedman, C., Roden, D. M., & Denny, J. C. (2014). Validating drug repurposing signals using electronic health records: A case study of metformin associated with reduced cancer mortality. *Journal of the American Medical Informatics Association : JAMIA*, 22(1), 179–191. DOI: 10.1136/amiajnl-2014-002649 PMID: 25053577

Xu, J., Biomedical, R., & Sciences, H. (2016). *Mapping SNOMED CT to ICD-10-CM*. https://rucore.libraries.rutgers.edu/rutgers-lib/49049/PDF/1/play/

Yang, S., & Kar, S. (2023). Application of artificial intelligence and machine learning in early detection of adverse drug reactions (ADRs) and drug-induced toxicity. *Artificial Intelligence Chemistry.*, 1(2), 100011. DOI: 10.1016/j.aichem.2023.100011

Yin, W., Ebert, S., & Schütze, H. (2016). *Attention-Based Convolutional Neural Network for Machine Comprehension.* DOI: 10.18653/v1/W16-0103

KEY TERMS AND DEFINITIONS

Real-World Evidence (RWE): RWE is the clinical evidence based on the analysis of real-world data (RWD) regarding actual use and the possible benefits or risks, associated with medical products. It shed light on the real world, regarding how therapies work beyond clinical trials.

Real-World Data (RWD): RWD is defined as health care data captured beyond the context of clinical trials that may include patient records and other forms of information harvested both within routine healthcare delivery settings (i.e., electronic medical records or EMRs), or in various sources such claims or billing activities for products dispensed to patients and machinery managing their ongoing treatment.

Electronic Health Record (EHR): EHRs are computerized reproductions of patient paper charts. They have a complete health record with the patient medical history, diagnoses, medications treatment plans, immunization dates, allergies, radiology images, and laboratory test results.

Adverse Drug Event (ADE): An injury resulting from medical intervention related to a drug. The risks to patient safety that may be present by ADEs are; side effects of high dose prescriptions, medication errors, allergic reactions and overdoses.

Artificial Intelligence (AI): AI refers to the simulation of human intelligence processes by computer systems. That is, AI has to learn (check a fact or rules acquisition perspective), reason (how can it be used by combining different facts and applying logical relationships between them) and relearn.

Machine Learning (ML): ML is a subset of AI which utilizes algorithms and statistical models to allow computers to execute specific tasks without using any explicit instructions but by relying on patterns and inference.

Deep Learning (DL): DL is the subset of ML that uses neural networks with multiple layers (hence "deep") to model high-level abstractions in data. One can see its superiority in tasks like image or speech recognition.

Natural Language Processing (NLP): NLP is another branch of AI that deals with the interaction between computers and humans using natural language. It encompassed building algorithms that enable computers to handle and study a large volume of natural language data.

Chapter 4
Revolutionizing Pharmaceutical Engineering:
A Deep Dive Into AI-Driven Drug Discovery and Development

Rawan Saleem
https://orcid.org/0000-0002-2475-2333
University of Sheffield, UK

ABSTRACT

The usual use of artificial intelligence (AI) in drug research and discovery is poised to usher in a revolutionary era for the pharmaceutical sector. This chapter examines the significance of artificial intelligence in pharmaceutical engineering, emphasising significant developments and approaches that are transforming the discipline. AI is also accelerating the time-to-time market and cutting costs in clinical trials by optimising patient selection, providing real-time monitoring, and designing adaptive studies. This chapter also explores the regulatory environment, ethical issues, and the potential applications of AI in the pharmaceutical industry. This chapter intends to educate and motivate researchers, business experts, and legislators to fully use AI's promise to transform pharmaceutical engineering by offering a thorough review of the technology's role in drug discovery and development.

DOI: 10.4018/979-8-3693-6270-9.ch004

INTRODUCTION

The pharmaceutical sector is about to undergo a radical change. Artificial intelligence (AI) is a revolutionary force that has the potential to completely change the pharmaceutical engineering field. Its incorporation into drug research and development is more than just a technical improvement (Iqbal et al., 2023). This significant change looks to address some of the longest-standing issues facing the sector, such as the need for more individualised and efficient therapies as well as the high cost and drawn-out process of introducing new medications to the market (Vora et al., 2023). A deeper exploration of the complexities of AI-driven pharmaceutical engineering reveals that this breakthrough has the potential to completely transform the global healthcare system (Niazi & Mariam, 2024).

Understanding the conventional approaches that have guided drug discovery and development for many years is crucial to understanding the entire impact of AI on pharmaceutical engineering (Vora et al., 2023). Traditionally the introduction of new medication onto the market has been an intricate, expensive, and time-consuming procedure (Deng et al., 2023). A new drug's path can cost billions and take over ten years from first discovery to final approval.

Target identification, in which scientists locate a biological target connected to a disease, is the first step in the conventional drug development process. High-throughput screening is the next step, in which thousands of chemical compounds are examined to see whether they can interact with the target (Fang et al., 2022). The next step for promising candidates is to lead optimisation, which enhances their safety and effectiveness characteristics. Following optimisation, a lead molecule moves on to preclinical testing, where both in vitro (in the lab) and vivo (in animal models) studies are conducted to determine its effects.

After that, the most promising candidate proceeded to the three-phase clinical trials. Phase I studies evaluate dose and safety in a limited number of well participants. Phase II studies assess the medication's effectiveness and adverse effects in a broader patient population. Phase III studies compare the medicine to current therapies, assess side effects, and include even bigger patient groups in an effort to establish the therapy's efficacy. If the trial is a success, the medication must first receive regulatory clearance before being made available for general sale (Mullowney et al., 2023).

The failure rate is considerable in spite of this process's strict requirements. A great deal of promising early-stage medications fails in clinical trials because of unanticipated toxicity, ineffectiveness, or other problems. These significant expenses and protracted lead times connected with conventional drug research and development are partly caused by this high attrition rate (Paul et al., 2021).

The development of AI provides a revolutionary answer to these problems. artificial intelligence is the umbrella term encompassing a wide range of technologies that allow computers to do activities that traditionally require human intellect, such as computer vision, natural language processing, machine learning, and deep learning (Gupta et al., 2021). artificial intelligence has the potential to improve drug discovery and development at every stage, resulting in a quicker, more cost-effective, and more efficient process in the field of pharmaceutical engineering (Bhattamisra et al., 2023).

The capacity of artificial intelligence to swiftly and reliably analyse enormous volumes of data is one of the technology's most important contributions to pharmaceutical engineering. The pharmaceutical sector produces vast amounts of data, ranging from real-world evidence and clinical trial outcomes to genetic and proteomic data (Alowais et al., 2023). The amount and complexity of this data make it difficult for traditional techniques to keep up with, but AI algorithms can process and analyse it in a fraction of the time, revealing patterns and insights that are impossible for people to see.

AI-driven drug development finds possible drug candidates more quickly than with conventional techniques by utilizing machine learning algorithms. Artificial intelligence is able to forecast which chemicals are likely to be successful against a given target by analysing vast databases of chemical and biological data (Hartl et al., 2021). By speeding up the early phases of drug research, this skill lowers the time and expense needed to find potential candidates.

Predicting chemical interactions using deep learning models is one of the most prominent uses of AI in drug development (Kolluri et al., 2022). Researchers may find possible medications with great precision thanks to these models, which can analyse the structure of millions of molecules and predict their binding affinity to certain targets. To dramatically expedite the drug development process. Atomise, a startup that specialises in AI-driven drug discovery, use deep learning to predict the binding affinity of tiny compounds to protein targets.

AI is useful not just for predicting chemical interactions but also for designing novel compounds. Generative models, such as generative adversarial networks (GANS) (Hartl et al., 2021), can generate unique chemical compounds with the necessary characteristics for a potential medicine. With this method, researchers may investigate a wide range of chemicals and locate substances that conventional techniques would have missed.

AI has the potential to be extremely important during the development stage of medicine once a viable candidate has been found (Kolluri et al., 2022). Optimising a compound's pharmacokinetic and pharmacodynamic features to guarantee safety and efficacy is one of the main problems in medication development. Based on the compound's chemical structure, AI systems can forecast these characteristics, empowering researchers to choose which options to move forward with (Iqbal et al., 2023).

AI can also track patients' responses in real-time during clinical studies, perhaps detecting negative reactions or side effects early on. With this flexibility, researchers may quickly modify the design of the study or the dosage schedule, enhancing patient safety and raising the likelihood of a favourable result (Niazi & Mariam, 2024). AI-driven solutions such as AiCure, for instance, employ computer vision to monitor patient adherence to drug regimens and give researchers and physicians immediate feedback.

Personalised medicine is one of the most exciting applications of AI in pharmaceutical engineering. Conventional medication research frequently takes a one-size-fits-all tack, with regimens created for typical patients (Fang et al., 2022). However, due to genetic, environmental, and lifestyle variables, each person's reaction to medicine might differ greatly. The goal of personalised medicine is to minimize therapeutic results by customizing care to each patient's specific needs (Sadee et al., 2023).

AI is essential to personalised medicine because it can analyse patient data individually and forecast a patient's response to various therapies. Clinicians can choose the most appropriate course of treatment for each patient by using machine-learning algorithms to find biomarkers that indicate a patient's propensity to react to a certain medication (Park et al., 2022). In addition to improving patient outcomes, this strategy lowers the prevalence of trial-and-error prescription, which occurs when a patient tries several different drugs before finding one that works.

Furthermore, by forecasting the ideal dosage and time for every patient, AI may help with the creation of customised medication regimens (Gupta et al., 2021). AI can suggest dosage regimens that optimise effectiveness and minimise negative effects by taking into account variables including metabolism, genetic profile, and illness progression (Alowais et al., 2023). This degree of personalisation offers the possibility of more accurate and efficient therapies, which is a big improvement in healthcare. Although AI has enormous potential in pharmaceutical engineering, there are significant ethical and practical concerns that need to be taken into account when integrating these technologies (Alowais et al., 2023). Security and privacy of data are two main issues. AI in medication research and discovery depends on having access to enormous volumes of private patient data (Nomura et al., 2021). Preserving patient confidence and adhering to legal mandates depend critically on protecting the confidentiality and integrity of this data.

AI algorithm research and implementation also need to be impartial and transparent. There's a chance that AI models would unintentionally reinforce preexisting prejudices in the medical field (Iqbal et al., 2023), which might result in unequal treatment outcomes, for example, the resultant algorithms could not work effectively for specific groups if the training data used to create the AI model is not representative of varied patient populations. Achieving fair healthcare outcomes requires addressing these biases and making sure AI models are trained on representative and varied datasets.

In order for regulatory frameworks to keep up with the quick advances in AI technology, they too must change (Niazi & Mariam, 2024). It's possible that conventional regulatory procedures are ill-suited to assess the security and effectiveness of AI-driven medication research and discovery techniques (Vora et al., 2023). Regulatory bodies will have to create new rules and guidelines in order to evaluate AI algorithms and make sure they satisfy strict requirements regarding transparency, accuracy and dependability.

Ultimately, the development implementation, and upkeep of these technologies call for a trained workforce, which is a prerequisite for the use of AI in pharmaceutical engineering. Continuous education and training programmes are required to give academics, physicians, and regulatory professionals the knowledge and abilities they need to use AI in their work (Paul et al., 2021).

The field of AI-driven pharmaceutical engineering has a bright future ahead of it. Together with developments in genetics and biotechnology, further advances in AI will improve our comprehension of complicated diseases and speed the creation of novel treatments (Mullowney et al., 2023). AI has the power to optimize clinical trials in ways that were previously unthinkable, find new therapeutic targets, and create safer, more effective medications (Paul et al., 2021).

To fully realise AI's potential and guarantee that these technologies are accessible in an ethical and fair manner, cooperation between academic institutions, businesses, and regulatory organisations will be crucial. Stakeholders may jointly create strong frameworks and standards that support innovation while preserving patient safety and privacy of data (Sadee et al., 2023).

DRUG DISCOVERY AND PREDICTIVE MEDICINE

The use of artificial intelligence (AI) in drug development has completely changed conventional approaches, especially when it comes to predictive modelling and virtual screening (Vora et al., 2023). This thorough investigation explores the ways in which these AI-driven methodologies are changing pharmaceutical engineering and offering hitherto unseen efficiency and insights.

In the preliminary phases of the drug discovery, virtual screening is a major advancement. In the past, finding promising drug candidates required time-consuming and labour-intensive high-throughput screening (HTS) techniques that examined hundreds of chemicals in relation to a biological target. On the other hand (Fang et al., 2022), virtual screening significantly expedites and lowers expenses by using computer methods to assess and rank compounds prior to their arrival in the laboratory (Vora et al., 2023).

Artificial intelligence and machine learning algorithms are used in virtual screening to stimulate the interactions between possible therapeutic compounds and their target proteins. These methods anticipate how well a chemical will bind to its target using a variety of computational methodologies, including pharmacophore modelling, and molecular docking (Paul et al., 2021).

Molecular docking is a method that replicates how tiny molecules dock into the target protein's binding site. AI systems generate a prioritised list of possible medication options according to their expected efficacy by predicting the most likely binding conformations and estimating the binding affinities (Paul et al., 2021).

QSAR models link a compound's biological activity to its chemical structure. AI systems can forecast the activity of novel compounds by using data that has already been collected. This capability helps to select viable candidates and optimise molecular structures for increased safety and efficacy (Park et al., 2022).

Pharmacophore modelling is a method that determines the spatial configuration of characteristics required for a molecule to interact with a particular target. In order to ensure that only molecules with the relevant properties are tested, AI algorithms can produce pharmacophore models that act as templates for screening vast chemical libraries (Sadee et al., 2023).

Virtual screening has many advantages. By concentrating trial efforts on the most promising candidates, it expedites the drug discovery process and saves time and money (Gupta et al., 2021). Compared to conventional techniques, the capacity to screen millions of molecules in silico allows researchers to conduct a more thorough exploration of chemical space (Bhattamisra et al., 2023).

Virtual screening can process large compound libraries in a fraction of the time compared to HTS experiments. This velocity enables the quick lead compound optimisation and iteration. Virtual screening dramatically reduces the cost of drug discovery by minimising the number of compounds that must be synthesised and evaluated in the lab (Alowais et al., 2023).

Computational screening can better investigate chemical variety by spotting new scaffolds and chemotypes that conventional approaches might miss. Several case studies demonstrate the effective use of virtual screening in the search for new drugs. For example, the identification of inhibitors for vital enzymes implicated in diseases such as cancer, HIV, and COVID-19 was made possible by the use of virtual screening. AI-powered virtual screening tools have proven useful in the real world by helping to find new antiviral drugs during the current pandemic (Kolluri et al., 2022).

Virtual screening has benefits, but it also has drawbacks, like forecast accuracy and the requirement for high-quality input data. It is anticipated that future developments in AI algorithms, more processing capacity, and improved experimental technique integration will raise the precision and dependability of virtual screening (Vora et al., 2023).

Another essential component of AI-driven drug development is predictive modelling, which provides strong instruments for predicting the pharmacokinetics, toxicity, and general efficacy of possible therapeutic options. By using AI to evaluate intricate biological data and forecast a drug's behaviour in the human body, this method greatly reduces the risk associated with the drug development process (Deng et al., 2023).

A variety of AI and machine learning techniques, each specifically designed to address different facets of drug behaviour and efficacy, are included in predictive modelling. Predictive models based on past data are constructed using methods like gradient boosting, random forecasts, and support vector machines (SVM) (Kolluri et al., 2022). These models are able to forecast the solubility, stability, and possible adverse effects of medication candidates, among other characteristics.

Neural networks in particular, which are algorithms for deep learning, have demonstrated impressive performance in predictive modelling. More accurate forecasts of medication toxicity and efficacy can be obtained by using convolutional neural networks (CNNs) and recurrent neural networks (RNNs), which are capable of capturing complicated relationships within the data (Kolluri et al., 2022).

Predictive performance can be improved by combining many machine-learning models into an ensemble. Ensemble approaches combine each model's advantage, lowering the possibility of overfitting and enhancing prediction robustness (Hartl et al., 2021).

Throughout the whole drug development process, from the early process, from early discovery to clinical trials, predictive modelling is used. An essential set of criteria in the development of new drugs is absorption, distribution, metabolism, excretion, and toxicity (ADMET) (Nomura et al., 2021). Artificial intelligence (AI) algorithms forecast these characteristics to guarantee that proposed medications are safe, bioavailable, and efficacious.

By examining genomic, proteomic, and pathway data, predictive modelling assists in the identification and validation of new therapeutic targets (Hartl et al., 2021). AI systems have the ability to identify previously unidentified connections between targets and illnesses, creating new opportunities for therapeutic intervention.

AI-driven predictive models play a key role in drug repurposing by finding current medications that can be modified for use in new therapeutic indications (Mullowney et al., 2023). This method expedites the development of licenced medications by discovering new uses for them using historical data and machine learning.

Predictive modelling has been successfully applied in drug discovery, as demonstrated by a number of case studies, AI models have been used, for instance, to discover biomarkers for early illness diagnosis, customise treatment regimens, and forecast the effectiveness of chemotherapy therapies for cancer patients (Park et al., 2022).

Predictive modelling made it easier to quickly identify medications that already have antiviral actions against COVID-19, which sped up the hunt for efficient therapies. Predictive modelling has many benefits, but it also has drawbacks, including issues with data quality, model interpretability, and regulatory acceptability (Sadee et al., 2023).

Ensuring the availability of annotated, high-quality datasets is essential for developing dependable models. Enhancing AI models' interpretability is also crucial to winning over regulators and medical professionals.

Future developments in AI algorithms, higher processing capacity, and the incorporation of multi-omics data are anticipated to improve predictive modelling's precision and usefulness. Predictive modelling in drug development will be important in the future because it can lead to more precise, effective, and personalised treatments, which will change pharmaceutical engineering as a whole (Deng et al., 2023).

The best results from virtual screening came from its integration with experimental procedures. The selection of chemicals for synthesis and biological testing is guided by AI-driven predictions (Paul et al., 2021), which lowers the rate of false positives and boosts the effectiveness of experimental validation.

Virtual screening has benefits, but it also has drawbacks, like forecast accuracy and the requirement for high-quality input data. Building trustworthy AI models requires making sure that a variety of valid training datasets are available (Gupta et al., 2021). Furthermore, winning over academics and regulatory agencies to AI predictions is contingent upon enhancing their interpretability.

It is anticipated that future developments in AI algorithms, more processing capacity, and improved experimental techniques integration will raise the precision and dependability of virtual screening (Bhattamisra et al., 2023). Novel approaches like hybrid artificial intelligence models and quantum computing have the potential to enhance virtual screening capabilities and open up new avenues for drug discovery.

Predictive modelling in therapeutic discovery is another essential component of AI-driven drug development, which provides strong instruments for predicting the pharmacokinetics, toxicity, and general efficacy of possible therapeutic options. By using AI to evaluate intricate biological data and forecast a drug's behaviour in the human body, this method greatly reduces the risk associated with the drug development process (Park et al., 2022).

Various AI and machine learning techniques, each designed to address particular elements of drug behaviour and efficacy, are included in predictive modelling, for example, Machine Learning models (Nomura et al., 2021). Predictive modelling as mentioned above, is based on past data are constructed using methods like gradient boosting, random forecasts, and support vector machines (SVM). These models are able to forecast solubility, stability, and possible adverse effects of medication candidates, among other characteristics. By determining the most pertinent factors, feature engineering and selection significantly increase the predictive potential of these models (Kolluri et al., 2022).

Another example of predictive modelling is the Deep Learning model. This includes Neural networks and other deep-learning algorithms that have demonstrated impressive predictive modelling performance. More accurate forecasts of medication toxicity and efficacy can be obtained by using convolutional neural networks (CNNs) and recurrent neural networks (RNNs), which are capable of capturing complicated relationships within the data (Hartl et al., 2021). Techniques for reinforcement learning and transfer learning are also being investigated to enhance predictive modelling skills.

The last example of predictive modelling is Ensemble learning. predictive modelling performance can be improved by combining many machine learning models into an ensemble. By combining the advantages of individual models, ensemble approaches lower the chance of overfitting and increase the accuracy of predictions. To build strong ensemble models, methods including bagging, boosting, and stacking are frequently employed (Park et al., 2022).

Predictive modelling has been successfully applied in drug discovery, as demonstrated by the following case studies (Park et al., 2022):

1- Cancer Treatment:

AI models have been used to discover biomarkers for early illness diagnosis, customise treatment regimens, and forecast the effectiveness of chemotherapy therapies for cancer patients. Predictive modelling, for instance, has aided in the identification of patients who are most likely to benefit from particular targeted medicines, enhancing treatment outcomes and minimising side effects.

2- COVID-19 Therapeutics:

Predictive modelling helped identify medications with potential antiviral activity quickly during the COVID-19 pandemic, which sped up the hunt for effective therapeutics. The development of COVID-19 therapeutics has been aided by the identification of multiple candidates for clinical study through AI-driven techniques.

3- Neurodegenerative Diseases:

Potential cures for neurodegenerative diseases including Parkinson's disease and Alzheimer's have been found through the use of predictive modelling (Fang et al., 2022). AI models have found new targets and pathways involved in the evolution of disease by analysing genetic and clinical data. This has led to the development of new therapeutic approaches.

Predictive modelling has many benefits and drawbacks as mentioned above, these challenges or drawbacks can be improved by ensuring the availability of annotated, high-quality datasets is essential for developing dependable models. Enhancing data quality is mostly dependent on data preparation methods including feature selection, imputation, and normalization (Iqbal et al., 2023). Enhancing AI models' interpretability is also crucial to winning over regulators and medical professionals. Predictive models' interpretability and transparency are being improved by employing strategies like LIME (Local Interpretable Model-agnostic Explanations) and SHAP (Shapley additive exPlanations) (Gupta et al., 2021).

Future developments in AI algorithms, higher processing capacity, and the incorporation of multi-omics data are anticipated to improve predictive medalling's precision and usefulness (Niazi & Mariam, 2024). Predictive modelling in drug development will be important in the future because it can lead to more precise, effective, and personalised treatments, which will change pharmaceutical engineering as a whole.

It is anticipated that cutting-edge technologies like explainable AI (XAI) and federated learning would improve predictive modelling even further, opening up more transparent and cooperative drug development procedures (Iqbal et al., 2023).

Clinical trials are being transformed by AI-driven advances, which are making them more patient-centred, economical, and efficient. Researchers can optimise a number of clinical trial processes, including patient recruitment, stratification, real-time monitoring, and adaptive trail designs, by utilizing AI technologies (Niazi & Mariam, 2024).

Recruiting and stratifying patients while getting and keeping the correct patients is one of the hardest parts of clinical studies. By examining genetic data, electronic health records (EHRs), and other pertinent data to find qualified applicants, AI can expedite this procedure (Sadee et al., 2023).

In order to guarantee that trials include patients who are most likely to benefit from the intervention, machine learning algorithms can predict patient eligibility based on inclusion and exclusion criteria.

AI also makes patient stratification possible, which divides patients into groups according to how likely they are to respond to a particular course of treatment. This division may be predicated on traits of the disease, genetic markers, or other variables (Park et al., 2022). Artificial intelligence assists in more successful clinical trials by identifying subgroups with comparable features.

Another area where AI is having a big impact is real-time monitoring. Large volumes of data about patients' health states are produced via wearable technology, smartphone health apps, and remote monitoring systems. In order to identify adverse events, track the effectiveness of treatment, and guarantee patient safety, AI systems evaluate this data in real-time (Paul et al., 2021).

The effectiveness and general quality of clinical trials are increased when prompt interventions and modifications are made possible by this ongoing monitoring. With the aid of AI, adaptive trial designs, which permit alternations based on interim data, are becoming increasingly widespread.

Researchers can make data-driven decisions on whether to continue, halt, or change the study by using AI-driven analytics to find trends and patterns in the data. Clinical trials are more flexible and efficient thanks to adaptive designs, which also lower costs and speed up the development process.

Predictive analytics powered by AI can anticipate trial results using real-time inputs and previous data. AI models can forecast the chance of success for various trial arms by examining variables including patient demographics, illness development, and therapy responses (Alowais et al., 2023). These forecasts assist researchers in making well-informed choices on the distribution of resources, the continuation of trials, and possible adjustments.

There are significant ethical and regulatory questions raised by the use of AI in clinical studies. In order to guarantee the ethical and safe application of AI in clinical research, regulatory organizations like the FDA and EMA are creating frameworks and guidelines. Data privacy, algorithm openness, and the requirement for thorough validation of AI models are important factors to take into consideration.

Crucial are the ethical ramifications as well, which include guaranteeing fair access to clinical trials and preventing prejudice in AI systems. Scientists need to make sure that AI-powered procedures don't unintentionally prejudice or exclude particular patient populations (Hartl et al., 2021). In order to persevere confidence and responsibility in clinical research, it is imperative that AI methodology and outcomes be reported transparently.

Precision medicine, another name for personalised medicine, tries to customise medical care for each patient according to their clinical, molecular, and genetic profiles. By making it possible to analyse intricate biological data and determine the best course of action for every patient (Park et al., 2022), artificial intelligence is a key factor in the advancement of personalised medicine.

AI's place in proteomics and genomics has been proven in the massive volumes of data on an individual's genetic and protein profiles are produced via proteomics and genomics. These data may be analysed by AI algorithms to find biomarkers, mutations, and genetic variations linked to certain diseases and how well they respond to therapy (Iqbal et al., 2023). AI contributes to better patient outcomes and treatment plan personalisation by identifying these biological fingerprints.

AI-powered technologies can forecast a patient's reaction to various treatments, allowing for more individualised treatment plans. AI algorithms, for instance, may evaluate genetic data to determine which patients are most likely to benefit from immunotherapies or targeted medicines (Niazi & Mariam, 2024). By guaranteeing that patients receive the best therapies possible, this individualised approach lowers the possibility of side effects and enhances overall results.

Measurable indications of biological processes or illnesses are known as biomarkers. Through the analysis of massive datasets from omics research, electronic health records, and clinical trials, AI is able to discover and variety of novel biomarkers (Vora et al., 2023). These biomarkers are useful in instruments for tracking the course of illnesses, forecasting treatment outcomes, and making diagnoses.

Tests known as companion diagnostics are designed to determine whether patients may most likely to benefit from a certain treatment. AI-powered companion diagnostics use prediction models and biomarkers to help in therapy selection. AI systems, for instance, are capable of analysing genetic and molecular data to assess a patient's suitability for a certain targeted medicine.

The process of finding and developing new drugs is being improved by the combination of AI with other cutting-edge technologies like big data, blockchain, and the Internet of things (loT). Innovations in manufacturing supply chain optimisation, pharmacovigilance, and medication safety are being propelled by these synergies (Niazi & Mariam, 2024).

Large volumes of data may be gathered, stored, and analysed from a variety of sources, such as omics research, clinical trials, EHRs, and empirical evidence, thanks to big data technology. AI systems are able to handle and examine this data in order to find hidden trends, produce new ideas, and assist in the decision-making process related to medication research and discovery.

Enhancing pharmacovigilance and drug safety can be ensured by improving the systems for pharmacovigilance powered by AI to track adverse drug reactions (ADRs) and guarantee medication safety, AI is able to recognise patterns in ADRs and identify possible safety warnings by examining data from social media, post-market surveillance, and clinical studies (Vora et al., 2023). By being proactive, pharmaceutical businesses and regulatory bodies can reduce risks and guarantee the safety of pharmaceuticals.

Through cost savings, quality control, and process optimisation, artificial intelligence is revolutionising the pharmaceutical manufacturing industry. Machine learning algorithms can increase manufacturing efficiency, optimise maintenance schedules, and forecast equipment breakdowns (Bhattamisra et al., 2023). Artificial intelligence (AI)-powered quality control systems examine sensor and production line data to find flaws and guarantee product consistency.

Artificial intelligence (AI) algorithms enhance supply chain logistics, demand forecasting, and inventory management. Artificial intelligence is able to minimise waste, forecast changes in demand, and optimise stock levels by examining data from distributors, retailers, and suppliers. This enhances patient access and lowers costs by guaranteeing that pharmaceuticals are available when and where they are required (Nomura et al., 2021).

Accountability and transparency are essential for building confidence in AI models used in medicines. It is imperative for researchers to guarantee the comprehensibility of AI systems and the transparency of their decision-making procedures. This entails giving thorough documentation of the techniques, data sources, and validation processes applied during the creation of AI models

The advancement of AI-driven drug discovery and development depends on cooperation between businesses, academia, and regulatory bodies. Data resources, and skills may be shared more easily through consortia, joint research efforts, and public-private partnerships. These initiatives promote creativity, quicken the creation of novel treatments, and guarantee the secure and efficient application of AI technology (Kolluri et al., 2022).

Several important areas will be the focus of future research and development in AI-driven pharmaceuticals:

1- Enhancing data quality and accessibility:

It is essential to make sure that top-notch, annotated datasets are available for AI model training. The objective will be supported by initiatives to standardize data formats, facilitate data exchange, and increase data interoperability.

2- Improving trust and interpretability of models:

Acquiring regulatory clearance and clinical acceptability of AI models will depend on developing methods to improve their interpretability and transparency. The use of Explainable AI (XAI) techniques will be crucial to this endeavour.

3- Progressing with integration with experimental methods:

The precision and effectiveness of drug discovery and development will be improved by further integrating AI with experimental procedures. High throughput screening, CRISPR-based gene editing, and other experimental method combined with AI-driven predictions will expedite the identification process, which will also expedite the handling of regulatory and ethical issues (Hartl et al., 2021). The safe and fair application of AI in medicines will be ensured by ongoing efforts to overcome ethical and regulatory constraints. To preserve public confidence and comply with regulations, strong frameworks for algorithm accountability, data protection, and AI validation must be developed.

THE ETHICAL CHALLENGES AND SOLUTIONS

Artificial intelligence (AI) in pharmaceutical research has the potential to revolutionize patient care, medication development, and discovery. Nonetheless, this shift also presents important ethical issues that need to be resolved to guarantee the ethical and fair application of AI technology. This chapter examines the main moral concerns surrounding artificial intelligence in pharmaceutical research and suggests solutions.

Artificial intelligence systems in pharmaceutical research frequently depend on enormous volumes of data, including private patient data like genetic information, medical records, and personal health histories. There are serious privacy and security hazards associated with the gathering, storing, and analysis of such data.

Identity theft, privacy violations, and breach of patient confidentiality can result from unauthorized access to this data. Further ethical issues are brought up by the possibility of patient data being misused by unauthorized individuals or for objectives other than those for which it was originally intended.

These concerns can be resolved by the following strategies:

1- Sturdy data security by using cutting-edge encryption methods:

Data is protected while it is in transit and at rest. This shields private data from potential breaches and stops unwanted access.

2- Identity and DE-identification and anonymization:

Before being employed in AI models, data should be de-identified or anonymized to preserve patient privacy. By removing personally identifying information, this procedure of privacy abuses.

3- Observance of data protection laws:

Pharmaceutical businesses are subject to data privacy laws, such as the Health Insurance Portability and Accountability Act (HIPAA) in the US and the General Data Privacy Regulation (GDPR) in Europe. These laws ensure that patient information is handled appropriately by establishing strict guidelines for data privacy and security (Hartl et al., 2021).

The quality of AI algorithms depends on the data they are trained on. Treatment and healthcare access inequities may result from AI models producing biased outcomes if the training data is biased or non-representative. An AI model may not function as effectively for other groups, for instance, if it was trained primarily on data from one demographic group. This might lead to unfair treatment and possibly exacerbate health inequalities (Deng et al., 2023).

Representative and diverse training data reduces bias and requires making sure that training data is representative of the whole population and varied. This entails gathering information from a range of demographic categories, such as age, gender, ethnicity, and socioeconomic status.

In the methods used for identifying and mitigating bias, it is crucial to have strategies in place for identifying and reducing bias in AI models. Fairness-aware algorithms, frequent bias audits, and the use of techniques like, resampling, re-weighting, or fairness requirements during model training are a few ways to achieve this (Iqbal et al., 2023).

To ensure accountability and transparency, it is essential that the creation and application of AI models be transparent. Businesses should make their AI systems techniques, data sources, and validation procedures available to the public by documenting and disclosing them. Putting in place explicit accountability procedures guarantees (Niazi & Mariam, 2024).

For the process of constant observation and assessment, for the AI models to continue operating fairly and properly, regular monitoring and assessment are required. This entails adding fresh data to models, assessing their effectiveness again, and modifying them as necessary to account for any biases that have surfaced.

A key ethical precept in medical research is informed consent, which states that subjects must be fully told about the purpose, advantages, and the dangers of a study before consenting to take part (Vora et al., 2023). Getting informed permission in the context of AI-driven pharmaceutical research can be difficult, particularly when working with intricate algorithms and huge datasets. Concerns around autonomy and permission may arise from patients' incomplete understanding of how their data will be utilised.

The technique that can be used to resolve informed consent issues is having open and intact communication It is crucial to make sure that patients are informed in a clear and honest manner about how their data will be utilised. This entails outlining the goal of the study, the function of AI, any possible advantages and disadvantages, and the security measures in place for personal data (Sadee et al., 2023).

Patients may comprehend the information being provided more easily if consent forms are made simpler and written in straightforward language. Videos and infographics are examples of visual aids that can improve understanding.

Artificial intelligence tools are being utilised more to aid in pharmaceutical research decision-making, from discovering potential drugs to forecasting patient outcomes. although AI can improve decision-making, depending too much on algorithms raises ethical questions. Recommendations from AI models might not always be accurate or trustworthy, and relying too much on AI could compromise human judgment and knowledge (Niazi & Mariam, 2024).

There are some ways to make sure AI is used ethically in decision-making, for example, the cooperation between AI and humans. It is crucial to encourage a cooperative strategy in which AI systems supplement human decision-making, not replace it. This guarantees that human judgment and knowledge play a crucial role in the decision-making process.

To achieve accreditation and confirmation and guarantee the correctness and dependability of AI models, thorough validation and verification are required (Gupta et al., 2021). This entails putting models to the test in practical situations, constructing expert judgment with AI-generated suggestions, and regularly assessing performance.

Having standards and guidelines for ethics ensures responsible practices in the use of AI in decision-making may be facilitated by creating and upholding ethical norms and guidelines (Iqbal et al., 2023). These rules ought to include matters like responsibility, openness, and the proper use of suggestions produced by AI.

Ongoing instruction and training are essential to give researchers and medical practitioners on the moral use of AI. This entails promoting awareness of the limitations, possible biases, and significance of human oversight that comes with AI.

The use of AI in pharmaceutical research has also raised questions about the potential workforce shifts and job displacement. AI systems have the potential to automate some jobs, which might result in job losses and workforce reorganisation (Niazi & Mariam, 2024). It is essential to make sure that these adjustments are handled morally and that employees are assisted through these changes.

The upskilling and reskilling of employers may assist the staff also in adjusting to new roles and responsibilities in an AI-driven workplace by funding workforce reskilling and upskilling initiatives. Employers can acquire new skills and maintain their competitiveness in the job market by receiving training in artificial intelligence and associated technologies.

AI systems have the potential to automate some jobs, which as mentioned, can result in job losses and workforce reorganization. It is essential to make sure that these adjustments are handled morally and that employees are assisted through these changes. AI has the potential to enhance human labour instead of displacing it, freeing up workers' time for more intricate and imaginative work (Mullowney et al., 2023). It is crucial to offer social and financial assistance to workers impacted by changes brought about by AI. To aid displaced workers in transitioning to new possibilities involves providing financial support, career counselling, and job placement services.

Employee participation in the decision-making process is guaranteed when workforce changes are approached with an inclusive and participative mindset. Getting employees involved in conversations regarding AI adoption and how it will affect their jobs will encourage a sense of ownership and teamwork.

When using AI in pharmaceutical research, it might be difficult to establish who is responsible and liable when the system malfunctions. It might be not evident who is at fault- the AI itself, its creators, or users- when an AI system malfunctions or causes harm. solve these issues, it is imperative to set up explicit accountability procedures.

Establishing precise accountability frameworks that specify the obligations of each party participating in the creation and application of AI systems is essential. This involves establishing who is responsible for the precision, security, and moral application of AI models (Bhattamisra et al., 2023).

Accountability may be improved by implementing legal and regulatory monitoring to control the application of AI in pharmaceutical research. This entails creating laws that specify who is responsible for mistakes and damages caused by AI as well as redress channels. Accountability depends on transparency in the design and implementation of AI systems. This entails revealing the sources of the data, recording the development process, and offering comprehensive details on the training and validation of AI models (Hartl et al., 2021).

Regularly conducting ethical audits and assessments of AI systems can assist in locating and resolving possible liability and accountability-related problems. The responsible and ethical application of AI systems can be ensured via independent oversight groups. artificial intelligence in pharmaceutical research has the potential to significantly affect treatment options, health outcomes, and healthcare access. AI technologies have raised worries that they may worsen already-existing health disparities and lead to unequal access to and management of healthcare(Kolluri et al., 2022) . For instance, AI models developed using data from wealthy nations would not function effectively in low- and middle-income nations, which could result in unfair treatment outcomes.

It is crucial to create AI systems that are inclusive and reflective of many communities. This involves making certain that a broad spectrum of demographic categories, medical problems, and geographical areas are included in the training data. AI models that are more equal can be produced via cooperative efforts among stakeholders in various geographic areas (Hartl et al., 2021).

In order to reduce inequities, international cooperation in AI research and development is encouraged. Assuring that AI technology benefits all populations may be achieved through partnerships between high-income and low-income nations these partnerships can allow the sharing of data, expertise, and resources.

Fair distribution of the advantages of AI may be ensured and ethical decision-making can be guided by the implementation of health equity frameworks in AI development and deployment. Improving underprivileged populations' access to care and tackling health inequalities should be given top priority in these frameworks.

Understanding the needs and concerns of the populations impacted by AI-driven developments in pharmaceutical research is essential. Participating community people in the planning and execution of AI projects helps guarantee that these tools are culturally and locally relevant and in line with health goals (Iqbal et al., 2023).

The creation of ethical and regulatory frameworks has lagged behind the quick growth of AI technology in pharmaceutical research. Uncertainty over how to guarantee the moral application of AI and safeguard patient interests results from this delay. The absence of set rules might result in unethical behaviour and inconsistent behaviour (Niazi & Mariam, 2024). Regulatory agencies and trade associations ought to create thorough policies for the moral use of AI in medical research. These policies should give researchers and developers a clear framework and handle concerns including data privacy, bias, informed consent, and responsibility.

Ensuring adherence to ethical norms in AI research projects can be facilitated by establishing ethical review committees. Experts in AI, ethics, laws, and patient advocacy should be on these boards to provide interdisciplinary viewpoints on moral dilemmas. It is also essential to provide researchers, developers, and healthcare practitioners with ongoing ethical ramifications should be the main topic of training programmes, giving participants the information and abilities they need to successfully handle moral dilemmas (Iqbal et al., 2023).

The effective use of AI in pharmaceutical research requires public confidence. Public trust may be damaged, though, by worries about algorithmic bias, data privacy, and the moral application of AI. More factors that fuel opposition and scepticism concerning AI technology include misinformation and ignorance of them. Establishing public trust in the use of AI in pharmaceutical research requires open and honest communication (Vora et al., 2023). This entails giving comprehensive explanations of the advantages and disadvantages of AI technologies as well as the security measures in place for patient data.

Educating the public and addressing concerns can be achieved by demystifying AI technologies. Opportunities for discussion and knowledge exchange can be found in public forums, workshops, and educational campaigns. Establishing public confidence requires a clear commitment to ethical AI activities. High ethical standards, patient welfare (Fang et al., 2022), and transparency about AI activities should be upheld by businesses and research institutions.

Maintaining public confidence in AI systems requires proactive efforts to correct disinformation. Building a better educated and supportive public impression of artificial intelligence in pharmaceutical research may be achieved via dispelling myths and providing factual facts (Mullowney et al., 2023).

As AI technologies advance, new moral quandaries will surface. It is imperative to anticipate and proactively tackle these issues in order to guarantee the conscientious and principled application of AI in pharmaceutical research (Niazi & Mariam, 2024).

Potential ethical issues with new AI technologies can be recognised and prepared for with the use of scenario planning and foresight (Fang et al., 2022). This entails investigating various future situations, evaluating any hazards, and creating plans to lessen them.

It is essential to create a flexible ethical framework that may change as technology advances (Fang et al., 2022). These frameworks ought to be adaptable and sensitive to emerging moral principles dilemmas so that moral principles continue to be useful and applicable.

Encouraging multidisciplinary cooperation among AI researchers, ethicists, lawyers, and medical practitioners can assist in resolving difficult moral dilemmas (Iqbal et al., 2023). Solutions that are more thorough and complex might result from collaborative efforts. Establishing systems for ongoing observation and input guarantees that moral dilemmas are found and dealt with promptly (Paul et al., 2021). Maintaining high ethical standards may be aided by iterative changes, stakeholder feedback, and regular ethics audits.

The Economic Consequences of the Use of AI in Pharmaceutical Research

Artificial intelligence (AI) has brought about revolutionary shifts in several industries, including pharmaceutical research. Because AI may improve precision, lower costs, and simplify workflows (Alowais et al., 2023). It is gaining a lot of interest as a possible revolution in drug research and development procedures. It is important to explore the financial effects of artificial intelligence on pharmaceutical research, looking at both present and potential future applications.

The conventional drug development process is infamous for being costly and time-consuming (Bhattamisra et al., 2023); it sometimes takes over 10 years and a significant amount of money to introduce a new medication to the market. AI has the ability to significantly lower these costs via a number of mechanisms:

1- Accelerated drug discovery:

Compared to conventional techniques, AI may uncover possible drug candidates more quickly by analysing large datasets. By predicting the interaction that various chemicals would have with biological targets, machine learning algorithms can considerably reduce the time required for lead discovery and optimisation.

2- Predictive modelling:

By predicting the safety and efficacy of novel drug candidates, AI-driven predictive models can lower the risks of expensive late-stage failures (Hartl et al., 2021). AI can assist in saving money by seeing possible problems early in the development process and avoiding wasting money on unpromising candidates.

3- Automation of routine processes:

AI can reduce the need for manual labour and related expenses by automating routine processes like data input, analysis, and report preparation (Kolluri et al., 2022). This frees up research to concentrate on more intricate and imaginative facets of medication creation.

AI improves productivity and efficiency in pharmaceutical research by:

1- High-throughput screening:

Compared to conventional techniques, AI algorithms can handle and analyse data from high-throughput screening trials more quickly and precisely. This makes it possible for researchers to swiftly choose interesting molecules from extensive libraries.

2- Clinical trial design optimisation:

AI can anticipate patient reactions and choose appropriate trial participants to optimise the design of clinical trials. This shortens trial times and raises the possibility of positive results, hastening the release of new medications onto the market.

3- Integrating data and analysing it:

AI is capable of integrating and analysing data from a variety of sources, including electronic health records, proteomics, and genomes. A better understanding of medication reactions and illness causes is made possible by this comprehensive approach, which speeds up the creation of more potent treatments.

The use of AI in pharmaceutical research is creating rivalry and changing market dynamics by a few methods, for example, reducing access hurdles. AI technologies are democratising drug discovery by reducing access hurdles for entrepreneurs and smaller biotech companies (Vora et al., 2023). By using AI to compete with long-standing pharmaceutical behemoths, these businesses may encourage innovation and diversity within the sector.

The second example is strategic alliances. In an effort to obtain a competitive advantage, pharmaceutical corporations are more frequently establishing strategic alliances with AI businesses (Deng et al., 2023). By combining the knowledge of the two industries, these partnerships quicken the development of new drugs and increase market potential.

The last example is intellectual property and patient landscape. An increase in patents pertaining to AI is being caused by the application of AI in medication development. As a result, businesses are forced to fight for intellectual property to protect their inventions and market positions (Hughes, 2012).

AI has a greater financial influence on pharmaceutical development than just cost savings. Reducing healthcare expenses can be achieved by using AI and hastening the creation of efficient treatments (Sadee et al., 2023). Early access to novel therapies can improve patient outcomes and reduce long-term illness-related healthcare costs.

The need for qualified workers in disciplines like data science, bioinformatics, and AI engineering is being driven by the use of AI technology. This promotes the development of skills and the production of jobs, which boosts economic growth (Iqbal et al., 2023). Enhanced allocation venture capitalists, private equity firms, and government agencies are making significant investments in pharmaceutical research because of the promising potential of artificial intelligence (Niazi & Mariam, 2024). This financial inflow is encouraging the industry to innovate and grow even more.

The use of AI in pharmaceutical research is creating rivalry and changing market dynamics, by reducing access hurdles, AI technologies are democratising drug discovery by reducing access hurdles for startups and smaller biotech companies (Ahmed et al., n.d.). By using AI to compete with long-standing huge pharmaceutical companies, these businesses may encourage innovation and diversity within the sector.

In an effort to obtain a competitive advantage, pharmaceutical corporations are more frequently establishing strategic alliances with AI businesses (Niazi & Mariam, 2024). By combining the two industries, these partnerships quicken the development of new drugs and increase market potential (Hughes, 2012).

Patents pertaining to AI are proliferating as a result of its application in medication research. As a result, businesses are forced to fight for intellectual property rights in order to protect their inventions and market positions.

With the development of AI algorithms and methodologies, there are intriguing prospects for the use of AI in pharmaceutical research. AI models can be made more accurate and predictive by utilizing deep learning and neural networks (Iqbal et al., 2023). By analysing intricate biological data, these tools can identify new drug targets and processes.

Transparency and interpretability are critical as AI systems get more complex. The goal of explainable AI approaches is to build regulatory compliance and trust by shedding light on how AI models make their predictions (Vora et al., 2023). By customising medicines for each patient based on their genetic profiles, lifestyle, and medical history, AI holds the potential to completely transform personalised medicine. This strategy can reduce side effects and maximise therapeutic results.

AI's influence on pharmaceutical research will be further amplified by its combination with other cutting-edge technologies (Niazi & Mariam, 2024). One of these technologies is called Blockchain Technology. In pharmaceutical research, blockchain can improve data security, traceability, and transparency. It can protect the integrity of study findings and enable a safe exchange of clinical trial data.

Another technology is Internet of Things (loT), its gadgets are able to gather patient data in real-time, which offers important insights for medication formulation and treatment efficacy monitoring (Fang et al., 2022). AI is capable of analysing this data to spot patterns and enhance treatment plans. Complex computational issues that are now unsolvable by conventional computers may be resolved by quantum computing. It can completely change the process of finding new drugs by making it possible to quickly stimulate chemical interaction and protein folding.

CONCLUSION

The use of artificial intelligence in pharmaceutical research is a revolutionary invention with great potential for the advancement of patient care, medication development and discovery. Artificial intelligence has several benefits, including faster drug development, precision medicine, better clinical trials, better medication repurposing, and higher operational efficiency (Mullowney et al., 2023). AI can handle enormous volumes of data at previously unheard-of rates. These developments have the potential to completely transform the pharmaceutical sector by cutting the time and expenses involved in introducing novel medications to the market, customising care, and eventually enhancing patient outcomes (Paul et al., 2021). researchers can find new medicinal compounds by more effectively identifying and validating pharmacological targets with the use of AI-driven high-throughput screening and predictive modelling (Kolluri et al., 2022). Furthermore, precision medicine is made possible by AI's contribution to genomic analytics, which enables the creation of personalised medicines based on the genetic profiles of specific patients. In addition to increasing therapeutic efficacy, this individualised strategy reduces side effects and promotes safer medical procedures (Nomura et al., 2021).

Enhancing clinical trials is yet another crucial area in which AI shows significant promise. AI contributes to the more successful and efficient execution of clinical trials by improving monitoring procedures, optimising trial design, and expediting patient recruitment (Hartl et al., 2021). This guarantees that innovative treatments get to patients faster and speeds up the entire drug development process.

Furthermore, AI makes it easier to repurpose pharmaceuticals by combining and evaluating various datasets to find novel therapeutic applications for already-approved medications. This method can save a great deal of money and time in the development process, making it possible to bring successful therapies to market more quickly (Niazi & Mariam, 2024). Before expensive clinical studies are conducted, AI's predictive modelling capability to mimic the effects of repurposed pharmaceuticals offers important insights into their prospective effectiveness and safety (Vora et al., 2023).

AI-driven workflow optimisation and regular job automation significantly increase operational efficiency in pharmaceutical research. For example, laboratory automation lowers the possibility of human mistakes and frees up researchers to concentrate on more intricate and imaginative parts of their job (Vora et al., 2023). AI can also improve supply chain management, lowering costs and guaranteeing the prompt delivery of research supplies.

Moving forward, AI-driven medication research and discovery have a bright future. Consistent progress in artificial intelligence, in conjunction with innovations in biotechnology and genetics, will augment our comprehension of intricate illnesses and expedite the creation of inventive treatments (Deng et al., 2023). To fully use AI while guaranteeing moral and fair access to these technologies, cooperation between academic institutions, businesses, and regulatory agencies will be crucial.

The application of artificial intelligence in pharmaceutical engineering has enormous potential going forward (Fang et al., 2022). Technological developments in computational biology, data analytics, and machine learning will improve our capacity to comprehend complicated illnesses and provide novel treatments (Paul et al., 2021). The integration of artificial intelligence with other cutting-edge fields like biotechnology and genomics may open up new avenues for medication research and discovery, providing hope for long-elusive illness solutions (Sadee et al., 2023). The revolution in pharmaceutical engineering that artificial intelligence has brought about is a major step forward in our efforts to enhance global health outcomes (Bhattamisra et al., 2023). rapid drug discovery and development, clinical trial optimisation, and personalised therapy delivery have the potential to revolutionise healthcare and improve its efficacy, accessibility, and efficiency (Hartl et al., 2021).

In conclusion, the pharmaceutical engineering revolution sparked by artificial intelligence is revolutionising the sector at a pace never seen before (Iqbal et al., 2023). Our mission is to enhance global health outcomes has advanced significantly with the capacity to quickly find and develop novel medications, optimise clinical trials, and provide individualised therapies. Even if there are still obstacles. AI technologies are continuing to advance and integrate (Niazi & Mariam, 2024).

REFERENCES

Ahmed, Z., & Barber, N., Yogini, Sara, J. ;, Bryony, G. ;, & Franklin, D. (n.d.). *Elsevier Editorial System(tm) for International Journal of Medical Informatics Manuscript Draft Title: Economic impact of electronic prescribing in the hospital setting: a systematic review*. DOI: 10.1186/s13195-021-00951-z PMID: 35012639

Alowais, S. A., Alghamdi, S. S., Alsuhebany, N., Alqahtani, T., Alshaya, A. I., Almohareb, S. N., Aldairem, A., Alrashed, M., Bin Saleh, K., Badreldin, H. A., Al Yami, M. S., Al Harbi, S., & Albekairy, A. M. (2023). Revolutionizing healthcare: the role of artificial intelligence in clinical practice. In *BMC Medical Education* (Vol. 23, Issue 1). BioMed Central Ltd. DOI: 10.1186/s12909-023-04698-z

Bhattamisra, S. K., Banerjee, P., Gupta, P., Mayuren, J., Patra, S., & Candasamy, M. (2023). Artificial Intelligence in Pharmaceutical and Healthcare Research. In *Big Data and Cognitive Computing* (Vol. 7, Issue 1). MDPI. DOI: 10.3390/bdcc7010010

Deng, S., Li, C., Cao, J., Cui, Z., Du, J., Fu, Z., Yang, H., & Chen, P. (2023). Organ-on-a-chip meets artificial intelligence in drug evaluation. In *Theranostics* (Vol. 13, Issue 13, pp. 4526–4558). Ivyspring International Publisher. DOI: 10.7150/thno.87266

Fang, J., Zhang, P., Wang, Q., Chiang, C. W., Zhou, Y., Hou, Y., Xu, J., Chen, R., Zhang, B., Lewis, S. J., Leverenz, J. B., Pieper, A. A., Li, B., Li, L., Cummings, J., & Cheng, F. (2022). Artificial intelligence framework identifies candidate targets for drug repurposing in Alzheimer's disease. *Alzheimer's Research & Therapy*, 14(1), 7. Advance online publication. DOI: 10.1186/s13195-021-00951-z PMID: 35012639

Gupta, R., Srivastava, D., Sahu, M., Tiwari, S., Ambasta, R. K., & Kumar, P. (2021). Artificial intelligence to deep learning: Machine intelligence approach for drug discovery. *Molecular Diversity*, 25(3), 1315–1360. DOI: 10.1007/s11030-021-10217-3 PMID: 33844136

Hartl, D., de Luca, V., Kostikova, A., Laramie, J., Kennedy, S., Ferrero, E., Siegel, R., Fink, M., Ahmed, S., Millholland, J., Schuhmacher, A., Hinder, M., Piali, L., & Roth, A. (2021). Translational precision medicine: an industry perspective. In *Journal of Translational Medicine* (Vol. 19, Issue 1). BioMed Central Ltd. DOI: 10.1186/s12967-021-02910-6

Hughes, D. A. (2012). Pharmacoeconomics. In *British Journal of Clinical Pharmacology* (Vol. 73, Issue 6, pp. 968–972). DOI: 10.1111/j.1365-2125.2012.04247.x

Iqbal, J., Cortés Jaimes, D. C., Makineni, P., Subramani, S., Hemaida, S., Thugu, T. R., Butt, A. N., Sikto, J. T., Kaur, P., Lak, M. A., Augustine, M., Shahzad, R., & Arain, M. (2023). Reimagining Healthcare: Unleashing the Power of Artificial Intelligence in Medicine. *Cureus*. Advance online publication. DOI: 10.7759/cureus.44658 PMID: 37799217

Kolluri, S., Lin, J., Liu, R., Zhang, Y., & Zhang, W. (2022). Machine Learning and Artificial Intelligence in Pharmaceutical Research and Development: a Review. In *AAPS Journal* (Vol. 24, Issue 1). Springer Science and Business Media Deutschland GmbH. DOI: 10.1208/s12248-021-00644-3

Mullowney, M. W., Duncan, K. R., Elsayed, S. S., Garg, N., van der Hooft, J. J. J., Martin, N. I., Meijer, D., Terlouw, B. R., Biermann, F., Blin, K., Durairaj, J., Gorostiola González, M., Helfrich, E. J. N., Huber, F., Leopold-Messer, S., Rajan, K., de Rond, T., van Santen, J. A., Sorokina, M., . . . Medema, M. H. (2023). Artificial intelligence for natural product drug discovery. In *Nature Reviews Drug Discovery* (Vol. 22, Issue 11, pp. 895–916). Nature Research. DOI: 10.1038/s41573-023-00774-7

Niazi, S. K., & Mariam, Z. (2024). Computer-Aided Drug Design and Drug Discovery: A Prospective Analysis. In *Pharmaceuticals* (Vol. 17, Issue 1). Multidisciplinary Digital Publishing Institute (MDPI). DOI: 10.3390/ph17010022

Nomura, A., Noguchi, M., Kometani, M., Furukawa, K., & Yoneda, T. (2021). Artificial Intelligence in Current Diabetes Management and Prediction. In *Current Diabetes Reports* (Vol. 21, Issue 12). Springer. DOI: 10.1007/s11892-021-01423-2

Park, S., Ock, C.-Y., Kim, H., Pereira, S., Park, S., Ma, M., Choi, S., Kim, S., Shin, S., Aum, B. J., Paeng, K., Yoo, D., Cha, H., Park, S., Suh, K. J., Jung, H. A., Kim, S. H., Kim, Y. J., Sun, J.-M., & Lee, S.-H. (2022). Artificial Intelligence-Powered Spatial Analysis of Tumor-Infiltrating Lymphocytes as Complementary Biomarker for Immune Checkpoint Inhibition in Non-Small-Cell Lung Cancer. *Journal of Clinical Oncology*, 40(17), 1916–1928. DOI: 10.1200/JCO.21.02010 PMID: 35271299

Paul, D., Sanap, G., Shenoy, S., Kalyane, D., Kalia, K., & Tekade, R. K. (2021). Artificial intelligence in drug discovery and development. In *Drug Discovery Today* (Vol. 26, Issue 1, pp. 80–93). Elsevier Ltd. DOI: 10.1016/j.drudis.2020.10.010

Sadee, W., Wang, D., Hartmann, K., & Toland, A. E. (2023). Pharmacogenomics: Driving Personalized Medicine. In *Pharmacological Reviews* (Vol. 75, Issue 4, pp. 789–814). American Society for Pharmacology and Experimental Therapy (ASPET). DOI: 10.1124/pharmrev.122.000810

Vora, L. K., Gholap, A. D., Jetha, K., Thakur, R. R. S., Solanki, H. K., & Chavda, V. P. (2023). Artificial Intelligence in Pharmaceutical Technology and Drug Delivery Design. In *Pharmaceutics* (Vol. 15, Issue 7). Multidisciplinary Digital Publishing Institute (MDPI). DOI: 10.3390/pharmaceutics15071916

Chapter 5 Drug Design and Discovery Through Artificial Intelligence: Concept of Drug Target Interactions

Zuber Peermohammed Shaikh
Savitribai Phule Pune University, India

Satish Balkrishna Bhise
Smt. Kashibai Navale Medical College and General Hospital, India

ABSTRACT

The pharmaceutical industry has seen a create powerful in data digitization in past few years. However, challenge of gathering, evaluating, and utilizing knowledge to solve complicated. Pharmaceutical problems arises with digitalization. This encourages the usage of AI, which can handle vast amounts of data for drug target interactions with greater efficiency. Artificial intelligence (AI) is a technology-based system that uses a variety of advanced tools and networks to simulate Drug Discovery and Design. At the same time, it does not pose complete threats to human physical presence. This chapter emphasizes importance of artificial intelligence (AI) in the pharmaceutical sector, including drug research and development, medication repurposing, enhancing pharmaceutical productivity, and clinical trials and its current and future applications in drug discovery development. To address a few of these problems, deep learning can be used to generate new compounds by selecting molecules from a known distribution and then designing fundamental distribution

DOI: 10.4018/979-8-3693-6270-9.ch005

INTRODUCTION

Drug discovery through Artificial Intelligence: The process of Drug Discovery affects the whole Pharmaceutical sector including all the phases such as a preliminary phase of research from target Discovery and validation to the discerning of molecules. A variety of streams can be used to initiate the identification of small therapeutic molecules. New research can lead to awareness of different diseases with different routes of drug administration and can be developed to take part in pharmaceutical companies to run large-scale trials and other waste programs, in order to identify the targeted molecular compounds. This process is mostly performed at the beginning of lead Discovery, with the prospect of taking identified compounds in the right way through preclinical and clinical trials. Artificial intelligence is an area of computer science that deals with the ability to solve problems using symbolic programming. Artificial intelligence can help solve health-care issues with large-scale applications. Expert system development is a significant and effective application of artificial intelligence. AI makes use of systems and software that can read and learn from data and to make independent judgments in order to achieve certain goals. Its applications in the pharmaceutical area are constantly being expanded, as discussed in this chapter. *(Ebhohimen IE,2020)*

Recently, healthcare sector is facing some complex challenges, such as the increased cost of drugs and therapies, and society needs specific significant changes in this area. Personalized medications with the necessary dose, release parameters, and other required aspects can be manufactured according to individual patient need with the use of AI in pharmaceutical product manufacturing. Using the latest AI-based technologies will not only reduce the time it takes for products to reach the market, but it will also improve product quality and overall safety of the manufacturing process, as well as provide better resource utilization and cost-effectiveness, emphasize the importance of automation.

Since 1960, medicinal chemistry has been applied to AI in different forms and with an assorted degree of progress in designing compounds. It involves supervised learning, in which labeled training datasets are used to train models broadly. One example is the quantitative structure-activity relationship (QSAR) approach, which is frequently used to predict properties, such as log P and solubility, for chemical structures. Unlike unsupervised learning, which is not based on labels, this is also popular within medicinal chemistry, with examples such as hierarchical clustering, algorithms, and principal components analysis used broadly to examine and break down large molecular libraries into smaller collections of indistinguishable compounds.*(Imam SS,2017)*

Figure 1. Artificial intelligence in drug design and discovery

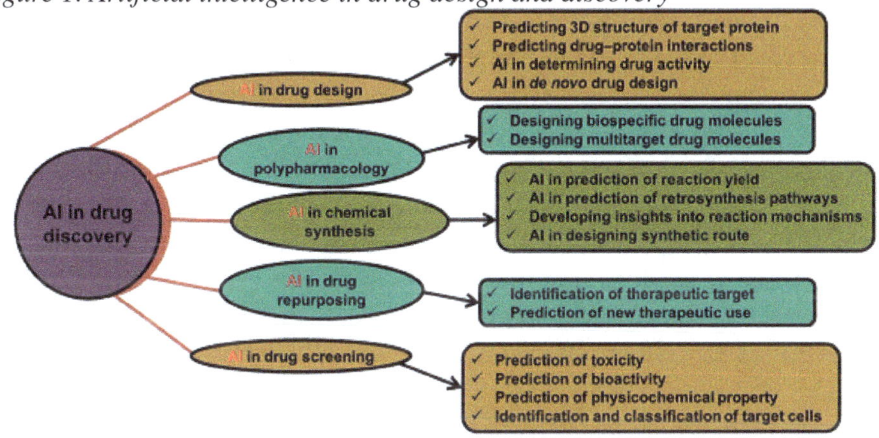

AI neural networks in drug discovery: The Research and Development (R and D) cycle that encapsulates: Problem analysis, grounding, design, implementation, and evaluation, for innovative small-molecule drugs as an example are required to overcome obstacles, such as high marketing cost, limited success rates in clinical trials, and overall prolonged R and D cycle time. The R and D productivity of drugs (for drugs of small-molecule) in the medical care industry continues to dwindle, despite expenditure records. In addition, partially because of the saturation of the market, it has been challenging to bring novel chemical matter through a complex approval process, and partly because people are willing to pay in both developed and developing markets. In recent times, scientists have more information than ever before on an assortment of topics that pertain to the subject, outperforming the ability of most to properly parse and amalgamate into their own workflows and research objectives. One solution to this kind of complication is to outsource our reasoning to machine intelligence when it comes to the analysis of multisource and multidimensional data. *(Miles J., 2006)*

Machine Learning for Drug Discovery: ML is a type of AI that enhances the accuracy of predictive outcomes and offers fresh opportunities for small-molecule drug discovery. ML approaches that might be considered instances of weak AI have made remarkable progress, with blossoming in their fundamental algorithms and application. AI has recently emerged as a hot topic in the pharmaceutical industry. AI in Biopharmaceutical Company's initiative subsistence rose at a summer workshop in 1956 at Dartmouth College, The Dartmouth Summer Research Project on AI was a groundbreaking event for AI. During the 1970s, a number of AI-based diagnostic tools were developed, such as PIP, Internist-1, MYCIN (an early expert system, or AI program, for treating blood infections), and Common Attribute Support

Network. In 1985, the R1 (eXpert CONfigurer, for expert configure) program was a production rule-based system that achieved 95–98% accuracy and was blown to a million-dollar industry. In the course of the early 1990s, AI exponentially grew in data communication (Internet), cloud technologies (Apps, Elastic Computing cloud, etc.), high-performance cloud computing, and big data storage. In the chess match between Garry Kasparov and an IBM supercomputer called Deep Blue, Deep Blue defeated Kasparov in 1997 which put AI in the limelight. Over the past decade, AI has expanded exponentially, and there has been a significant increase in investments in AI for drug discovery. A firm in Silicon Valley called Andréessen Horowitz recently announced a 450-million-dollar bio investment fund, with AI as a major focus area. *(Yang Y.,2018)*

LITERATURE REVIEW

De novo drug design with AI In drug discovery, one of the most challenging computer-aided tasks is the creation of new molecules with desired pharmacological properties from scratch. This is due to the unique chemical space of molecules with such properties. In de novo molecule generation, there is a danger of a series of combinative explosions because of the enormous amount of different atomic types and molecular topologies a researcher could explore. As a result, ligand-based approaches, structure-based approaches, or a combination of both approaches may be used based on the information aided to guide the de novo design process. The ligand-based methodology can be grouped into two main categories:

A rule-based approach consists of a set of rules for building molecules from reagents or molecular fragments. For the process of stepping through analogs of active leads to their maximum potency, the Topliss scheme is one of the forerunners of modern rule-based de novo design. Modern approaches to optimization use a set of molecular transformations, such as matched pairs of molecules, or rules-of thumb for functional groups, and molecular framework modification. Synthesis-oriented approaches include rules for building block assembly and ligand generation in particular. These approaches can be used to design synthetically accessible libraries, such as BI CLAIM and CHIPMUNK. Hybrid approaches such as Testing Operations Provisioning and Administration System, Difference of Gaussian, and DINGOES, have been developed to guide the generation of novel compounds, since the late 1990s, by concurrently maximizing both, their similarity to known bioactive ligands and the chemical synthesizability of the designs. *(Abdullahi, M.,2020)*

Rule-free approaches have no rigid construction rules, but rather aim to generate molecules with desired properties without the need for molecular construction rules. Molecular representations are learned by learning generative deep-learning models, which sample new molecules from the latent molecular representation. Although these approaches have gained popularity within a previous couple of years, the concept of sampling from a numerical presentation of molecules for de novo design goes back to the "inverse QSAR" problem formulated in the pioneering work of Skvortsova and Zefirov in the early 1990s. The present QSAR model, anchored by inverse QSAR, not only detects the descriptive values which correlate to the desired property but also utilizes this information for molecule production. In contrast, the latter method poses several obstacles, such as the existence of multiple solutions for each property and the difficulty of reverse-decoding cogent structures from molecular descriptors. The most common implementation is Simplified Molecular Input Line Entry System (SMILES) paired with generative models borrowed from natural language processing. It teaches them how to use the SMILE "syntax" (i.e., create a chemically valid string), based on chosen "semantics" (e.g., bioactivity or other desired molecular property). They generally rely on recurrent neural networks, combined with transfer or reinforcement learning. There have also been a variety of other deep-learning-based generative learning models reported, such as variational autoencoders and generative adversarial networks, as well as graph-convolution models. Some recent papers have proposed conditional generative design approaches, which take advantage of supplementary factors steering the design, such as three dimensional shape, drug-likeness, synthesizability, and molecular descriptor values. Elucidating balanced objective functions that enable intricate and constrained multi-parameter optimizations will be a major challenge in the future, analogous to those found in Pareto or desirability-based approaches that are classic in drug discovery. As a result of the rapid development of generative neural networks, the number of ligand-based design methods has risen dramatically. In addition to neural generative models, GuacaMol and MOSES provide a set of metrics that can compare them, as well as more traditional models (like genetic algorithms). *(Mohsin NuA, 2022)*

de novo design tools are generally more difficult to evaluate retrospectively than predictive methods, but some of the most commonly used metrics include: 1. Rationality of the created molecular representations and novelty of the simultaneous molecules 2. Chemical and biological resemblance with the known compounds, and 3. Scaffold and fragment diversity. The advantages of rule-based and rule-free approaches differ. The rule based methods use preexisting knowledge, such as building blocks and reaction rules, to generate molecules that are often freely synthesizable and have the desired physicochemical properties. Hard-coded rules and library selections, however, play a role in influencing the chemical diversity of the designs. Theoretically, rule-free approaches learn straight from the data without requiring hard-coded design or similarity rules, thereby permitting a wide exploration of the chemical space. But to the disadvantage, this freedom of exploration endangers the generation of compounds that are more difficult, if not impossible, to synthesize. Lately, a combined strategy was demonstrated to be feasible for designing bioactive molecules in a rule-free fashion, while simultaneously retaining synthesizability within a microfluidics system, using predefined virtual reactions. The majority of deep-learning-based de novo design studies, till now, have concentrated on ligand-based approaches. Research directed at orphan receptors and hitherto unexplored macromolecules through structure-based generative design has great potential. Based on the best knowledge known, deep learning has not yet heavily invaded these approaches that utilize information about the ligand-binding site (e.g., fragment linking or growing). In the meantime, prime developments in ligand design have been made based on the shape and properties of the binding pocket. (*Vosooghi, M.;2014)*

Kumar et al. used 745 compounds to train six predictive models [SVMs, ANNs, k-nearest neighboring algorithms, LDAs, probabilistic neural network algorithms, and partial least square (PLS)] that were then applied to 497 compounds to predict their intestinal absorptivity based on parameters such as molecular surface area, molecular mass, total hydrogen count, molecular refractivity, molecular volume, logP, the sum of E-state indices, the solubility index (log S), and rotatable bonds[36]. In a similar line, RF and DNN-based in silico models for predicting human intestinal absorption of a variety of chemical substances have been developed. As a result, AI plays an important role in drug development, predicting not only the drug's desired physicochemical properties, but also its desired bioactivity.

Guo et al. combined Expert Systems (ES) and Artificial Neural Networks (ANN) to establish a hybrid system for the development of direct-filling hard gelatin capsules containing piroxicam which satisfy the dissolving profile specifications. Based on the input parameters, the MODEL EXPERT SYSTEM (MES) makes formulation development decisions and recommendations. To ensure hassle-free formulation development, ANN uses backpropagation learning to link formulation parameters to the desired response, which jointly regulated by the control module[43].CFD can also be used to investigate how tablet geometry affects the dissolving profile[46]. The combination of these mathematical models with AI could be extremely useful in accelerating pharmaceutical product development. (*Kang, S.N.;2012)*

THE RISE OF AI IN THE DRUG DISCOVERY MARKET: The biopharmaceutical sector offers stimulating opportunities for advancements in AI. It is no secret that the biopharmaceutical industry is working hard to leverage AI to improve drug discovery, decrease costs for R and D, reduce failure rates, and ultimately develop superior drugs. Recent years have seen an evolution of AI-based start-up companies devoted to drug discovery as a result of the fast development of ML algorithms and the availability of immense statistics in life sciences. Several notable AIbio pharmaceutical alliances were announced in 2016-2017, such as Pfizer and IBM Watson, AstraZeneca, Abbvie, Merck, Novartis, GSK Sanofi Genzyme, and Recursion Pharmaceuticals, and Exscientia. The top biopharmaceutical company's current AI initiatives include: a. Mobile platforms - the caliber to recommend patients, by the means of real-time data collection and thus improving patient outcomes b. Personalized medicine - the capability to evaluate a big database of patients so as to recognize cure alternatives using a cloud-based system as personalized medicine c. Acquisitions galore - new startups are combining AI and healthcare to foster the innovation requirements of large biotech firms d. Drug Discovery - in conjunction with software companies, pharma companies are trying to implement the most cutting-edge technologies in the costly and extensive process of drug discovery. Based on the growth of deep learning applications in drug discovery and the fact that these methods avail from large training sets, conscientious data curation and proper benchmarking of newly developed models are mandatory. The availability and size of chemical compound libraries have improved over the past few years, with databases such as ZINC and European Molecular Biology Laboratory representing a commonly-used starting point for ligand-based projects. A similar trend was observed for structure-based modeling, for which databases such as protein database bind and binding database provide highly detailed structural information on protein-ligand complexes, as well as their associated bioactivity data.*(Xu, H.-B.;2015)*

BACKGROUND

AI makes use of systems and software that can read and learn from data in order to make independent judgments in order to achieve certain goals. Its applications in the pharmaceutical area are constantly being expanded, as discussed in this chapter. The McKinsey Global Institute predicts that significant developments in AI-guided automation would fundamentally alter society's work culture. Machine learning (ML) is an area of AI that employs statistical methods with the ability to learn with or without being explicitly programmed. There are three types of machine learning: supervised, unsupervised, and reinforcement learning. Classification and regression methods are used in supervised learning, and the prediction model is built using data from input and output sources. Under the subgroup classification, supervised ML produces disease diagnosis, and under the subgroup regression, it produces drug efficacy and ADMET prediction[9]. Clustering and feature-finding methods are used in unsupervised learning to group and analyze data based purely on input data. Disease subtype discovery via clustering and disease target discovery from feature-finding approaches can both be achieved using unsupervised ML. Reinforcement learning is primarily driven by decision-making in a given environment and the execution of those decisions in order to maximize performance. De novo drug design under decision making and experimental designs under execution are two examples of outputs from this sort of ML, both of which may be achieved using modelling and quantum chemistry.

The big data and associated data mining and algorithm methods can provide us with the capacity to discover new compounds that can potentially be new drugs, uncover or repurpose drugs that could be more potent when used individually or in combination and improve the area of personalized medicine based on genetic markers. The emergence of DL was observed with the increasing amount of data and the continuous growth of computer power. *(Wirtz B.W.; 2019)*

FUTURE BEHOLD: Reports have shown that a few companies are engaging in silico synthetic planning into their whole course, accessing target molecules through the use of AI and ML; this has proven to be a beneficial technique in predictive chemistry and synthetic planning of small molecules. ML for Pharmaceutical Discovery and Synthesis (MLPDS) consortium, composed of MIT and 13 chemical and pharmaceutical companies, is developing and evaluating a data-driven synthesis planning program. The integration of predictive models into the medicinal chemistry synthesis workflow, the use of these models in MLPDS member companies, and the outlook for this field. Predictive deep learning tends to require significantly more human expertise in many practical scenarios compared to other, more thoroughly tested approaches. While one can train a well-performing random forest model with a relatively small effort for hyperparameter tuning, our understanding of contemporary deep learning approaches is not yet at the level of reliable defaults, although recent theory suggests that this may change soon. Deep neural networks might provide the right answers for misleading reasons and tend to produce overly confident predictions, even when these are evidently wrong. This is further exacerbated in the context of property prediction in drug discovery, as experiments under similar conditions can provide significantly different measurements. This drawback might be alleviated in the next few years with the wider adoption of uncertainty estimation techniques, either with deep learning approaches that have uncertainty directly embedded into their design, such as Bayesian neural networks, or post hoc techniques such as ensemble learning. Chemical reaction prediction problems can be viewed as graph transformation problems as a way to directly rank products. In recent years, quantum mechanics has led to the development of approaches that make use of first-principle calculations (e.g., density functional theory) to assess the energy barrier of a reaction. The accurate prediction of energies and forces through quantum-mechanical ML might help bridge this gap soon. Concerning template-free forward synthesis prediction, natural language processing approaches based on the transformer or recurrent neural network architectures are also becoming popular. These have reported a top-1 reactant accuracy above 90%. In terms of the future, Friedrich Rippmann sees the greatest opportunity as drug discovery and attrition rates being reduced. This would result in more novel drugs being available to patients faster.

AI has great prospects for drug discovery, but for now, the cost of implementing it is prohibitive. Increasing competition will bring down costs, opening up exciting possibilities for discoveries in a variety of fields. (*Smith R.G., 2000)*

The newfound interest in explainable AI, with methodologies such as feature attribution, instance-based molecular counterfactual explanation, and uncertainty estimation, will increase the acceptance of AI-supported drug discovery. AI is still far from perfect, and there are still areas in which data cannot be analyzed, which makes combining human and machine intelligence an effective strategy. The current trend suggests that these methods will be increasingly accessible in the coming future, with the continued development of general high-level research and deployment software packages, as well as comprehensible documentation. Recently, AI has captured the attention of many people and has been extensively used in drug discovery. It is possible to expect improvement in the future if the chemical representation can be adapted to the problem at hand. AI for drug discovery is strongly benefited from open source implementations, which allow access to software libraries that allow neural networks to be implemented. The development of robotics will be particularly vital to this progress. (*Lamberti M.J. 2019)*

AI in understanding the pathway or finding molecular targets (Drug Target Interaction: In the area of drug development, AI has revolutionized the methodologies for identifying disease pathways and targets. This was made achievable by combining genetic data, biochemical characteristics, and target tractability. The plausibility of predicting therapeutic targets using a computational prediction application known as 'Open Targets' a platform consisting of gene disease association data was probed in one study, and it was discovered that animal models exhibiting a disease-relevant phenotype with a neural network classifier of >71 percent accuracy provided the most predictive power. AI can be used in the drug development process. IBM Watson for Drug Discovery, an AI platform, has discovered five new RNA-binding proteins (RBPs) connected to the pathophysiology of amyotrophic lateral sclerosis, a neurodegenerative disease (ALS). (*Bishop, C.M.2013)*

Figure 2. Artificial intelligence in lead and hit optimization of drug

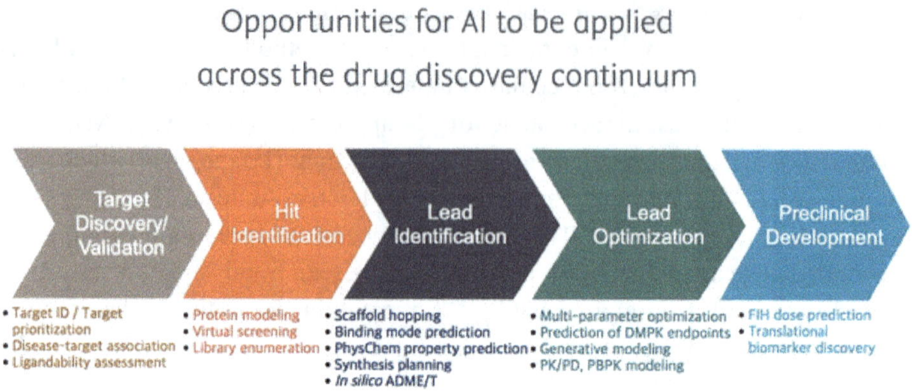

AI in finding the hit or lead: Use of AI in the discovery of small drug-like molecules is focused with chemical space use. Because it is possible to computationally enumerate the potential organic compounds, chemical space provides the stage for identifying unique and high-quality molecules. Furthermore, machine learning techniques and predictive model software assist in the identification of target-specific virtual molecules and their association with their particular targets, all while improving the safety and efficacy qualities. By decrease the quantity of synthesized compounds that are then examined in either in vitro or in vivo systems, AI systems can reduce attrition rates and R&D expenditure. With the available data on small-molecule modulator probes or their structural biology, a variety of in silico techniques for profile selection, such as virtual ligand or structure-based design approaches, can be used. In cases where structural data is insufficient, DL comes in very handy. Phenotypic data, disease, biology, or molecule network-based algorithms can all be used in this way. Validated AI techniques can be used to improve drug development success rates, but AI techniques under development must be validated before being used in drug development process. The synthesis of selected compounds is the most important step in the medication development process. As a result, AI is useful because it can prioritize molecules based on their ease of synthesis or design tools that are effective for the best synthetic route (Lee, *J.-G. et al., 2017)*

AI in synthesis of drug-like compounds: Drug-like molecules are those that follow Lipinski's five-step rule: (l) 500< Da molecular weight; (ii) H-bond donors: < 5; (iii) H bond acceptor: < 10; and (iv) computed Log P (cLogP): <5. Retro synthesis is widely used by chemists for the synthesis of drug-like molecules. The target compounds are recursively analyzed and sequentially converted into smaller fragments or building blocks that can be easily acquired or made in the retrosynthetic approach. The next stage is to figure out how these fragments will be converted into target compounds. The second step is the most difficult because it is difficult for the human brain to sort through the vast number of relevant organic reactions in the literature to identify the most plausible ones. By filling the voids that cause high failure in predicted organic synthesis (often known as 'out of scope' molecules), AI may help predict the best sought-after reactions. Unpredictable steric and electronic effects, as well as an insufficient understanding of the reaction process, are the main causes of voids in organic synthesis. Several computers aided organic compound synthesis (CAOCS) systems are currently available to assist chemists choose the best synthesis method; however, CAOCS is not part of the computer-aided drug discovery (CADD) workflow. *(Guncar, G. et al; 2018)*

Predicting the mode-of-action of compounds using AI: Those involved in the drug development process, particularly medicinal chemists, are excited by the idea of having an AI platform that can predict on- and off-target effects as well as in vivo safety profiles of compounds before they are created. Drug development time, R&D costs, and attrition rates are all reduced when such platforms are available. DeepTox (which predicts the toxicity of novel chemicals) and PrOCTOR (which predicts the probability of toxicity in clinical trials) are two examples of such platforms. If a larger and more precise dataset on toxicity and therapeutic profile of a diverse set of compounds is made available, the predictive accuracy of these platforms can be improved. However, this can only be accomplished if the industry is prepared to exchange data. SPiDER, a new AI tool designed as an alternative to chemoproteomics to improve natural products for drug discovery, was recently developed[73]. SPiDER was used to predict the molecular target of b-lapachone, a clinical-stage natural naphthoquinone with anticancer activity, as a proof-of-concept. B-lapachone was predicted to be an allosteric and reversible regulator of 5-lipoxygenase by the platform (5-LO). A 5-LO functional assay is used to verify the prediction. Another AI tool, read-across structure–activity relationships (RASAR), was shown to accurately predict the toxicity of unknown compounds by connecting molecular structures and toxic properties by mining a large database of chemicals. *(Koohy, H.; 2017)*

METHODOLOGY

Methodology of AI in Drug Discovery and Design is elaborated as follows:

Dataset ChEMBL is an open-source database that includes data on the biological properties of small molecules. It stands for "Chemical Biology Information Resource for Lead Discovery." ChEMBL is widely used in drug discovery and pharmaceutical research to access and explore data related to drug targets, compounds, and their activities. The bioactivity data of compounds against our target, Cyclooxygenase-2 (COX-2) using ChEMBL web service package. The target with ChEMBL id as CHEMBL230 of the selected dataset included characteristics such as, target type was 'single protein' and target organism was 'Homo sapiens'. A standard type with an IC50 value for its inhibitory concentration was used to filter the specified target ID. Initially, the dataset had 7430 rows of compunds and 45 columns of data for each compound, including the canonical smiles, assay chembl_id, standard upper value, molecule's chembl_id, standard units, assay description, etc. for each molecule.

Data Preprocessing: Data preprocessing is an essential step in preparing datasets for use in machine learning models. In the context of drug discovery, several preprocessing steps were taken to clean and prepare the dataset for use in a QSAR model. Firstly, any compounds with missing values for the standard value and canonical smiles columns were removed from the dataset. This was necessary because missing values can lead to errors in the machine learning models and can result in inaccurate predictions. Secondly, any duplicate canonical smiles were removed from the dataset. This was done to ensure that each compound in the dataset is unique and to prevent any biases in the machine learning models. The required three columns (molecule_chembl_id, canonical_smiles, and standard_value) were combined into a DataFrame. This was done to create a dataset that can be used to train a machine learning model for predicting bioactivity. Lastly, the compounds were labeled as either being active, inactive or intermediate according to their IC50 values. This labeling was done to classify the compounds based on their bioactivity and was used to train a classification machine learning model. After all the preprocessing steps were completed, the dataset contained 4671 rows and 4 columns, which was used to train a QSAR model for predicting the bioactivity of new compounds.

Descriptor calculation: The first step in this process involves the calculation of Lipinski descriptors for each compound in the dataset. Lipinski descriptors are an amalgam of four physicochemical parameters that are frequently utilized for evaluating compound drug likeness. To allow IC50 data to be more uniformly distributed, the IC50 values are converted to PIC50 values, which are simply the negative logarithm of the IC50 values. This conversion allows us to convert IC50 values that range over several orders of magnitude to a more uniform scale, and to facilitate data analysis and comparison. After performing exploratory data analysis (EDA) using Lipinski descriptors, the data is balanced by removing the values with intermediate PIC50 values. This ensures that the data is representative of both active and inactive compounds, and not biased towards compounds with intermediate bioactivity. About 2045 instances were active and 1537 cases were inactive to account for the bioactivity class distribution result. Further, around 881 descriptors are calculated using PaDEL Descriptor software, which calculates a wide range of molecular descriptors that capture different aspects of molecular properties such as electronic, structural, and topological properties. However, not all of these features are useful in predicting bioactivity, and so low variance features are removed. After balancing and removing low variance features, the dataset consists of 3582 rows × 235 columns. This preprocessed data can now be used to train a machine learning model for predicting the bioactivity of compounds. In the QSAR analysis, the input features are the calculated descriptors and the output feature is the PIC50 value. The data is first split into train and test sets in an 80:20 ratio. A random forest model is built on the training set, and the model's performance is evaluated using the R-squared value. In this case, the random forest model achieved an R-squared value of 0.89 on the training set and 0.48 on the test set. Approximately 39 machine-learning models from the lazypredict Python framework were utilized for model analysis. These models are initially examined on the preprocessed COX-2 inhibition dataset with the default parameters. Decision Tree Regressor performed the best with R-Squared value of 0.92 and RMSE value of 0.42. These results can be visualized for better understanding. (*Young, J.D. et al.; 2017)*

Deployment of model using a web application: After building a QSAR model to predict PIC50 values, the next step is to develop a web application that makes use of this model. In this case, the web app was built using Streamlit, a Python library for creating interactive web apps. The aim of the app is to provide a user-friendly interface for users to predict the PIC50 values of new or existing drug molecules for the target enzyme. To use the web app, the user is required to upload a text file containing the canonical smiles and ChEMBL ID for the compounds they wish to predict. The app then processes this input data using the QSAR model to predict the corresponding PIC50 values. The output is presented in a table that displays the predicted PIC50 values for each compound, along with their respective ChEMBL IDs

The steps involved in the process of drug discovery:

- ***Step 1 – Target identification and validation:*** The first step involves target identification and validation as it starts the whole drug discovery process. The basic targets for therapeutic use are cellular on modular structures which materialize naturally and take part in prime roles in pathogenicity. The target molecule should be conveniently safe and efficacious and should meet the clinical demands of the patient to get the desired drug molecule after identification of the drug target system approach should be performed in the mode of action of the API to be qualified for efficacy.
- ***Step 2 – hit identification and validation:*** The next step is to recognize whether the small molecule leads have the desired effect against the identified targets. Hits can be identified using several techniques, such as high-

throughput screening, knowledge based approaches, and virtual screening. Validation of hits is important during the initial stage of screening.

- ***Step 3 – moving from a hit to a lead validation:*** The aim now is to clarify each hit series to develop more selective compounds based on the various series of hits introduced so far. It is particularly important to work on multiple series in random order since some successful series will fail due to unique characteristics. Focusing on multiple series structurally, different sets of hit series will help to offset this possibility.
- ***Step 4 – lead optimization:*** To develop a preclinical drug candidate, it is necessary to improve on the deficiencies of lead compounds and maintain their desired properties. Using this step, you can determine whether your drug metabolizes in the right area of your body, or whether you have any current side effects of concern. An integrated approach is recommended for the same. Bringing together experts in computational chemistry, medical chemistry, drug metabolism, and other fields will allow them to provide unique insight into this late stage of the process.
- ***Step 5 – late lead optimization:*** Before progression to preclinical and clinical trials, late-stage optimization, in which further pharmacological safety of a lead compound is assessed, is a vital step. A drug's efficacy, pharmacokinetics, and safety will be more likely to be compromised later in development if this phase is ignored. As part of safety optimization, the aim is to identify and progress leads with the best overall safety profile, remove the most toxic leads, and establish a well-defined hazard and translational risk profile necessary for further in vitro testing. By thoroughly calculating the risks at this point, more opportunities can be taken when investments are made into leads. Further, if the drug is approved for development it is passed to perform preclinical and clinical trials.*(Chen, H. et al.; 2018)*

Automated synthesis planning with AI: The fragments of today, the drugs that treat diseases, the fertilizers that safeguard our crops, the products that make life accessible are becoming rapidly worldly-wise and refined thanks to advancements in chemical synthesis. As tools for synthesis upgrades, molecular designers can be valiant and innovative in the way they outline and put together the molecules. A variety of devices combining chemical synthesis and data science have come to the forefront in recent years, including robotics for autonomous or high-throughput synthesis, as well as algorithms for retrosynthesis and reaction prediction. Recently, progress has been made in retro-synthesis logic, predicting reactivity, and chemistry automata, with assurance from contributors in several fields. Chemical synthesis in the information era guarantees to increase the quality of the molecules of the future with help of data harnessing and automation. Automation molecule synthesis involves three main components: Retrosynthesis, reaction prediction, and automated synthesis. The following topics describe how the strategy of multistep synthesis can be distilled into a logic that can be taught to a computer. Various tools and models are implemented in the part on reaction prediction, including those for developing reaction conditions, catalysts, and even the most recent alterations based on the abundance of data sets and census tools such as ML. *(Grys, B.T. et al.;2017)*

- ***Synthesis planning with AI*** has a well-of past, in 1970 in the field of computer-aided retrosynthetic prediction. Improved computational facilities, the surfacing of big data, and the advancement of novel algorithms for deep learning and expansion have arisen in a revival of AI for synthetic organic chemistry.
- ***In retrosynthesis,*** where the main aim is to periodically design efficient synthetic pathways for a molecule of the concert, rule-based techniques are undoubtedly beneficial. These aim to stipulate retrosynthetic pathways with the help of reaction mechanism encoding and skeletal building. One of their main curbs is their reliance on direct chemical changes/reactions. These generally demand physical establishment and administration. The latest drawn inspiration of the field is from natural languages processing techniques, such as sequence-to-sequence models and transformer models. Forward synthesis planning differentiates itself from retrosynthesis. While the final might be explainable with the help of existing reaction databases, forward synthesis would be in need of data from reactions that give no product though. The present chemical reaction databases are heavily distorted regarding productive reaction data. There is an essential call for additional data, like experimental conditions (e.g., solvent and temperature) or side-product information. With the goal of addressing some of these disadvantages, several measures have been taken to develop known reaction databases with negative reaction results, and therefore, design the latest customized data collection for automated synthesis planning.*(Labovitz, D.L. et al.;2017)*

RESULTS

Results for Artificial Intelligence of Drug Discovery

The bioactivity predictor app for COX-2 was developed using QSAR modelling to predict the bioactivity of new compounds. The molecular descriptors were calculated for chemical compounds using PaDEL software, and the noninformative and low variance descriptors were removed. The bioactivity predictor app designed specifically for COX-2 demonstrated an impressive accuracy rate of 85%. This indicates that the app's predictions align closely with the actual experimental PIC50 values of the compounds being analyzed. To further assess the reliability and performance of the app, a scatter plot was generated, plotting the standardized residual (the difference between the predicted and experimental values, normalized) against the experimental PIC50 values. The scatter plot revealed a scattered pattern of data points distributed randomly above and below the zero baseline of the standardized residual. This pattern is indicative of the absence of any systematic error in the predictions made by the app.

Artificial intelligence in drug discovery with QSAR: The enormous chemical space, which contains over 1060 compounds, encourages the synthesis of several drug molecules. The lack of new technology, on the other hand, affects drug development, making it a time-consuming and costly that can be addressed by using AI. AI can determine hit and lead compounds, leading to faster drug target validation and structural design optimization. Despite its benefits, AI has significant data challenges, including the data's scale, growth, diversity, and uncertainty. Pharmaceutical companies' drug development sets of data can contain millions of molecules, and typical machine learning algorithms may not be able to handle them. A computational model based on the quantitative structure-activity relationship (QSAR) can quickly predict huge numbers of compounds or simple physicochemical parameters like log P or log D. However, these models are a some way from predicting complicated biological features like chemical efficacy and side effects. Small training sets, experimental data error in training sets, and a lack of experimental validations all are problems which QSAR-based models face. To overcome these issues, recently developed AI technologies, such as deep learning (DL) and relevant modelling studies, can be used to evaluate the safety and efficacy of drug molecules using big data modelling and analysis. Merck sponsored a QSAR ML challenge in 2012 to investigate the benefits of DL in the pharmaceutical industries or in drug discovery process. DL models showed significant predictivity compared with traditional ML approaches for 15 absorption, distribution, metabolism, excretion, and toxicity (ADMET) data sets of drug candidates. By illustrating the distributions of molecules and their properties, the virtual chemical space provides a geographical map of molecules. The goal of the chemical space illustration is to gather positional information about molecules inside the space in order to search for bioactive compounds, and therefore virtual screening (VS) helps in the selection of relevant molecules for further testing. PubChem, ChemBank, DrugBank, and ChemDB are just a few of the chemical spaces that are accessible to the public.

Numerous in silico methods for virtual screening compounds from virtual chemical spaces, as well as structure and ligand-based approaches, provide better profile analysis, faster elimination of nonlead compounds, and drug molecule selection at lower cost. To select a lead compound, drug design algorithms like coulomb matrices and molecular fingerprint recognition take in consideration of physical, chemical, and toxicological properties. To predict the desired chemical structure of a compound, a variety of parameters can be used, including predictive models, molecule similarity, the molecule generation process, and the use of in silico approaches. When 95 000 decoys were tested against these receptors, Pereira et al. presented a new system, DeepVS, for the docking of 40 receptors and 2950 ligands, which demonstrated remarkable performance. Another method used a multi-objective automated replacement system to examine the form similarity, biochemical activity, and physicochemical features of a cyclin-dependent kinase-2 inhibitor to enhance its potency profile.

Artificial intelligence in drug screening: A drug discovery and development can take more than a decade and cost an average of US$2.8 billion. Even still, nine out of 10 medicinal compounds fail to make it through Phase II clinical trials and receive regulatory approval. Algorithms like Nearest-Neighbor classifiers, RF, extreme learning machines, SVMs, and deep neural networks (DNNs) are used to predict in vivo activity and toxicity in VS based on synthesis feasibility. Several biopharmaceutical companies, including Bayer, Roche, and Pfizer, have collaborated with IT companies to establish a platform for drug discovery in areas including immuno-oncology and cardiovascular diseases. The aspects of VS to which AI has been applied are discussed below.

Prediction of the physicochemical properties: Physicochemical properties of drug, such as solubility, partition coefficient (logP), degree of ionization, and intrinsic permeability, have an indirect effect on its pharmacokinetic properties and target receptor family, and must be considered while developing a new drug. Physicochemical properties can be predicted using a variety of AI-based methods. For example, to train the program, ML makes advantage of vast data sets produced from previous compound optimization. Molecular descriptors, such as SMILES strings, potential energy measurements, electron density around the molecule, and atom coordinates in 3D, are used in drug design algorithms to generate feasible compounds using DNN and predict their attributes.

Prediction of bioactivity: The affinity of drug molecules for the target protein or receptor determines their efficacy. Drug molecules that do not interact with or have a high affinity for the targeted protein will not be able to provide a therapeutic response. It's also possible that produced therapeutic molecules interact with unintended proteins or receptors, resulting in toxicity in rare cases. As a result, DTBA (drug target binding affinity) is critical for predicting drug–target interactions.AI-based methods can assess a drug's binding affinity by considering at the features or similarities between the drug and its target. To determine the feature vectors, feature-based interactions recognize the chemical moieties of the drug and the target.

In a similarity-based interaction, on the other hand, the similarity between the drug and the target is considered, and it is assume for predicting drug target interactions. web applications such as ChemMapper and the similarity ensemble method (SEA) are available[38]. KronRLS, SimBoost, DeepDTA, and PADME are a few of the ML and DL algorithms that have been usedto determine DTBA. To determine DTBA, ML-based approaches such as Kronecker-regularized least squares (KronRLS) assess drug and protein molecular similarity. SimBoost, on the other hand, uses regression trees to predict DTBA and considering both feature-based and similarity-based interactions. SMILES drug features; ligand maximum common substructure (LMCS), extended connectivity fingerprint, or a combination of thereof can be considered[39] that similar drugs will interact with similar targets.

Prediction of toxicity: To avoid hazardous effects, it is critical to predict the toxicity of any drug molecule. Preliminary studies using cell-based in vitro assays are frequently employed, followed by animal studies to determine a compound's toxicity, increasing the cost of drug research. LimTox, pkCSM, admetSAR, and Toxtree are some of the web-based solutions that can assist cut costs. Advanced AI-based techniques search for similarities among compounds or predict the compound's toxicity based on input features. The Tox21 Data Challenge, sponsored by the National Institutes of Health, the Environmental Protection Agency (EPA), and the United States Food and Drug Administration (FDA), evaluated several computational techniques for forecasting the toxicity of 12 707 environmental compounds and drugs[41]. An ML algorithm called DeepTox outperformed all methods by identifying static and dynamic features within the data. The safety target prediction of 656 marketed drugs was evaluated using SEA against 73 unintended targets that might cause adverse effects. eToxPred was developed using an ML-based approach and was used to assess the toxicity and synthesis feasibility of small organic molecules with a 72 percent accuracy. Similarly, open-source toxicity prediction algorithms like TargeTox and PrOCTOR are used.

Figure 3. Artificial intelligence in toxicology of drug

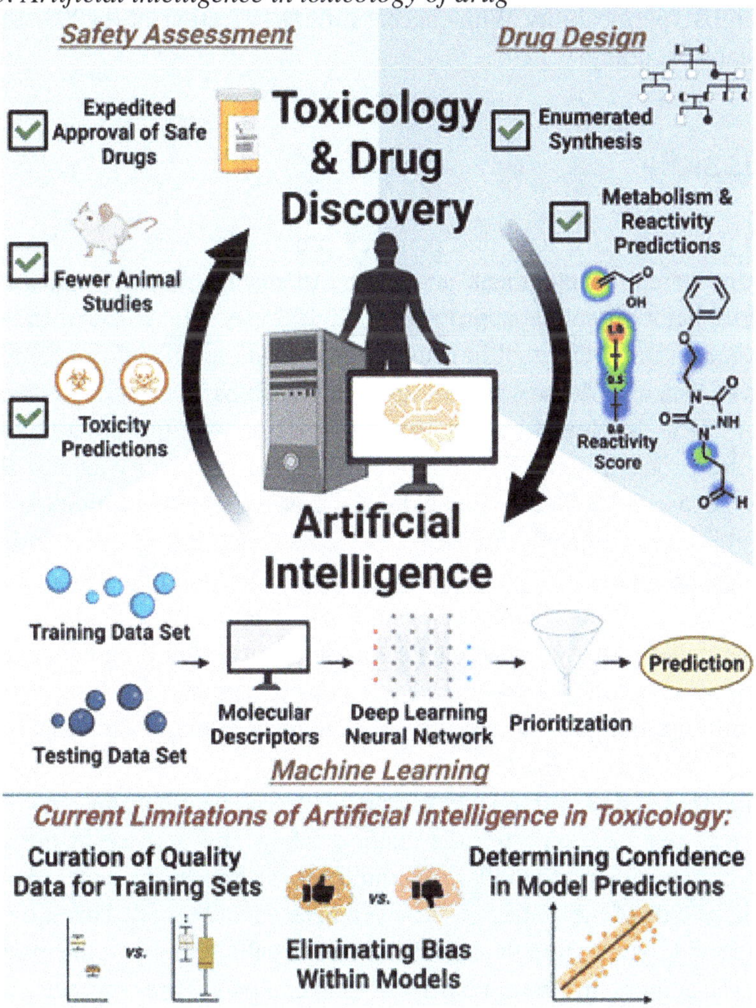

Prediction of blood brain barrier permeability: Using 67–199 descriptors, the penetration of the blood–brain barrier (BBB) can be predicted computationally with 75–97% accuracy (for penetrating and non-penetrating molecules). Although the accuracy for non penetrating molecules is lower (60–80 percent), Zhao et al. reported that this bias in statistical learning methods might be overcome by using recursive feature elimination to extract the features from only 19 molecular descriptors, including polarizability, polarity-related properties, hydrogen bond properties, volume, weight, surface area, bond rotations, and pKa.. The molecules in their training set were classified with an accuracy of over 90%. The accuracy of their model in predicting the BBB penetration of molecules in a test set as greater than

95%. A decision tree induction ML method was developed in another investigation to predict BBB permeability. With a successful classification rate of 90%, this model has a greater accuracy.

DISCUSSION

Drug discovery is a long and complex process because it involves multiple stages of research, development, and testing to ensure the safety and efficacy of a new drug before it can be approved for clinical use. AI (Artificial Intelligence) has become an important tool in drug discovery due to its ability to analyze vast amounts of data and identify patterns and relationships that might not be apparent to humans. The developed bioactivity predictor app uses Quantitative Structure-Activity Relationship (QSAR) model to predict the bioactivity against the target Cyclooxygenase-2 (COX-2) which helps to identify potential drug molecules that may be effective in treating diseases. COX-2 has been identified as an important target in QSAR studies due to the potential for COX-2 inhibitors to treat a variety of diseases such as cancer, Alzheimer's disease, and cardiovascular disease. By using AI, drug discovery researchers can identify potential drug candidates more efficiently and at a lower cost compared to traditional methods. This can accelerate the lead optimization process and reduce the number of compounds that need to be tested *in vitro or vivo. (Mak K.-K., 2019)*

The **process of discovering a new drug** is time-consuming and expensive, with several steps required to ensure the quality, safety, and potency of the marketed drug. To achieve a slight number of candidates who meet the necessary requirements, thousands of molecules must be synthesized and tested. This process takes an average of 12 years from the initial stage of target discovery to the marketing of the drug. To address this issue, pharmaceutical companies are constantly exploring methods for predicting the properties and activities of molecules before they are synthesized. The usage of Qualitative Structure Activity Relationships (QSAR) models is one such approach that has proven to be a useful tool for comprehending drug action, synthesizing compounds, and analyzing chemical libraries. The paper focuses on the development and implementation of a web application specifically designed to assist in the identification of potential drug molecules that target the COX-2 enzyme using artificial intelligence (AI). The traditional process of drug discovery involves basic research to identify targets susceptible to attack. Further testing is then conducted to optimize the structure of the compound or evaluate its various characteristics, including its ability to effectively reach and interact with the target within a living organism. QSAR models attempt to associate a compound's properties obtained from its structure to its chemical or bio activity.

These models begin with the obtaining of input data from databases, then define molecular descriptors that contain information about the molecular structure. The most effective descriptors are then determined, and models describing the explicit relation between the structure and the targeted feature or activity are created using chemoinformatic methods. In conclusion, the time and expenditure associated with drug discovery could be reduced dramatically by using QSAR models and AI. The integration of these methodologies will enable the identification of more potent and selective molecules that meet the essential criteria for drug development COX-2 (Cyclooxygenase-2) has been identified as an important target in QSAR studies due to the potential for COX-2 inhibitors to treat a variety of diseases such as cancer, Alzheimer's disease, and cardiovascular disease. Prostaglandins, which play a major role in inflammation, are produced by COX-2 enzymes. COX-2 inhibitors primarily reduce inflammation, without affecting the COX-1 enzyme that is responsible for maintaining the normal physiological functions of the gastrointestinal tract, kidneys, and platelets.

The potential of COX-2 as a target for inhibition lies in its role in the inflammatory process and the development of selective inhibitors that can provide therapeutic benefits without causing the gastrointestinal side effects associated with traditional NSAIDs, which inhibit both COX-1 and COX-2 enzymes. The process of early drug discovery in the pharmaceutical industry is essential. Trials take a long time because there are so many different testing phases, such as Phase 1, Phase 2, and Phase 3. Testing of drug compounds in phases 2 and 3 frequently ends in failure. The traditional approach entails carrying out fundamental research to pinpoint potential attack targets, like a disease-related protein receptor on a specific cell's surface. Then, to determine which compounds bind the target, scientists employ strategies like high throughput screening. The structure is then tweaked or other features, such as a compound's ability to reach its target in an organism, are tested using various biological and chemical testing techniques. Scientists and biologists believe that using machine learning techniques will speed up the process into more rigorous testing because the starting target is crucial for drug discovery. We will be able to produce more medicines and better medicines by using cutting edge computational tools, simulations, faster processing, and AI to create new molecules. Regarding drug discovery. This methodology will assist us in locating novel medications and virtual molecules. The objective is to create virtual molecules on demand, identify them, and classify them appropriately. (*Vyas M.; 2018)*

AI in advancing pharmaceutical product development: The subsequent incorporation of a novel drug molecule into a suitable dosage form with desirable delivery characteristics followed the discovery of a novel drug molecule. In this case, AI can take the role of the classic trial-and-error approach. With the use of QSPR, various computational tools can handle problems encountered in the formulation design area, such as stability concerns, dissolution, porosity, and so on. Decision-support tools employ rule-based systems to select the type, nature, and quantity of excipients based on the drug's physicochemical characteristics, but they use a feedback mechanism to constantly monitor and modify the process. (*Mak K.-K., 2019)*

APPLICATIONS OF AI IN DRUG DEVELOPMENT: Finding successful new drugs is a demanding task, and it is the most difficult aspect of drug research. The huge extent of what is known as chemical space, which is estimated to be in the order of 1060 molecules, is the source of this. AI-enabled technologies have evolved into versatile tools that can be used at various stages of drug development, including drug target identification and validation, drug design, drug repurposing, R&D efficiency, aggregating and analyzing biomedicine information, and refining the decision-making process to recruit patients for clinical trials. These AI applications have the potential to mitigate the inefficiencies and uncertainties that afflict traditional drug development methods while also reducing bias and human intervention. Prediction of feasible synthetic routes for drug-like molecules, pharmacological properties, protein characteristics as well as efficacy, drug combination and drug–target interaction, and drug repurposing are a few of the applications of AI in drug development. The discovery of novel biomarkers and therapeutic targets, personalized medicine based on omic markers, and discovering the connections between drugs and diseases all are examples of how omic analysis can be used to identify new pathways and targets. DL has a track record of identifying promising drug candidates and properly predicting their qualities as well as potential toxicity hazards. Using AI methods[61], it is now possible to avoid prior challenges in drug development, such as analysis of enormous datasets, laborious screening of compounds while reducing standard error, and requiring large amounts of R&D cost and time of over US$2.5 billion and more than a decade. New research can be conducted using AI technology to aid in the identification of new drug targets, rational drug design, and drug repurposing.(*Sellwood M.A.; 2018)*

Figure 4. Application of artificial intelligence in pharmaceutical research and development

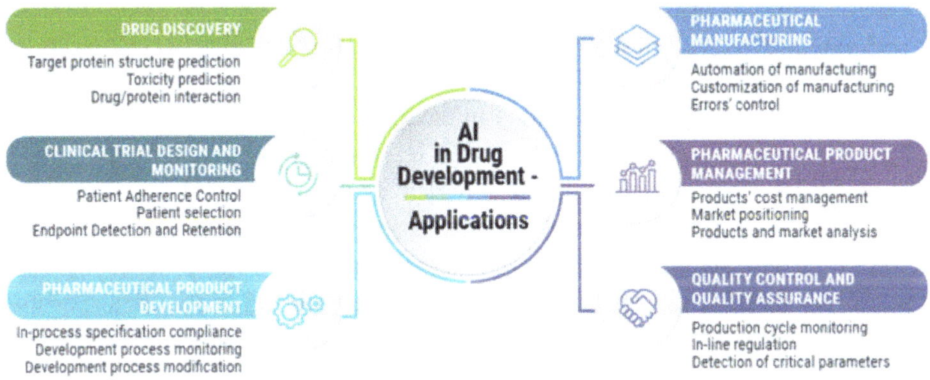
DRUG DISCOVERY
Target protein structure prediction
Toxicity prediction
Drug/protein interaction
CLINICAL TRIAL DESIGN AND MONITORING
Patient Adherence Control
Patient selection
Endpoint Detection and Retention
PHARMACEUTICAL PRODUCT DEVELOPMENT
In-process specification compliance
Development process monitoring
Development process modification
AI in Drug Development - Applications
PHARMACEUTICAL MANUFACTURING
Automation of manufacturing
Customization of manufacturing
Errors' control
PHARMACEUTICAL PRODUCT MANAGEMENT
Products' cost management
Market positioning
Products and market analysis
QUALITY CONTROL AND QUALITY ASSURANCE
Production cycle monitoring
In-line regulation
Detection of critical parameters

AI in selection of a population for clinical trials: An ideal AI tool for clinical trials may identify patients' disease, identify gene targets, and predict the effect of the drug designed, including on- and off-target effects. In a Phase II trial of schizophrenic patients, a novel AI platform called AiCure was developed as a mobile application to monitor medication adherence, and it was claimed that AiCure increased adherence with 25% compared to traditional modified directly observed therapy'[75]. The process of selection of patients for a clinical trial is critical. Examining the relationship between human-relevant biomarkers and in vitro phenotypes allows for a more predictable and measurable assessment of therapeutic response uncertainty in a specific patient. The advances in artificial intelligence (AI) technologies to detect and predict human-relevant disease biomarkers enables for the recruitment of a specific patient population in Phase II and III clinical trials. Use of AI predictive modelling in the selection of a patient population may improve clinical trial success rates. *(Zhu H.; 2020)*

AI in drug repurposing: The process of drug repurposing becomes more appealing and feasible using AI. Applying an existing treatment to a new disease has the advantage of allowing the new drug to proceed directly to Phase II studies for a different indication without having to go through Phase I clinical trials and toxicology testing again. DL applications were used to develop in silico methods for predicting drug pharmacological properties and drug repurposing using transcriptomic data from various biological systems and conditions. The methods described are based on high-level representations of data using DNNs. DNNs were seen in a study by Aliper et al. to be able to classify complex drug action mechanisms on the pathway level, enabling drugs to be categorized into therapeutic categories based on their functional class, efficacy, therapeutic use, and toxicity.

AI in polypharmacology: Because of a deeper understanding of pathological processes in diseases at the molecular level, the 'one-disease–multiple-targets' paradigm currently reigns over the 'one-disease–one-target' paradigm. Polypharmacology is the study of a single disease with several targets. Molecular pathways, crystal structures, binding affinities, drug targets, disease relevance, chemical properties, and biological activities can be found in databases like ZINC, PubChem, Ligand Expo, KEGG, ChEMBL, DrugBank, STITCH, BindingDB, Supertarget, and PDB, among others. To design polypharmacological agents, AI could be utilized to examine these databases. The authors developed a computational platform, DeepDDI, for better understanding of drug–drug interactions and associated mechanisms, as well as prediction of alternative drugs for intended clinical use without negative health effects[82], which was recently published in the literature as a big success of an AI application in designing polypharmacological agents. *(Ciallella H.L.,2019)*

CONCLUSION AND FUTURE SCOPE/ PERSPECTIVES:

The advancement of AI, along with its remarkable tools, is constantly aimed at reducing obstacles faced by pharmaceutical companies, affecting the drug development process as well as the total lifespan of the product, which may explain the rise in the number of start-ups in this sector. The contemporary healthcare sector is confronted with a number of complex challenges, such as increasing drug and treatment costs, and society need significant changes in this field. Personalized medications with the necessary dose,'release characteristics, and other required aspects can be made according to individual patient demand using AI in pharmaceutical product manufacturing. Using the latest AI-based technologies will not only reduce the time it takes for products to reach the market, but it will also improve product quality and overall safety of the manufacturing process, as well as provide better resource utilization and cost-effectiveness, thereby increasing the importance of automation.

In conclusion, the developed bioactivity predictor app for COX-2 using QSAR modeling has shown good accuracy and has the potential to identify potential drug candidates more efficiently and at a lower cost compared to traditional methods. COX-2 inhibitors have shown promising therapeutic benefits in various diseases such as cancer, Alzheimer's disease, and cardiovascular disease. From lead identification and optimization through lead development, QSAR models have become indispensable tool in the pharmaceutical industry. The use of AI in drug discovery can accelerate the lead optimization process and reduce the number of compounds that must be examined in vitro or in vivo. The bioactivity predictor app for COX-2 could help researchers identify potential COX-2 inhibitors with improved efficiency.

REFERENCES

Abdullahi, M., Adeniji, S. E., Arthur, D. E., & Musa, S. (2020). Quantitative structure-activity relationship (QSAR) modelling study of some novel carboxamide series as new anti-tubercular agents. *Bulletin of the National Research Center*, 44(1), 136. DOI: 10.1186/s42269-020-00389-7

Bishop, C. M. (2013). Model-based machine learning. *Philosophical Transactions. Series A, Mathematical, Physical, and Engineering Sciences*, •••, 371. PMID: 23277612

Chen, H., Engkvist, O., Wang, Y., Olivecrona, M., & Blaschke, T. (2018). The rise of deep learning in drug discovery. *Drug Discovery Today*, 23(6), 1241–1250. DOI: 10.1016/j.drudis.2018.01.039 PMID: 29366762

Ciallella, H. L., & Zhu, H. (2019). Advancing computational toxicology in the big data era by artificial intelligence: Data-driven and mechanism-driven modeling for chemical toxicity. *Chemical Research in Toxicology*, 32(4), 536–547. DOI: 10.1021/acs.chemrestox.8b00393 PMID: 30907586

Ebhohimen, I. E., Edemhanria, L., Awojide, S., Onyijen, O. H., & Anywar, G. (2020). Advances in computer-aided drug discovery. In *Phytochemicals as Lead Compounds for New Drug Discovery* (pp. 25–37). Elsevier. DOI: 10.1016/B978-0-12-817890-4.00003-2

Grys, B. T., Lo, D. S., Sahin, N., Kraus, O. Z., Morris, Q., Boone, C., & Andrews, B. J. (2017). Machine learning and computer vision approaches for phenotypic profiling. *The Journal of Cell Biology*, 216(1), 65–71. DOI: 10.1083/jcb.201610026 PMID: 27940887

Guncar, G. et al. (2018) An application of machine learning to haematological diagnosis. *Sci. Rep.* 8, 411DOI: 10.1083/jcb.201610026 PMID: 27940887

Imam, S. S., & Gilani, S. J. (2017). Computer aided drug design: A novel loom to drug discovery. *Organ Med Chem Int J*, 1, 113–118.

Kang, S. N., Hong, S.-S., Lee, M.-K., & Lim, S.-J. (2012). Dual function of tributyrin emulsion: Solubilization and enhancement of anticancer effect of celecoxib. *International Journal of Pharmaceutics*, 428(1-2), 76–81. DOI: 10.1016/j.ijpharm.2012.02.037 PMID: 22405988

Koohy, H. (2017). The rise and fall of machine learning methods in biomedical research. *F1000 Research*, 6, 2012. Advance online publication. DOI: 10.12688/f1000research.13016.1 PMID: 29375816

Labovitz, D. L., Shafner, L., Reyes Gil, M., Virmani, D., & Hanina, A. (2017). Using artificial intelligence to reduce the risk of nonadherence in patients on anticoagulation therapy. *Stroke*, 48(5), 1416–1419. DOI: 10.1161/STROKEAHA.116.016281 PMID: 28386037

Lamberti, M. J., Wilkinson, M., Donzanti, B. A., Wohlhieter, G. E., Parikh, S., Wilkins, R. G., & Getz, K. (2019). A study on the application and use of artificial intelligence to support drug development. *Clinical Therapeutics*, 41(8), 1414–1426. DOI: 10.1016/j.clinthera.2019.05.018 PMID: 31248680

Lee, J.-G., Jun, S., Cho, Y.-W., Lee, H., Kim, G. B., Seo, J. B., & Kim, N. (2017). Deep learning in medical imaging: General overview. *Korean Journal of Radiology*, 18(4), 570–584. DOI: 10.3348/kjr.2017.18.4.570 PMID: 28670152

Mak, K.-K., & Pichika, M. R. (2019). Artificial intelligence in drug development: Present status and future prospects. *Drug Discovery Today*, 24(3), 773–780. DOI: 10.1016/j.drudis.2018.11.014 PMID: 30472429

Mak, K.-K., & Pichika, M. R. (2019). Artificial intelligence in drug development: Present status and future prospects. *Drug Discovery Today*, 24(3), 773–780. DOI: 10.1016/j.drudis.2018.11.014 PMID: 30472429

Miles, J., & Walker, A. The potential application of artificial intelligence in transport. IEE Proc.-Intell. Transport Syst. 2006; 153:183–198 DOI: 10.1049/ip-its:20060014

Mohsin, N. A., Aslam, S., Ahmad, M., Irfan, M., Al-Hussain, S. A., & Zaki, M. E. A.Mohsin NuA. (2022). Aslam S, Ahmad M, Irfan M, Al-Hussain SA, Zaki MEA. Cyclooxygenase-2 (COX-2) as a Target of Anticancer Agents: A Review of Novel Synthesized Scaffolds Having Anticancer and COX-2 Inhibitory Potentialities. *Pharmaceuticals (Basel, Switzerland)*, 15(12), 1471. DOI: 10.3390/ph15121471 PMID: 36558921

Sellwood, M. A. (2018). Artificial intelligence in drug discovery. *Fut. Sci.*, 10, 2025–2028. PMID: 30101607

Smith, R. G., & Farquhar, A. (2000). The road ahead for knowledge management: An AI perspective. *AI Magazine*, 21, 17–17.

Vosooghi, M., & Amini, M. (2014). The discovery and development of cyclooxygenase-2 inhibitors as potential anticancer therapies. *Expert Opinion on Drug Discovery*, 9(3), 255–267. DOI: 10.1517/17460441.2014.883377 PMID: 24483845

Vyas, M. (2018). Artificial intelligence: The beginning of a new era in pharmacy profession. *Asian Journal of Pharmaceutics*, 12, 72–76.

Wirtz, B. W., Weyerer, J. C., & Geyer, C. (2019). Artificial intelligence and the public sector—Applications and challenges. *International Journal of Public Administration*, 42(7), 596–615. DOI: 10.1080/01900692.2018.1498103

Xu, H.-B., Shen, F.-M., & Lv, Q.-Z. (2015). Celecoxib enhanced the cytotoxic effect of cisplatin in drug-resistant human gastric cancer cells by inhibition of cyclooxygenase-2. *European Journal of Pharmacology*, 769, 1–7. DOI: 10.1016/j.ejphar.2015.09.025 PMID: 26407653

Yang, Y., & Siau, K. MWAIS; 2018. A Qualitative Research on Marketing and Sales in the Artificial Intelligence Age. DOI: 10.1016/j.ejphar.2015.09.025 PMID: 26407653

Young, J. D., Cai, C., & Lu, X. (2017). Unsupervised deep learning reveals prognostically relevant subtypes of glioblastoma. *BMC Bioinformatics*, 18(S11), 381. DOI: 10.1186/s12859-017-1798-2 PMID: 28984190

Zhu, H. (2020). Big data and artificial intelligence modeling for drug discovery. *Annual Review of Pharmacology and Toxicology*, 60(1), 573–589. DOI: 10.1146/annurev-pharmtox-010919-023324 PMID: 31518513

KEY TERMS AND DEFINITIONS

Artificial Intelligence (AI): Is a technology-based system that uses a variety of advanced tools and networks to simulate human intelligence in drug discovery.

Deep Learning (DL): Is a subfield of machine learning that use artificial neural networks to adapt and learn from huge amounts of data. The ability to discover new compounds that could potentially be new drugs, uncover or repurpose drugs that could be more potent when used individually or in combination, and improve the area of personalized medicine based on genetic markers could be provided by big data and associated data mining and algorithm methods. With the increasing amount of data and the continuous expansion of computer power, the emergence of DL was observed.

Data-Driven Approaches: For molecular predictions of properties are in contradiction to techniques that are physics-based and are also fundamentally limited in their ability to extrapolate and make reliable predictions for the unseen classes of compounds.

Deep Neural Networks (DNNs): These are a highly adaptive multilayer network consisting of connected and interacting artificial neurons that perform various data manipulations.

QSAR Modelling Tools: Such as ***linear discriminant analysis (LDA),*** support vector machines (SVMs), random forest (RF), and decision trees, have been used to identify prospective drug candidates and have evolved into AI-based QSAR approaches that can be used to speed up QSAR analysis. When King et al. examined the capacity of six AI systems to rank anonymous compounds in terms of biological activity to that of traditional techniques, they found a negligible statistical difference.

AI in Clinical Trial Design: Clinical trials, which take 6–7 years and a significant financial investment, are developed to assess the safety and efficacy of a drug product in humans for a particular disease condition. However, just one out of every ten molecules that enter these trials gets cleared, resulting in a huge loss for the industry. Inappropriate patient selection, a lack of technical requirements, and poor infrastructure all can lead to these failures. However, with the vast amount of digital medical data available, AI can be used to reduce these failures.

Chapter 6

Exploring the Role of Digital Biomarkers and Artificial Intelligence in Precision Therapeutics

Abdullah Saeed
https://orcid.org/0000-0002-2021-1089
Ministry of Health, Saudi Arabia

Sarah A. Alajlan
https://orcid.org/0000-0003-0050-4164
Almaarefa University, Saudi Arabia

ABSTRACT

This chapter discusses the roles of digital biomarkers and artificial intelligence in enhancing precision therapeutics, which is the adaptation of treatments to a person's biomarker patterns for improving an individual's health. Digital biomarkers are collected from wearable technology and other digital devices that record variations in physiological and behavioral indexes thus improving disease diagnosis and treatment. This AI augments these biomarkers' prognostic accuracy and unearths patterns within large datasets within clinical settings; a major change to individualized care. This chapter in the book describes passive and active data acquisition in actual clinical scenarios and offers a conceptual foundation for employing digital biomarkers and artificial intelligence in trials. It also examines diagnostic image analysis and more specifically, the use of MRI to monitor Parkinson's disease, and EEG in managing mental health.

DOI: 10.4018/979-8-3693-6270-9.ch006

1. INTRODUCTION TO PRECISION THERAPEUTICS

Recent advances in digital technologies used at personal and population scales have led to an increase in interest in patient-specific or precision therapeutics. Biomarkers are central to the selection of suitable patients for targeted treatments in the precision therapeutics paradigm, which includes personalized medicine, adaptive care, and integrative therapy. As health care moves from personalized to broader precision therapeutics, the role of increasingly available digital data from mobile health and consumer health wearables, social media, the internet, and applications, along with artificial intelligence algorithms and tools, becomes prominent. In particular, digital biomarkers have the potential to provide new ways to measure patient status and response to therapy in wide patient populations during real-world use and to deliver these new capabilities inside increasingly useful monitoring, prognostic, diagnostic, and therapeutic digital health feedback loops. In this position paper, we review the multiparametric nature of precision therapeutics and the principles behind the emerging field of digital biomarkers. Summarize common statistics for clinical evaluation of digital biomarkers, look at examples from different chronic disease domains, and discuss key challenges to enabling the deployment of effective digital biomarkers at scale for precision therapeutics. We conclude with a discussion of constructs for evaluating digital therapeutics during their development and use. (Manta et al., 2020) (Alonso et al., 2023)

1.1. Definition and Significance

Personalized, high-efficiency, and legitimate medical treatments, which are the primary goals of precision therapeutics in the 21st century, have driven the rapid development of various diagnostic tests during the process of diagnosis and treatment. The concept of traditional diagnostic tests, such as digital or virtual biomarkers, has always been associated with specific biochemical substances. In recent years, rapid growth in the research and development of digital medicine has given rise to new diagnostic tests for measuring physiological and pathological parameters. The diagnostic test combined from traditional and digital or virtual biomarkers is the first generation of combinatorial diagnostic technologies used in cognitive digital medicine. The approach has simplified the processes of examination and verification by connecting disease-specific symptoms with the prediction model output, thus making it a valuable tool in the construction of exponential medicine. (Wang & Wang, 2023)

As a term that is frequently mentioned in the field of predictive medicine, digital biomarkers demonstrate their potential efficacy in many diseases in aspects such as disease detection, prediction, and treatment monitoring. In addition to the diagnostic tests, the technologies supporting the diagnostic tests of precision therapeutics, comprising big medical data and the cloud electronic medical data system, have also improved the capacities of clinical decision-making and researchers working on the software and hardware required for cognitive digital medicine. The new term 'precision therapeutics' reveals an emerging trend in contemporary neurological and psychiatric therapeutic development. Notably, the relevant research and applications in cognitive digital neurology and psychiatry from both industry and academia are far from intensive. As a result, finding specific clinical phenotypes for the development of cognitive digital medicine has become essential for a deeper and broader understanding, diagnosis, and treatment of indication-specific neurological and psychiatric diseases. (Akhoon, 2021)

1.2. Evolution and Advancements

New types and a higher volume of health data are generated in the present epoch of constant connection and the Internet of Things. As we can see, AI is already revolutionizing the consumer tech sphere; and in the same vein, it can be a very powerful disruptive technology helping to unlock and scale this goldmine of health information. Machine and deep learning computer science are contributing much in many aspects of health care industry such as risk assessment of clinical incidents using EHR data, precision medicine, and accelerating drug discovery process. The context today, however, is very different from that which existed in the past and which has been described above. Apart from AI and machine learning, drug research and development pipelines are frequented by other revolutionary science and technology advancements such as nanomedicine and its drug delivery capabilities in precision therapeutics. Traditional symptom-based diagnoses and assessments are increasingly being supplanted by quantitative, objective data that is continuously generating greater resolution and accuracy, leading to a more complete picture. Furthermore, in a digital fabric, these different disciplines are converging and leveraging each other. As a result, they are lifting higher into a reinforcing cycle. The theme paper for this Special Issue provides an overview of one aspect: the exploration of the role of digital biomarkers and AI in changing not only precision medicine but disease therapeutics in general. (Bashraheel et al., 2020)

2. DIGITAL BIOMARKERS: CONCEPT AND APPLICATIONS

Anatomic, physiological, and clinical characteristics of the human body play the critical role in the drive towards advancements in medical knowledge, enhancing pharmaceutical treatments, making managerial decisions, and monitoring product safety and efficacy after the drugs have been approved for use. Consequently, those measurements are usually collected from the tests administered by the healthcare providers in clinical context. However, this approach can restrict the number of samples and their collection frequency and also become problematic in assessing acute or intermittent or chronic structural and functional changes associated with disease processes. On the other hand, digital biomarkers are such indicators that are obtained from digital devices to capture these difficulties, and their usage has recently gained emerging interests by regulatory organizations, companies, and scholars. With improvements in sensing technology and an increased understanding of population health, we expect an upsurge in the use of digital biomarkers and other real-world digital measures in drug development and regulatory decision-making in the future. To understand how digital biomarkers can provide new insights into the use of therapeutic products, we provide definitions and clarifications related to digital biomarkers and other digital real-world measures, along with supportive applications and future considerations for the use of digital biomarkers and digital health technology in the context of therapeutic product development and evaluation. The emergence of digital biomarkers is a critical innovation in patient phenotyping paired with rising breakthroughs in therapeutic products and landmark advances in advanced computational science. Digital biomarkers are measures derived from digital devices, such as smartwatches, smartphones, or sensors in pill bottles, that are used in clinical studies to improve measurement, detection, and monitoring of a patient's clinical outcomes. Therefore, intra-therapy measurement instruments like digital biomarkers can help improve precision medicine and also determine the predictive measure of the therapeutic product. But care should be taken in handling the various challenges which arise when validating and supervising the digital biomarkers. (Wahida et al.2023)

2.1. Definition and Types

There is no accepted universal definition of digital biomarkers. Some definitions refer to the types of data used by digital biomarkers—for example, "quantifiable behavioral data associated with the manifestation of health"—whereas other definitions refer to the use of such data—for example, "objective, quantifiable physiological and behavioral data that are collected and measured by means of digital devices such as portables, wearables, implantables, or digestibles."In this document, we use the term "digital biomarker" to refer to "objective, quantifiable physiological and behavioral data that are collected and measured by means of digital devices such as portables, wearables, implantables, or digestibles" or "quantifiable behavioral data associated with the manifestation of health," but not "digital measurements of biological markers." (De et al.2021)

Digital biomarkers can be divided into passive and active digital biomarkers. "Passive digital biomarkers" are a type of driver data that is always generated in contrast to active measurements, which are taken only at certain defined times and are thus not continuous. The widest range of data is generated by everyday activities that are mainly spontaneous, such as walking, eating, or speaking. This does not require the patient to act or interact with any diagnostic or monitoring equipment. Many diseases are characterized by a constant presence of certain signs or symptoms, which are often not easy to perceive by patients. In contrast to passive digital biomarkers, the second type, "active digital biomarkers," involve active or intentional interactions of the patient with diagnostic or monitoring devices, such as during medical tests, so that specific measurements can be made. The main types of data are mostly provided by specific action. For example, in a cognitive test, the data will be mainly the interaction of the patient with the stimulus and the patient's responses to questions. This type of data may concern activities that are defined by time. For example, the frequency of blood glucose concentration measurement. (Wick et al.2021)

2.2. Role in Disease Monitoring

Smartphone and wearable data collection and subsequent analysis of the selected digital biomarkers comprise an essential end for the health tech system. It describes how continuously monitored digital biomarkers may eventually facilitate the early diagnosis of a disease, while not only changes in value with time can predict the individual dose and treatment efficacy in drug development. By combining multimodal data with other patient context and clinical data, the full range of patient cellular and biological antibody levels highlighted by the pandemic will enable actionable insights for the wider treated patient and also enable a significant advancement in public health monitoring. Despite the obvious benefits, few commercial applications and technical challenges exist in collecting, processing, analyzing, and interpreting digital biomarkers. Tools that can effectively handle large-scale digital biomarker data across devices without inappropriately hampering user consent are required. In addition, as established biomarkers used in clinical settings, new digital biomarker endpoint qualifications are critical to establishing use and trust. (Darwich et al.2021)

Digital biomarkers may profoundly affect several clinical care preparation considerations, including direct benefits associated with the relative ease of data collection as well as the provision of continuous and real-world patient data. As these digital biomarkers graduate from sensors to diagnostic evidence, AI models, such as the detection of a digital biomarker of depression, acknowledging issues through algorithm causality and real-world data identification, are critical in ensuring safety and effectiveness. The digital biomarker-derived endpoint would have the same key important attributes as the biomarker collected in a research environment, including epidemiological and psychobiological characteristics: clinical treatment relevance, confidence in accuracy and reproducibility, relevance to population diversity and especially to subgroups, applicability sensitivity, ability to track change and identify treatments with different potencies, interpretability, and feasibility of resulting clinical study control moments and associated costs. Rich and tailored information will affect patients in a realistic way. For AI, the improvement of the overall system through real-world data will be assessed. As part of this rollout, efforts beyond the classic patient journey to inference of quality and monitoring associated with digital platforms such as equity, infrastructure, and process responsibility are important to the concept of digital biomarkers as well. (Akhoon, 2021)

2.3. Integration with AI

The utilization of digital data and artificial intelligence (AI) appears to offer significant opportunities with regard to differentiating, discriminating and identifying patient subgroups on the basis of which precision medicines might be appropriate. The combination of smart device and digital health data and other real-world data streams for AI augmented applications offers core possibilities of optimization, prediction and identification of ideal treatment targeting and patient management across multiple and diverse clinical trial environments and other healthcare domains. AI can handle tremendous amounts of largely incomplete, noisy, and biased data. Furthermore, linking an AI-based classification to deep learning could also help infer the underlying mechanistic components of poorly understood rare diseases. AI can also automate the execution of personalized treatment protocols in clinical trials and healthcare settings, potentially more rapidly and cost-effectively than traditional approaches while providing individual-level, objective, and personalized insight into symptoms and functional change. Given the ubiquity of AI in a variety of other industries, this approach could be more approachable for clinicians than traditional clinical trial approaches. (Wahida et al.2023)

However, there are many challenges to overcome in integrating digital data and AI into precision therapeutics. Rules and methods need to be developed in order to efficiently handle the messy, complex data that comes from smart devices for use in AI applications. Importantly, other aspects of patient and disease status beyond what can be easily captured in device-level data must also be reliably integrated into linked patient-device data sources. Specific evaluation criteria will be to sustain data confidentiality and accuracy and to guarantee the interpretability and external validity of group- and individual-level conclusions together with conforming to rules. It will be necessary to build instruments that would turn AI-produced knowledge into usable information, that would interpret the knowledge obtained by an AI-driven model to clinicians, and that would show clinicians how knowledge can be applied to enhance the quality of the decision made. These cases showcase the significant of effectively leveraging digital data and Artificial Intelligence in PDX for the non-cancer drug pipeline and for patients with limited or no disease awareness; a category of illness that bears a very heavy social cost. (Wahida et al.2023) (Naithani et al.2021)

3. ARTIFICIAL INTELLIGENCE IN HEALTHCARE

Healthcare is one of the biggest challenges in the contemporary world. At stake is the assurance that people can be free from disease, can benefit from the best preventive, diagnostic, and therapeutic medicine of the highest standard and personalization, and also avail themselves of safety, efficacy, efficiency, and accessible competent personalized healthcare services. Artificial intelligence is being widely adopted in healthcare for a variety of applications. Available computing power, the improvement of big data storage, the exponential growth of AI research papers, applications, and implementations are fostering AI to surpass conventional medical tools. As AI in healthcare continues to grow and develop, it is vital to understand its future impacts and devise plans for how we can responsibly adopt AI and shape its evolution to deliver trustworthy, equitable, and beneficial medicine. (Bizzarri et al.2021)

We review a variety of AI techniques and applications in healthcare. Among them, we discuss how several learning techniques including deep neural networks, reinforcement learning, and unsupervised learning, as well as important AI applications in medical image analysis, prognosis, precision therapeutics, and disease prevention. Digital biomarkers - data traces from personal devices - stand as a unique source of personalized healthcare data. User data can help redefine our understanding of disease and management, as well as lead to the discovery and development of transformative therapies. With that, personality traits data traces become the real currency to accurately predict, preemptively change your health destiny, and the way you actually live, manage, and optimize the belief in yourself and lead fulfilling and happy lives. (Hassan et al.2022)

3.1. Overview of AI Technologies

Traditional AI means coding decision-related framework that ensures the likelihood of desired outcome by employing decision ladders. AI modeling in the context of this paper means the active acquisition of pattern, motion, and results in electronic information using a predefined mathematical structural model. Machine learning, a method of computational learning in which a model uses algorithms and statistics to learn from patterns in data, connects the value dots and performs many complex calculations. As a result, gains from information do the talking, not the machines. Machine learning evaluates data and studies to feed the resulting experience into the algorithm for subsequent training. The outcome is exact predictions. Deep learning is a subfield of AI that focuses on the theorized learning of multiple levels of accumulated values. Instead of passing implications from input to output, as is typical in most algorithmic calculations, deep learning assesses abstract data, mimicking the speech and visual processing of the decision-making process in brains, also known as neural networks. The process is based on a layered organization of algorithms called neurons, which work in a similar way to human brain cells. (Strianese et al.2020)

The artificial neural network is the basic block of deep learning. Complicated operations enable pattern recognition, which allows machines to improve decision-making by continuously adding new knowledge and revising algorithms to determine significance. Deep learning as self-programming is referred to as unsupervised learning. AI technologies include various types of mathematical equations, such as statistical regression, which is a linear technique used to identify a relationship between a dependent variable and a series of independent variables. The purpose is to define a linear equation that predicts the dependent variable as a function of one or more independent variables. Regression is an approach often used in finance for making predictions and, to a greater extent, in healthcare, where it models behavior and sets advanced analysis surfaces. Gaussian process regression is a non-parametric modeling technique. Data are not predefined, and the prior probability of the parameters is created based on a flat distribution, giving the data prominence to influence the predictions. Gaussian can be directly computed through a pair of prior and pair rule and has only two parameters, although it can technically fit any dataset without unreasonable modifications. (Fountoulakis & Stahl, 2021)

3.2. Applications in Diagnostics and Treatment

This is even more critical for psychiatry, as by 2030, mental and substance use disorders are going to become the leading cause of disability in the world, contributing substantially to the increasing burden of non-communicable diseases. Over the past few years, an increasing number of studies have demonstrated the value of digital biomarkers in collecting real-world evidence in the diagnosis and management of diseases. Digital phenotypes that characterize a patient's daily life experiences in real cultural contexts of care have begun to have importance as a signature of meaningful clinical outcomes. The availability and data sharing of remote real-world patient data, such as digital biomarkers that passively and actively monitor specific behavioral traits, have led to the optimization of treatment development, evaluation, and post-labeled use. Opportunities provided by AI should be harnessed and improved upon to catalyze rapid learning about patient digital phenotypes and prompt the development of precise and more effective personalized treatments. The most salient advance of deploying digital biomarkers in precision therapeutics is their ability to non-intrusively monitor patients while obtaining an unprecedented amount of individual behavioral data needed to create new psychiatric phenotypes and subtypes. The frequent capturing of highly varied data provides a timely assessment. With richer individual-level data, there is an opportunity to develop precision diagnostics and interventions for patient subtypes. Moreover, advances in sensors will allow psychiatrists to capture more objective data in real time, diminish recall bias, and provide more reliable planning and monitoring, including early identification of relapse symptoms. Results from digital biomarkers can be used to inform bi-directional feedback to patients via a smartphone or computer device that can make sense of real-time personal health information and suggest personalized treatment options, contingencies, and resources. (Tyson et al.2020)

4. CONVERGENCE OF DIGITAL BIOMARKERS AND AI

Digital biomarkers have the potential to transform precision therapy development. Indeed, in many cases, traditional accuracy and confirmatory clinical endpoints will be replaced by digital markers reflecting improvements in clinical efficacy. Major catalysts include artificial intelligence and silico disease modeling. Consequently, an alliance is formed between digital biomarkers, artificial intelligence, and precision therapeutics. This chapter explores evolving developments and the likely impact on research and development. New data sources, artificial intelligence, and advances in knowledge of disease pathways are providing opportunities to develop digital biomarkers for many diseases. These digital endpoints can substantially reduce the cost and patient exposure required to determine clinical trial success. As drug development slows and costs surge, this is a game changer. (Yuan, 2022)

There are major incentives to develop digital biomarkers offering substantial benefits compared with traditional clinical trial endpoints. They enable trials to be conducted rapidly in smaller numbers of patients and predominantly in more relevant trial populations. This accelerates new treatment launch and lowers development costs. In silico endpoints can also contribute to the evaluation and registration pathway for companion diagnostics and help to improve the value proposition of kits, reagents, and instrument platforms in personalized medicine. (Carmo-Fonseca, 2021)

4.1. Synergistic Benefits

The vision of precision therapeutics, targeted at the unique combination of characteristics present in individual patients, stands to benefit greatly from the combination of digiceutical products and associated methods of clinical translation and biomarker-based progression markers. Each perspective profits synergistically from the homes possessed by the other: digiceuticals that exhibit patient benefits will not only provide targeted relief but also, in doing so, will inherently provide treatment feedback; quantitatively monitoring how a patient responds to treatment using continuously collected digital biomarkers will enable faster, more accurate precision biomarker development. This perspective explores the questions that arise from the interfacing of digiceuticals and precision biomarker development; the possibilities for progression to enable standalone digiceutical development; and the implications for the precision opioid crisis and treatment challenges in central nervous system drug development. The digital age is reimagining therapeutics; wearables are permitting longer, more objective insights into patient states. Indeed, the digiceutical revolution has the promise of providing drug-like benefits through a continual treatment philosophy underpinned by a high degree of personalization based on patient condition, context, historical treatment efficacy, and incremental disease progression. There is already much research on the potential impact of digiceuticals on the patient burden. In this work, the focus is on digital metrics that monitor digitized activity, so-called digital biomarkers, which are of collective utility to both precision therapeutics and digiceutical perspectives. The digiceutical synergy viewpoint argues that while digiceuticals will likely possess individual patient benefits for easily studied treatments, the digiceutical will simultaneously be a tool for treatment monitoring; namely, that if a patient is on such a device, there is no need to send the patient for expensive lab-based tests or independent remote monitoring via the standard of care, at least for the purpose of monitoring the ongoing therapy. (Bustin & Jellinger, 2023)

4.2. Challenges and Ethical Considerations

Health information elicited from human behaviors and lifestyles using smart devices is also in contrast to the laboratory and clinical health information. Through the years, there has been a need to have an interface in describing biological characteristics, and digital biomarkers have been seen to meet this need. However, in the process, the nature and sources of digital biomarkers have made it quite challenging. It has drawn extensive attention to the ethical issues or moral paradoxes of big data produced in this context. Such digital biomarkers allow identifying, for the first time, a potential range of changes or disruption of a disease network. For achieving the comprehensive, perfect, and dynamic balance between health and disease, digital biomarkers must first characterize the systems in the dynamics of living organisms. In the era of intelligence, more and more intelligent Medical Devices using artificial intelligence could upload data to the cloud, thus users change the figure and speed of pathogen in medical environment, but also possibly use the data continuously to observe the health condition, so that prevention becomes a new mode. Nevertheless, the difficulties that digital biomarkers entail stem from the same issues arising from any markers employed for diagnostic, staging and prognosis. New potential problems may be installed by the person himself, due to intentional or accidental changes in body function through psychical processes. Ethical questions concerning patients' self-determination, consent, and privacy linked with digital biomarker surveillance are complex. Potential ethical questions regarding wearable health monitoring technologies and infrastructure are changes brought about by use of the device, privacy, confidentiality, handling of data interpretation and querying, and consent documentation and dissemination. Today, society has yet to accept a formal body of human rights and duties where such rights might be brainstormed and discussed. (Assidi et al., 2022)

5. CASE STUDIES AND SUCCESS STORIES

To motivate the role of digital biomarkers and artificial intelligence in therapeutics, we present assorted practical success stories of using digital biomarkers and big data. A unique conception of using visuomotor statistics to provide quantitative measurements of vision function in children is illustrated. A pilot study of exploiting smartphone accelerometer time series of volunteers to discriminate patient groups due to chemo-induced peripheral neuropathy is demonstrated. Patients with Parkinson's disease were asked to use a smartphone app to test device-captured voice characteristics, showing that the voice app could classify different disease severities. In an effort to use AI in improving the well-being of patients, a new standard human emotion classification protocol was revealed, and the empathic robot interactively adjusted its routine assignment.

In the Offices of Mental Health, the aim was at reducing both the cost and duration of psychiatric testing by employing machine scoring of the Psychodynamic Diagnostic Manual. Spearheaded by recent progress in using digital biomarkers and AI in precision therapeutics, we hope this review can lay the basis to celebrate digital biomarker discovery in clinical applications. As scientists dive deep into the mystery of such digital biomarkers with new continuous and wearable devices, we anticipate the emergence of a much more concrete understanding of the human body and human behavior in health and disease. To develop the conceptual breakthrough strategy of using merely quantifiable signals of human behavior, signals that can be completely collected by digital devices, to classify and score both structural and dynamic characteristics of pathoetiological conditions, we first must understand what is a so-called digital biomarker. (Al-Dewik et al.2022)

5.1. Real-World Examples of Precision Therapeutics

We will provide some real-world examples as to how A.I. is guiding us with therapeutics. First, using single-cell RNA-seq data in multiple sclerosis, it was found that several immune cell types substantially increase in the optic nerve and the spinal cord—two major regions of the CNS—but not in the cerebellum. They performed an extra newly developed algorithm to identify pathways, which were activated in microglia and astrocytes experimentally. Our takeaways are twofold: single-cell RNA-seq data can reveal a highly detailed atlas of cell type and state changes in disease-damaged organs, and a new development to identify pathway activations within immune cell populations improves the interpretability of analyzing single-cell RNA-seq in complex tissues and diseases. Finally, we want to round off quickly with some more excellent work looking at various therapeutic solutions. For a variety of movement disorders, a developed ML-guided treatment can decode a patient's natural movement from local field potentials, infer a patient's intention in advance of physical movement, and interface with an external device to produce a sub-thalamic nucleus deep brain stimulation signal. Their patient successfully managed his sitting stance using the technique, recovered from his off period, and improved his activities of daily living. Currently, there are poor, if any, effective treatments of disorders like dystonia or basal ganglia impairment. Through integrating biology and technology, A.I. is now inaugurating a new epoch to restore volitional movement in these rare diseases. In the last part, a new dilution mass spectrometry protocol showed that DMS could detect, in an effective manner, whether the concentration of potential targeted imaging ligands was right or not. While this study focuses on a particular biomedical modality, its speed and accuracy have implications across diseases and therapeutic modalities. Reflecting that not all effective quantitative biological tools need to be computational, we wanted to share this case of a new rapid assay that could help evaluate potential imaging cue-based drugs. (Naithani et al.2021)

6. REGULATORY LANDSCAPE AND FUTURE DIRECTIONS

In this manuscript, we reviewed the landscape of AI and A/B testing of digital biomarkers, working with the definition of the clinical use of digital biomarkers as 'clinical measurements derived from digital health tools used as diagnostic tests', and reflected on the relevant regulatory issues. From a regulatory perspective, we consider fitness trackers or measurements derived from mobile phones or other wearable and home-based sensors as interventions that provide 'supportive, non-diagnostic information.' Nevertheless, the use of digital biomarkers generated from real-world data as diagnostic tools can ultimately serve as supporting evidence in registrational clinical trials or interact with regulatory agencies on different pathways to drug development.

The number of digital biomarkers that have clearance to be used in regulated clinical trials has been growing. We designed and assembled a chart summarizing the scientific level of evidence of registered digital biomarkers generating real-world data, as reported in the registry. Among those, quite a few are performing A/B experiments powered by AI algorithms, enabling evidence generations to follow the pace of technological innovation.

6.1. Current Regulations and Guidelines

It is important to understand that digital measurements of all kinds are increasingly being used to assist in diagnosis, treat patients, and measure the outcomes of various interventions. However, most digital measurements, particularly those that involve the use of sensors, have not yet been rigorously thresholded such that they are equivalent to the information obtained from a laboratory measurement that has been validated and can generally be relied upon to be accurate and robust. When assessments are made with sensor readouts, the inclusion of a feature with an origin primarily related to the assessment of the state of a living organism is termed a biomarker. These digital biomarkers are of increasing interest and have notable applications in a variety of areas. Ease of collection is an asset, as is the ability to monitor the markers on a near-continuous basis. These measurements can be made remotely, and the digital information can be easily transmitted so that measurement is feasible without requiring the subject to be present in a physician's office.

The use of digital features in healthcare is becoming very popular, but so far society has done a relatively modest job related to establishing standards and regulations to ensure that the digital measurements are accurate and reliable. This is very important to remember since definitions of data validity include accuracy and precision of the specific measurements. Guidelines should be developed so that it is clear what is required by the owners of the measurement algorithms to establish a specific measurement in an individual who has a disease. Of interest is that someone who is apparently healthy may not generally be the appropriate target if the true goal is to manage a particular form of morbidity. In the US, the standard may be the comparison to a traditional biomarker or that the diagnosis of the pathology in concern should be sufficient. These assays are performed in a laboratory, and results are taken as the "gold standard." International standards organizations have already developed guidelines to ensure that medical data is reliable and can be stored in a manner that respects the privacy of the subjects on whom the tests are conducted. (Bashraheel et al., 2020)

6.2. Emerging Trends and Opportunities

One way to break away from the trend in predicting near-term adherence to drug therapies is to look at new forms of data about patient health beyond the two-second taps, background of the patients, and exposure to interventions. Increasingly, research using smartwatch and wearable sensor data— traditionally used for health monitoring, as opposed to disease diagnosis—has demonstrated how fine-grained inferences of patient identity, emotional state, stress levels, substance use, sleep onset, and inclusion in a clinical study can leak from such real-time sensing signals. We posit that an opportunity exists to repurpose the bio-behavioral insights generated from smartwatch or wearable sensor data for the secondary purpose of enhancing the measurement of the effects of biologically active agents on human subjects.

Interpreting the potential relationships between these signal characteristics and both patient health and drug effects is still replete with confounding factors and non-trivial challenges, and implementing the recommendation to collect these measurements in precision therapeutic trials warrants caution and the exercise of ethical diligence. Notwithstanding, increasingly advanced bio-behavioral measurement capabilities may help mitigate some of these sociotechnical and epistemic challenges currently affecting precision training studies by enhancing not only controlled but also long-term, longitudinal, and minimally obtrusive assessments of the true effects of precision therapeutic interventions in freely moving patients. The early history has shown that statistically significant evidence of the efficacy of many gene-gene, protein-protein, pathway-pathway, or multi-disciplinary omic overweight studies often fails to replicate when tested in a clinical setting. (Carmo-Fonseca, 2021)

7. CONCLUSION AND IMPLICATIONS FOR HEALTHCARE

The healthcare industry is in the midst of a transformation guided by precision medicine. Within this broader trend, we are witnessing the nascent stages of the uptake of digital biomarkers, powered by data acquisition from biosensors and passively through smartphones and wearables, for monitoring human physiology. These biomarkers, when combined with additional health data and metadata to provide a better understanding of population risk, can help in more continuous and objective monitoring and lead to better-informed decision-making. We believe that, through creating continuous digital biomarker data, precision medicine will be enabled to move beyond acute intervention and into precision therapeutics, intervening earlier in disease progression, before the onset of symptoms and disease manifestation. This requires close collaboration between technology companies, research infrastructure, and all the stakeholders in the sciences to ensure correct governance of data and affordability within the traditional reimbursement models. In this chapter, we set out some underlying problems that need to be solved to enable this vision. We argue that industry must support the generation of dense and scalable phenotypes and demonstrate value in topics, patient cohorts, and diseases across the continuum of care. This will require investment in technology, data management, and analysis to monitor and model an increasing number of parameters at an individual level while also showing that it is possible to empower patients with their data, including data generated using smartphones and wearables. The patient narrative is always key to these success stories. The more data that is collected, the better the model for understanding and predicting the escalations and de-escalations becomes. In such a precision model, even for diseases with stable phenotypes, understanding variation is critical. Ultimately, markets and reimbursement models need to be addressed, following effective demonstrations of clinical outcomes and the ability to demonstrate additional value by influencing quality of life and clinical pathways. All disease research is driven and bounded by the available investment. For common preventable diseases, we must invest in prevention strategies rather than ongoing symptom management. We believe digital biomarkers can help in this endeavor.

7.1. Key Takeaways

Digital phenotyping and biosensing devices, combined with machine learning techniques, can form digital biomarkers to enable precise and personalized treatments for mental health disorders. This is the first initiative leading to the development of precision therapeutics. With the use of standardized datasets, AI models could learn about relations between each proprietary measurement, questionnaires, and diagnosis outcomes, which ultimately result in developing more valid measurements covering neurocognitive aspects as well. NGN is the largest smartphone study utilizing digital markers and analyzing the clinical application of pre-existing AI models. Using standardized and data-privacy-respecting procedures, Next Generation Neurometrics aims to contribute to biomarkers for psychiatric disorders. There are numerous important open questions and challenges within this new field that are only beginning to be addressed, from ethical data collection and integration of subjective and objectively measured data to the different aspects of representativeness. Only if these research gaps can be resolved, digital phenotyping is a promising tool to progress in understanding and thereby improving the treatment of mental disorders.

7.2. Future Outlook and Potential Impact

The therapeutic benefits of the precision therapeutics approach to both health and wellness have the potential to be disruptive. In addition to preventative interventions, precision therapeutics focuses on novel diagnostics and treatments based on comprehensive individual health records. These records, consisting of DNA, RNA, protein, and the applicable relevant phenotypic data, can be empowering for both individuals and data-driven medical researchers. Unlike current state-of-the-art electronic health records, these records, or some combination of them adapted to personal medical needs, are ideally the result of a consortium of responsive individuals and their caregivers working in collaboration with seed data from the research community that can identify when current diseases and future syndromes actually manifest in the individual.

A significant research investment should focus on developing and integrating technologies aimed at simultaneously capturing the individual's epigenomic and other biological signals integral to maintaining a healthy life. The combination of these signals immersed in specific environmental and social contexts, for an individual or a cohort of individuals, could provide a new data resource to potentially optimize the questions that explore the roots of health and wellness. In addition to potentially improving individual health, such data collection efforts are likely to accelerate research and the introduction of new scientific discoveries and intellectual opportunities. Moreover, intellectual value could also be provided to those who contribute their own data either through the quality of health care they receive or some other benefit.

REFERENCES

Akhoon, N. (2021). Precision medicine: a new paradigm in therapeutics. International journal of preventive medicine. lww.comDOI: 10.3390/pr10061107

Al-Dewik, N. I., Younes, S. N., Essa, M. M., Pathak, S., & Qoronfleh, M. W. (2022). Making biomarkers relevant to healthcare innovation and precision medicine. [mdpi.com]. *Processes (Basel, Switzerland)*, 10(6), 1107. DOI: 10.3390/pr10061107

Alonso, A. K. M., Hirt, J., Woelfle, T., Janiaud, P., & Hemkens, L. G. (2023). Definitions of digital biomarkers: a systematic mapping of the biomedical literature. *medRxiv. medrxiv*.org DOI: 10.1101/2023.09.01.23294897

Assidi, M., Buhmeida, A., & Budowle, B. (2022). Medicine and health of 21st Century: Not just a high biotech-driven solution. Npj genomic medicine. nature.comDOI: 10.3390/pr10061107

Bashraheel, S. S., Domling, A., & Goda, S. K. (2020). Update on targeted cancer therapies, single or in combination, and their fine tuning for precision medicine. Biomedicine & Pharmacotherapy. sciencedirect.comDOI: 10.3390/pr10061107

Bizzarri, M., Fedeli, V., Monti, N., Cucina, A., Jalouli, M., Alwasel, S. H., & Harrath, A. H. (2021). Personalization of medical treatments in oncology: Time for rethinking the disease concept to improve individual outcomes. [springer.com]. *The EPMA Journal*, 12(4), 1–14. DOI: 10.1007/s13167-021-00254-1 PMID: 34642594

Bustin, S. A., & Jellinger, K. A. (2023). Advances in molecular medicine: unravelling disease complexity and pioneering precision healthcare. International Journal of Molecular Sciences. mdpi.comDOI: 10.3390/pr10061107

Carmo-Fonseca, M. (2021). *Precision Medicine: Enabling Healthcare Progress in the Twenty-First Century*. Precision Medicine in Stroke. [HTML]

Darwich, A. S., Polasek, T. M., Aronson, J. K., Ogungbenro, K., Wright, D. F., Achour, B., Reny, J.-L., Daali, Y., Eiermann, B., Cook, J., Lesko, L., McLachlan, A. J., & Rostami-Hodjegan, A. (2021). Model-informed precision dosing: Background, requirements, validation, implementation, and forward trajectory of individualizing drug therapy. [diva-portal.org]. *Annual Review of Pharmacology and Toxicology*, 61(1), 225–245. DOI: 10.1146/annurev-pharmtox-033020-113257 PMID: 33035445

De Maria Marchiano, R., Di Sante, G., Piro, G., Carbone, C., Tortora, G., Boldrini, L., Pietragalla, A., Daniele, G., Tredicine, M., Cesario, A., Valentini, V., Gallo, D., Babini, G., D'Oria, M., & Scambia, G. (2021). Translational research in the era of precision medicine: Where we are and where we will go. [mdpi.com]. *Journal of Personalized Medicine*, 11(3), 216. DOI: 10.3390/jpm11030216 PMID: 33803592

Fountoulakis, K. N., & Stahl, S. M. (2021). Precision and personalized assessment, diagnosis and treatment in psychiatry. [HTML]. *CNS Spectrums*, 26(4), 326–332. DOI: 10.1017/S1092852920000139 PMID: 32228728

Hassan, M., Awan, F. M., Naz, A., deAndrés-Galiana, E. J., Alvarez, O., Cernea, A., Fernández-Brillet, L., Fernández-Martínez, J. L., & Kloczkowski, A. (2022). Innovations in genomics and big data analytics for personalized medicine and health care: A review. [mdpi.com]. *International Journal of Molecular Sciences*, 23(9), 4645. DOI: 10.3390/ijms23094645 PMID: 35563034

Manta, C., Patrick-Lake, B., & Goldsack, J. C. (2020). Digital measures that matter to patients: a framework to guide the selection and development of digital measures of health. Digital Biomarkers. karger.comDOI: 10.1186/s13054-021-03822-z PMID: 34814925

Naithani, N., Sinha, S., Misra, P., Vasudevan, B., & Sahu, R. (2021). Precision medicine: Concept and tools. medical journal armed forces india, 77(3), 249-257. nih.govDOI: 10.1186/s13054-021-03822-z PMID: 34814925

Strianese, O., Rizzo, F., Ciccarelli, M., Galasso, G., D'Agostino, Y., Salvati, A., Del Giudice, C., Tesorio, P., & Rusciano, M. R. (2020). Precision and personalized medicine: How genomic approach improves the management of cardiovascular and neurodegenerative disease. [mdpi.com]. *Genes*, 11(7), 747. DOI: 10.3390/genes11070747 PMID: 32640513

Tyson, R. J., Park, C. C., Powell, J. R., Patterson, J. H., Weiner, D., Watkins, P. B., & Gonzalez, D. (2020). Precision dosing priority criteria: Drug, disease, and patient population variables. [frontiersin.org]. *Frontiers in Pharmacology*, 11, 420. DOI: 10.3389/fphar.2020.00420 PMID: 32390828

Wahida, A., Buschhorn, L., Fröhling, S., Jost, P. J., Schneeweiss, A., Lichter, P., & Kurzrock, R. (2023). The coming decade in precision oncology: Six riddles. [HTML]. *Nature Reviews. Cancer*, 23(1), 43–54. DOI: 10.1038/s41568-022-00529-3 PMID: 36434139

Wang, R. C., & Wang, Z. (2023). Precision medicine: disease subtyping and tailored treatment. Cancers. mdpi.comDOI: 10.1186/s13054-021-03822-z PMID: 34814925

Wick, K. D., McAuley, D. F., Levitt, J. E., Beitler, J. R., Annane, D., Riviello, E. D., Calfee, C. S., & Matthay, M. A. (2021). Promises and challenges of personalized medicine to guide ARDS therapy. [springer.com]. *Critical Care*, 25(1), 1–15. DOI: 10.1186/s13054-021-03822-z PMID: 34814925

Yuan, B. (2022). What personalized medicine humans need and way to it——also on the practical significance and Scientific Limitations of Precision Medicine. Pharmacogenomics and Personalized Medicine. tandfonline.comDOI: 10.1186/s13054-021-03822-z PMID: 34814925

Chapter 7
AI-Powered-IoT (AIIoT)-Based Decision-Making System for BP-Patient Healthcare Monitoring:
BP-Patient Health Monitoring Using KSK Approach

Kutubuddin Sayyad Liyakat Kazi
https://orcid.org/0000-0001-5623-9211
Brahmdevdada Mane Institute of Technology, India

ABSTRACT

The KSK approach to BP patient healthcare monitoring, which is powered by AI and IoT, has the potential to completely transform the way hypertension is treated. It makes it easier for healthcare providers to make decisions based on exact information, as well as to monitor patients accurately and in real time, customise treatment plans, and empower patients. We anticipate a major improvement in the management of hypertension and other chronic disorders with additional technological developments. Three measures are used to evaluate classifier performance. Accuracy, precision, and recall are all measured. The KSK technique used in the BP healthcare industry currently achieves an accuracy rate of 89% to 93% for each condition.

DOI: 10.4018/979-8-3693-6270-9.ch007

INTRODUCTION

The term "blood pressure," or BP, refers to a health problem that affects millions of people all over the world. High blood pressure is the main basis of death around the World, accounting for 13% of all deaths, as stated by the World Health Organisation (WHO (World Health Organization). According to Neeraja et al. (2024), patients and medical professionals alike have to be particularly concerned about it because it is associated with a significant risk of cardiovascular disorders such as heart disease, stroke, and other forms of cardiovascular diseases.

In order for those who have high blood pressure to successfully handle their condition, they require the assistance of a qualified medical professional. The importance of providing healthcare to patients with high blood pressure is examined in Figure 1, along with the different factors that must be taken into consideration for the patients' overall health.

- **Accurate Diagnosis:** Accurate diagnosis and consistent monitoring are the two most important aspects of diabetes management. Accurate diagnosis and frequent monitoring are the fundamental tenets for handling high blood pressure. Because they take the patient's blood pressure on a regular basis and identify hypertension if it is present, healthcare practitioners play an essential role in this process. In addition, they provide patients with information on how to take their blood pressure at home and advise them on how frequently they ought to check their blood pressure considering their condition, as stated by Sunil Kumar et al (2022).
- **Medication:** The majority of people who suffer from high blood pressure need to take medication in order to keep their blood pressure under control. After doing a comprehensive assessment of the patient's condition, medical professionals will prescribe the proper prescription at the suitable dosage. For the purpose of determining whether or not their treatment is working, patients are required to take their prescription exactly as directed and to visit their physician on a regular basis.
- **Lifestyle Modifications:** Modifications to one's lifestyle are required to bring down high blood pressure. Patients are educated by healthcare benefactors about the need of upholding a healthy diet, likable in consistent physical activity, and learning how to effectively manage stress. Additionally, they keep track of the patient's weight and offer advice on how to lose weight when it is required. These modifications in lifestyle, in addition to the use of medication, have the potential to assist in lowering blood pressure and reducing the probability of experiencing additional health problems, as stated by Kazi K (2024).

- **Regular Checkups and Screenings:** Patients with high blood pressure should have routine checkups and screenings in order to keep track of their status and identify potential problems that may arise. In order to properly evaluate the patient's general health and identify any anomalies in blood pressure, medical professionals conduct routine testing on their patients. According to Wale et al. (2019), these tests serve the additional purpose of identifying any additional illnesses that may be caused by high blood pressure. These illnesses include diabetes, heart disease, and kidney disease.

Figure 1. Aspects of healthcare for BP patients

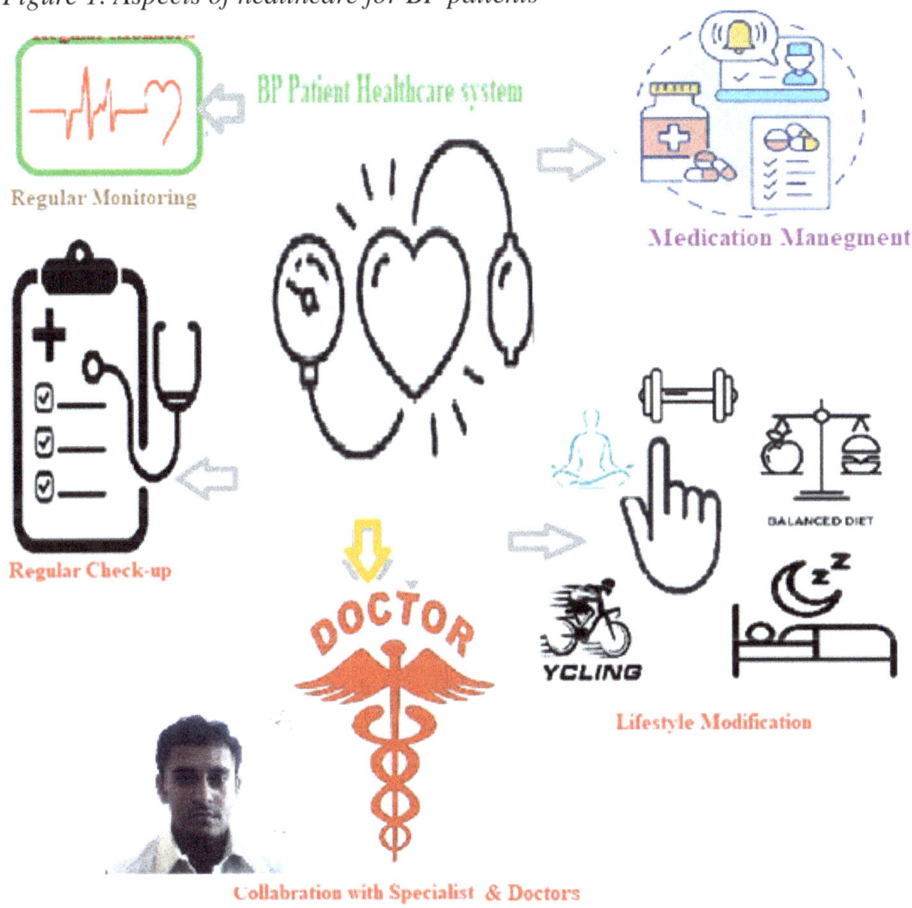

- **Education and Support:** In order to effectively manage their condition, people who suffer from high blood pressure need to receive the required education and support. When it comes to educating individuals regarding hypertension, its root cause, and the significance of following to treatment plans, the role that healthcare professionals play should not be underestimated. In addition to this, they offer patients counsel and support regarding the management of stress as well as the required alterations to their lifestyle. In addition, according to Liyakat et al. (2024), physicians offer patients advice on how to safely and effectively manage the probable adverse effects of their prescriptions.
- **Utilizing the Services of Specialists:** Some people with high blood pressure may require the assistance of a medical professional due to the presence of underlying medical issues. In these kinds of situations, medical professionals work along with experts like cardiologists, nephrologists, and endocrinologists in order to give patients comprehensive care. Through this teamwork, it is ensured that all elements of the patient's health have been taken care of, and that Kazi K S L (2018) will immediately identify and report any potential issues that may arise.
- **Innovative Technologies for Monitoring and Management:** As a result of technical breakthroughs, a wide range of instruments and apparatuses are now available for the purpose of monitoring and managing high blood pressure. Patients, for instance, have the option of using blood pressure monitors that they can use at home to assess their blood pressure on a regular basis. Additionally, there are applications for smartphones that offer users insights connected to their health and assist them in recording current blood pressure readings by providing it. Not only do these technologies help people better manage their ailments, but they also provide healthcare personnel with the ability to remotely monitor patients, as stated by Sultanabanu et al. (2024).
- To control their high blood pressure and lessen the likelihood of consequences, those who suffer from high blood pressure need to receive the appropriate medical attention. It is necessary for patients and healthcare practitioners to work together in order to handle it, with the primary focus being on education, regular monitoring, medication management, and lifestyle adjustments. Patients who suffer from high blood pressure may successfully manage their disease and lead healthy lives if they adhere to these instructions.
- Due to the increasing number of cases of high blood pressure (BP), it is imperative that the circumstances of patients be monitored on a continuous basis. The condition known as hypertension, which is synonymous with high blood pressure, can lead to significant health problems if it is not managed. It is a condition that persists over time. As a result of this, it is absolutely nec-

essary to adequately monitor individuals with high blood pressure in order to ensure their well-being and prevent any complications from occurring.

- One of the primary objectives of monitoring is to ensure that patients with high blood pressure continue to have their blood pressure under control. It is of the utmost importance to take measurements of their blood pressure on a regular basis in order to determine whether taking medicine or making changes to their lifestyle have contributed to the effective prevention of their disease. It is recommended that patients who have high blood pressure have their blood pressure measured at least every month, or regularly if it is appropriate.

Also, keeping a close eye on people who have high blood pressure helps in determining whether or not the sickness has any potential adverse repercussions. The heart, the brain, the kidneys, and the eyes are just some of the organs that can be harmed by high blood pressure. There is a possibility that it could lead to blindness, heart attacks, strokes, and renal failure. By administering blood pressure measurements to their patients on a regular basis, medical professionals are able to detect and treat potential early indicators of organ damage, as well as prevent any complications from occurring.

In addition, measuring blood pressure gives medical practitioners the ability to assess the effectiveness of a treatment strategy. Patients who suffer from high blood pressure often need to take medicine, make adjustments to their lifestyle, and have routine examinations in order to bring their condition under control. The monitoring process allows medical professionals to decide if the current treatment plan is effective or whether it needs to be updated. Patients diagnosed with high blood pressure are assured of receiving the most effective and individualized treatment for their illness as a result of this. Patients who are frequently checked for their blood pressure have the ability to reveal vital details about their general well-being if they are given the opportunity to do so. The presence of high blood pressure is frequently linked to a number of other illnesses, including diabetes, obesity, high cholesterol, and others. Frequent monitoring can be helpful in identifying certain coexisting conditions, which enables medical practitioners to treat both diseases simultaneously and improve the patient's overall health.

Monitoring a patient's blood pressure has become more accurate and feasible thanks to technological advancements in recent years. The advancements that have been made in wearable technology and home blood pressure monitors have made it possible for patients to check their blood pressure readings in a short amount of time. Using the data that these devices offer in real time, patients are able to keep a closer eye on their blood pressure and make adjustments to their lifestyle as required in order to effectively manage their condition. In addition to self-monitoring, cardiovascular disease (BP) patients are monitored by medical experts through the use of electronic health records (EHRs). EHRs are able to provide a comprehensive account of a patient's medicinal history, which includes the results of tests, the history of prescriptions, and measures of blood pressure. It is because of this that medical professionals are able to monitor changes in blood pressure over time and select the most appropriate treatment for their patients.

In addition to having their blood pressure checked on a regular basis, people who have high blood pressure may benefit from making changes to their lifestyle at the same time. The management of stress, the consumption of a balanced diet, the regular exercise, the abstinence from alcohol and tobacco, and the regular exercise are all factors that might contribute to a reduction in blood pressure. Together with monitoring blood pressure, keeping an eye on these lifestyle factors can provide a holistic approach to the management of hypertension.

For this reason, it is absolutely necessary to keep a close eye on patients who have high blood pressure in order to protect their overall health and shield them from any potential effects which may arise as a outcome of the disease. In recent eras, technological advancements and the accessibility of a wide range of monitoring technologies have made it possible for individuals who suffer from high blood pressure to become more capable of managing their disease. Patients who have high blood pressure are required to take an active role in their own care and work closely with their medical providers in order to maintain control of their blood pressure. In spite of their disease, individuals are able to live a life that is full of joy and good health by continuing to adhere to this.

BACKGROUND

The combination of Artificial Intelligence (AI) and Internet of Things (IoT) results in the creation of a revolutionary paradigm that is referred to as AI-Powered IoT(AIIoT). This paradigm has enormous implications for the healthcare industry, notably in the supervision of patients who have issues related to their blood pressure (BP). Increasingly, decision-making tools that are based on AI and IoT are altering the way in which healthcare providers monitor and manage chronic illnesses such as hypertension. This is improving both patient outcomes and operational efficiency.

AIIoT systems make use of devices that are connected to one another in order to gather data on health in real time, carry out trend analysis, and make it easier to make informed decisions. Those individuals who are experiencing blood pressure anomalies can benefit from these systems since they provide continuous monitoring tools that measure blood pressure readings through the use of connected health devices and smart wearables. The information that is gathered by these devices is then sent to a centralized platform, where it is analyzed by artificial intelligence algorithms, which then provides healthcare practitioners with insights that can be put into action.

AIIoT's Advantages in Blood Pressure Monitoring:

- Real-Time Monitoring: Conventional techniques of blood pressure monitoring frequently take the form of irregular checkups, which can result in delays in the implementation of intervention. AI and IoT solutions provide continuous tracking, which enables the rapid identification of harmful tendencies, which is essential for making appropriate adjustments to treatment.
- Analysis and Prediction of Data: AI systems have the ability to recognize trends and irregularities in blood pressure measurements that may not be obvious to clinical professionals. The utilization of machine learning techniques enables these systems to forecast the occurrence of possible health emergencies, which in turn enables proactive patient treatment.
- AIIoT has the potential to improve patient assignations by giving patients access to their own health data through mobile applications or web platforms. This can give patients more control over their own health. A better awareness of their diseases is fostered as a result of this transparency, which also encourages patients to adhere to their treatment regimens.
- Personalized Treatment Plans: With the availability of extensive datasets, medical professionals are able to personalize treatment regimens to the specific needs of individual patients, taking into consideration the distinctive health patterns and lifestyle aspects of each patient.

The deployment of AIIoT in blood pressure patient monitoring is not without its hurdles, despite the fact that it offers a number of promising advantages. Due to the fact that sensitive health information is sent and kept digitally, data privacy and security are of the utmost importance. Interoperability problems can arise as a result of the incorporation of a wide diversity of devices and platforms, which can make it more difficult to share data between different systems. Furthermore, it is of the utmost importance to guarantee the precision and dependability of AI algorithms, as any instances of inaccuracy could have serious repercussions for the treatment of patients.

The introduction of AI-powered-IoT in the healthcare industry, in particular for the purpose of monitoring blood pressure patients, represents a noteworthy step advancing in the management of chronic diseases. AI and IoT systems not only make it easier to make decisions based on data in real time, but they also encourage a collaborative environment between patients and providers. When it comes to completely realizing the potential of AI and IoT in terms of altering healthcare, it will be vital to overcome the problems related with data security, interoperability, and algorithmic accuracy as technology continues to improve. When seen as a whole, the continued development of AIIoT solutions provides a potential frontier in the pursuit of more efficient and patient-centered healthcare delivery.

LITERATURE SURVEY

Plant ailments are the primary focus of the research, according to Sunil Kumar (2022), because they seriously jeopardized food production and moderate farmers' means of subsistence. In conventional farming, it is routine practice for knowledgeable laborers to examine every row to check for plant ailments. This labor-intensive and time-consuming method is flawed by nature because it is done by people. The objective of this research is to develop an automated exposure model for the 3 most prevalent diseases that harm maize plants: Northern Leaf Blight, Cercospora Spot, and Frequent Rust. This will be accomplished by merging deep learning (Faster R-CNN+ResNet50) and image recognition techniques to evaluate real-time photographs. With a 93.5% accuracy rate, the offered approach successfully identified 3 illnesses that impact maize.

According to Pradeepa (2022), IoT technologies for the creation of physiological and behavioral monitoring systems—specifically, IoT-based student's medicinal management systems—have evolved swiftly in recent years in tandem with the advancement of sensor technology. Monitoring the health function status of the growing quantity of students living independently and spread over wide geographic areas is becoming more and more important. The number of single students has increased, which is the cause of this. The proposal of an IoT-based methodology to student health management is the goal of this study. This approach aims to continuously monitor children's vital signs and identify biological and behavioral changes using modern medical tools. According to this notion, the IoT module is in charge of obtaining crucial data, which is then evaluated using ANN models. These models are then used to examine the data in order to identify any possible dangers associated with the physiological and behavioral changes in youngsters. The results of the studies demonstrate the accuracy and effectiveness of the projected model in determining the conditions of the learners. After evaluating the proposed model, the SVM achieved a maximum performance of 99.1%, which is good considering our goals. Furthermore, the outcomes were able to outsmart algorithms for multilayer perceptron neural networks, random forests, and decision trees.

According to Kazi K (2024) the purpose of this study is to provide a comprehensive but succinct analysis of the benefits and challenges accompanying the application of AI and IoT in the healthcare industry. Included are an overview of AI and IoT, their applicability, some views on recent advancements, a look ahead, and the challenges that healthcare systems are currently facing. The integration of medical gadgets, advanced sensors, and remote monitoring are just a few of the many applications of IoT in the healthcare sector. In any case, technology can support practitioners in better conveying ideas while safeguarding the security and well-being of patients. The IoT can help human establishments achieve fulfilment and accountability by encouraging patient engagement with qualified medical providers. This is accomplished by promising patients to work with medical professionals more.

In this chapter, Kazi K S (2024a, 2024b) analyses the growing uses of deep learning (DL) in the field of ophthalmology. In particular, it examines how well DL systems may be integrated to enhance patient outcomes, especially with regard to the diagnosis and management of diseases like retinopathy of prematurity, diabetic retinopathy, and age-related macular degeneration. It also describes how deep learning algorithms are used to analyze retinal images and complicated datasets, enabling early detection, accurate diagnosis, and efficient treatment options. This chapter also discusses the difficulties in integrating artificial intelligence into clinical practice. Among these obstacles are data bias, algorithmic reliability, ethical concerns, and the requirement for various datasets that accurately reflect the community. It draws attention to ethical concerns, the significance of ongoing research and development, and offers guidelines for the proper application of DL in ophthalmology. In the discipline of ophthalmology, this chapter attempts to depict a future in which these technologies improve clinical practice and patient outcomes.

Priya (2023) claims that this cutting-edge technology forecasts future patterns and results in using data gathered from past occurrences, assisting heart-care organizations in making better decisions about how to best serve their clients. But, like any other data-driven technology, forecasting needs to be used properly to ensure that corporate operations are both practically and morally good. Because of the growing applications of AI and ML, healthcare forecasting has become increasingly important in recent years. Forecasting has uses in medicine as well, assisting medical professionals in diagnosing patients more quickly and accurately. Medical personnel can identify and treat patients more precisely and quickly when they plan ahead for potential medical events and make the necessary preparations. It's possible that patients will gain more from this and that costs may be reduced. Because these systems replicate human cognition, they are able to identify disorders and provide necessary support for treatment. They might also be applied to medical diagnosis. This topic includes studies that use machine learning (ML) methods to forecast the heart healthcare system (HHS). During system implementation, a DT was utilized for health and human services, MySQL was used for vaccine reminders, and the K-means Elbow method was employed for registration and notification.

The convergence of artificial intelligence (AI) with the internet of things (IoT) has resulted in revolutionary improvements in the field of healthcare, particularly in the treatment of chronic illnesses such as hypertension. The persistence of this review is to examine a Problem Statement, Goal, and Objective pertaining to the creation of an AI-Powered Internet of Things (AIIoT) based decision-making system that is specifically designed for the monitoring of blood pressure (BP) in healthcare patients.

PROBLEM STATEMENT

There are millions of people throughout the world who are affected by hypertension, also known as high blood pressure. Hypertension is a significant precursor to a variety of cardiovascular disorders and consequences. When it comes to preventing severe health emergencies, effective monitoring and management of blood pressure are absolutely necessary. The conventional methods of monitoring, which include going to the doctor on a regular basis and performing manual blood pressure checks, can be ineffective and may result in a delay in responding to potentially harmful variations in blood pressure. Furthermore, the absence of data that is updated in real time can be a barrier to individualized treatment techniques. In order to facilitate continuous monitoring and prompt interventions, which will ultimately lead to improved patient outcomes, there is an immediate requirement for a system that is both robust and automated.

GOAL

The creation of a complete healthcare monitoring platform that enables real-time tracking of blood pressure levels and delivers actionable insights to both patients and healthcare professionals is the fundamental objective of the decision-making system that is established on the Internet of Things (IoT). The purpose of the system is to support proactive healthcare management by utilizing the power of artificial intelligence to evaluate data received from IoT-enabled devices. This will ensure that patients adhere to the treatments that have been prescribed to them and will enable healthcare providers to make educated decisions in a timely manner.

OBJECTS

- Continuous Monitoring: Create an IoT infrastructure that continuously collects real-time data on patients' blood pressure readings using wearable devices. This will ensure that the data is always up to date and accurately reflects the patient's actual state of health.
- Implementing AI algorithms that not only evaluate current blood pressure measurements but also analyze previous data in order to forecast patterns and potential dangers is an important step in the process of data analysis and prediction. When it comes to identifying individuals who are at risk of hypertension-related problems, this predictive skill could prove to be quite important.
- An alarm system that warns both patients and healthcare providers in the case of abnormal blood pressure readings or adverse trends should be developed as part of the personalized alerts program. The purpose of this feature is to make it possible to take prompt action before a potentially dangerous situation emerges.
- Patient Empowerment: Empower patients by providing them with insights into their health data, medication adherence, and lifestyle suggestions through the use of user-friendly interfaces on mobile or web platforms. In order for patients to take an active role in their own care, it is necessary to encourage self-management.
- Integration with Healthcare Systems: Ensure that the AIIoT system is seamlessly integrated with the Electronic Health Records (EHRs) that are already in place. This will enable healthcare practitioners to have a more comprehensive perspective of patient health, which will improve the quality of care that is provided in collaboration.
- Privacy and Security: Address the essential issues of data privacy and security, adopting rigorous mechanisms to protect sensitive health information collected through the AIIoT platform. Additionally, ensure that the data is protected from unauthorized access. For Security purpose, we suggests KK approach for Security of IoT devices.

The most important needs in the management of hypertension is addressed by the creation of an artificial intelligence-powered IoT-based decision-making system for monitoring blood pressure in patients. This approach to the IoT promises to greatly enhance patient outcomes and the quality of care by utilizing continuous monitoring, powerful data analytics, and personalized interventions by harnessing these technologies. As technology continues to advance, the incorporation of artificial intelligence and the IoT into healthcare will significantly contribute to the development of healthcare monitoring solutions that are more intelligent and efficient, which will eventually be of benefit to patients as well as the healthcare ecosystem as a whole. It is possible that the effective implementation of this effort would prepare the groundwork for future breakthroughs in the management of chronic diseases and care that is centered on the patient.

AIIOT SCENARIO

As a result of the constant evolution of technology, the combination of AI and IoT is currently a trend that is gaining popularity all over the world. Currently, the IoT presents opportunities. It was the combination of two exceedingly complicated technologies that gave rise to the idea of AIIoT scenarios. According to Dhanwe et al. (2024), this idea has the potential to revolutionize the way in which we live, work, and engage with the world around us.

To what does the phrase "AI-driven-IoT (AIIoT) scenario" refer? In a nutshell, it is the utilization of artificial intelligence in order to analyze and make smart decisions regarding the enormous amounts of data that are generated by IoT devices. In light of this, it can be deduced that IoT devices, in addition to having the capability to collect and send data, may now use data to learn and make decisions on their own, without the need for human intervention. According to Mishra et al. (2024), this has the potential to fetch momentous changes in a wide variety of enterprises and to improve the efficiency, convenience, and safety of our day-to-day lives. There is an in-depth understanding of the AIIoT scenario for the year 2024 presented in Figure 2, which is based on information gathered from literature in a number of different journals.

Figure 2. AIIoT scenario 2024

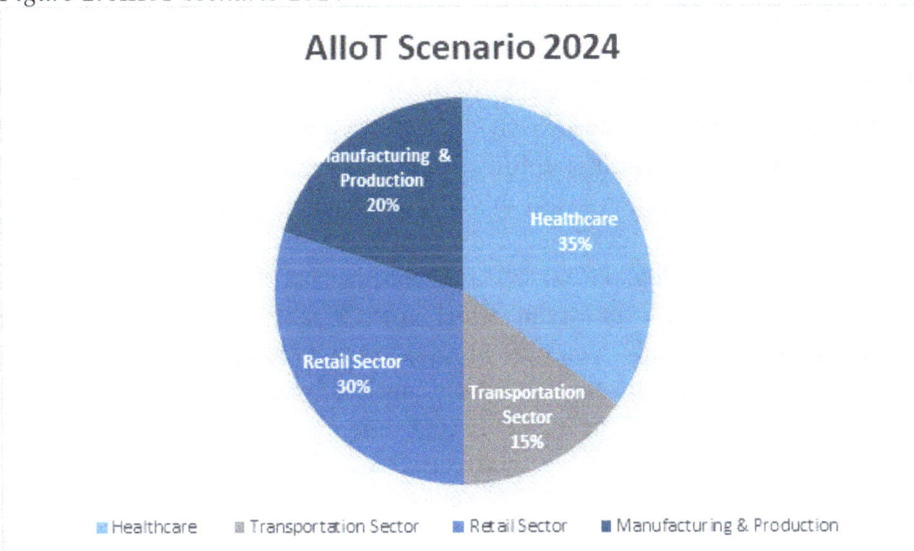

A huge impact could be made by AI and IOT situations in the healthcare industry. Through the utilization of wearable technologies and sensors, it is feasible to perform monitoring and evaluation of patient data in real time. In this way, artificial intelligence algorithms are able to detect any inconsistencies or changes in the data and alert medical professionals. The ability to recognize and prevent potential health problems at an earlier stage is made possible by this. The quality of care provided to patients is enhanced, while at the same time the strain placed on healthcare systems is reduced. This is Kutubuddin's 2023. In the transportation industry, scenarios involving the IoT and AI have the possibility to greatly increase both efficiency and safety. The utilization of real-time data from connected vehicles, for example, can be utilized by intelligent traffic management systems in order to enhance the flow of traffic and decrease congestion. A further benefit of predictive maintenance that is powered by artificial intelligence is that it can help identify and resolve possible problems with automobiles before they get serious, hence reducing the likelihood of crashes. In addition, it is feasible to implement this technology into public transportation systems, which would significantly improve their dependability and provide passengers with additional benefits (Liyakat, 2023).

The industrial and production sector is yet another application that stands to gain a great deal from the use of AI, IoT scenarios. It is possible for manufacturers to obtain real-time data on their operations if they connect their production gear and equipment to the internet. It is possible for artificial intelligence systems to use this data in the future to identify trends and anomalies, which will make it possible to do predictive maintenance and reduce the likelihood of equipment failures. Not only does this save time and money, but it also lessens the likelihood of accidents occurring in the workplace.

Similarly, situations involving the IoT have the potential to revolutionize the retail industry. Retailers are able to provide customers with individualized shopping experience and discounts utilizing IoT devices. These discounts are based on the customers' activities and interests. AI-driven inventory control solutions can also help merchants optimize their stock levels and reduce waste, both of which are important business goals. According to Kazi (2017), businesses benefit from increased sales and revenue in addition to an overall improvement in the quality of the interaction between the customer and the company during the purchasing process.

These developments, on the other hand, are followed by concerns regarding the privacy and security of the data collected from customers. In order to protect against any potential cyber-attacks, thorough security measures need to be put into place. This is because of the enormous amount of data that is being captured and transmitted continuously. Halli et al. (2022) and Liyakat (2024) state that IoT and AI professionals need to collaborate in order to build secure solutions that can protect sensitive data. In order to solve the security problem, we recommend utilizing the KK approach for WSN and IoT security.

In an instant, the marriage of artificial intelligence and the IoT has increased the efficiency, convenience, and safety of our day-to-day lives. Additionally, it has opened up a wide range of possibilities and has the potential to fundamentally transform a number of different industries. All things considered, the benefits of AIIoT scenarios far outweigh any potential negatives, despite the fact that there are challenges to overcome. In light of the rapid pace at which technological advancements are being made, we are only able to conjecture about the infinite possibilities that this convergence may bring about in the years to future (Neeraja et al., 2024).

KSK APPROACH: AI-POWERED DECISION-MAKING SYSTEM BUILT ON IOT

AI and IoT have enabled an emerging generation of decision-making systems. With the help of AI and the broad network of connected devices, businesses and organizations are able to make decisions with greater speed and accuracy, which in turn increases their output and efficiency. An AI-driven-IoT)-based decision-making system that has the prospect of significantly amending both industry and civilization is the KSK approach, which was inspired by Dr. K. S. Kazi.

To be more specific, what exactly is an IOT-based artificial intelligence-driven decision-making system (KSK method)? To put it succinctly, it is a system that uses artificial intelligence algorithms to analyze and make sense of data that has been acquired from various IoT sensors. These decisions could be as simple as turning on or off the lights, or they could be more complex, such as Liyakat's (2023) forecasting of market trends or other business decisions. Any of these decisions could be made.

Creating a network of linked devices is the first step in the process of constructing an artificial intelligence-powered-IoT decision-making system (KSK Approach). The devices in question could be cameras, home appliances, sensors, or any number of other sophisticated devices. Artificial intelligence algorithms review and analyze the data that is gathered by these devices, which then transfer it to a server on the cloud or a central hub.

Because it processes enormous amounts of data at a far faster rate than humans can, artificial intelligence is an indispensable component of this system. In addition, it has the potential to recognize patterns and trends that individuals would overlook, which would result in an increase in the accuracy and efficiency of decision-making, as stated by Praasd et al (2024).

The KSK Approach offers a number of innovative benefits, one of which is task automation. For instance, the system of a smart house is able to adjust the lighting, temperature, and other settings in line with the routines that the people of the home follow on a regular basis. This results in a reduction in energy use, which, when paired with time savings, leads to cost savings. Businesses have the ability to automate tasks and estimate the amount of maintenance that is required by utilizing this technology. For instance, artificial intelligence systems can analyze immediate sensor data on machine performance in a production facility to determine when a machine will require maintenance, thereby preventing costly downtime (Megha, 2024).

Another advantage of using this KSK technique is that it allows for decisions to be made in real time. As a result of the continuous flow of data from IoT devices and the swift processing of artificial intelligence algorithms, decisions can be established in a matter of seconds. When it comes to industries such as healthcare and transportation (Kasat et al., 2023), where delaying decisions might result in catastrophic consequences, this is especially useful.

The KSK Approach has the prospect of improving the experience of the clientele as well. By S L (2022), businesses will be able to better understand the interests and behaviors of their customers by taking advantage of the data that is gathered from IoT devices and using it to adapt their offerings. Customers that are more satisfied and loyal to the brand could be the result of this.

Even with all of these benefits, there are still concerns regarding the privacy and security of one's data when using a (KSK Approach). As a result of the fact that these systems are so dependent on data, there is a possibility that confidential information could be compromised. Therefore, in order to protect data and ensure that privacy is maintained, it is necessary to implement stringent security measures. Therefore, we advocate the KK technique for ensuring the safety of every IoT and wireless sensor network.

Now that AI and the IoT are connected, there are several chances to make decisions more rapidly and accurately. Inferences can be made more quickly and accurately. The implementation of this technology has the potential to enhance customer satisfaction, productivity, and efficiency in both residential and commercial settings. Security and privacy concerns need to be addressed before this great technology can be utilized to its full potential. With the further development of AI and IoT, we are expecting substantially more cutting-edge application and technology from Sultanabanu (2023, 2023b, 2023c) in the near future.

METHODOLOGY

Internet of Things (IoT) is a process that integrates millions of different somatic methods for the delivery and collection of data over the internet. Internet of Things is comprised of a vast assortment of software and sensors. Through the use of wireless communication protocols, it is currently possible to facilitate interaction among mobile devices, various physical objects, and machines that is located in faraway locations. Models of healthcare are considerably improved by IoT. For the purpose of collecting patient data, a wide variety of sensors, both internal and external, are utilized. Body-implanted sensors are assigned the responsibility of collecting the patient's internal data, whilst the everlasting sensor is in charge of collecting the patient's data on their surroundings and the environment around them. The information that is provided to the physicians is evaluated by them in order to make predictions regarding probable ailments.

The data that was collected is classified by the model that was developed using a variety of different machine learning classification approaches. Consequently, the framework has the capacity to differentiate between people who are physically healthy and people who don't seem healthy in terms of their physical condition. A dependable and efficient method of disease classification can be achieved through the application of machine learning. Three separate types of patient data have been collected through the IoT in accordance with the approach that has been suggested:

- Information concerning the patients who are currently under quarantine Patients that fall into this data group have IoT sensors installed that are readily available and within a reasonable price range. Using these IoT sensors, patients' health data is collected and then transmitted to an IoT assistant for further study.
- Information about the patient from a clinical or laboratory setting: In this scenario, the patient visits clinics and laboratories; yet, despite having access to all of the resources accessible to them, there is no doctor available to see them.
- Information pertaining to the patient who lives in a foreign location: On this particular occasion, the patient lives in a remote region or in an isolated area that is not in close proximity to any hospitals. The staff members working on the medical assistance programs were the ones who obtained this information. Doctors are able to provide better care for their patients by utilizing contemporaneous patient information from sensors that are connected to the IoT.

Each and every IoT device has the capability to gather data, which can then be sent to a cloud server for further examination. With the help of categorization algorithms, the fog server does an analysis on the data. For the purpose of providing rapid diagnoses to patients, the information is distributed to medical professionals and power storage facilities. According to Veena et al. (2023), this is accomplished through the utilization of the cloud server. For the purpose of developing medical models, the primary focus of research is on the application of artificial intelligence algorithms for categorization inside the KSK methodology. The Decision Tree (DT), the K-Nearest Neighbor (KNN), and the Artificial Neural Network (ANN) are some of the techniques employed in this classification.

Some of these methods are used in a dataset that includes information about blood pressure figures. It is illustrated in Figure 3 that the framework of the suggested model is constructed. Both AI and IoT play significant roles in the paradigm that has been presented. Anything can be connected to the internet through the use of the initial parameter, that somewhat can also be referred to as the Internet of Things (IoT). Information pertaining to patients is gathered and processed in real time. This ensures that the information is processed in a timely manner and that it is delivered to the appropriate individuals. The subsequent parameter, machine learning, makes use of the data that has been gathered in order to generate results in a short amount of time. With the assistance of AI and IoT technology, enormous quantities of data might be managed effectively. The work can be broken down into three distinct components and sections. The second stage consists of acquiring the data, preparing it, and performing the calculations on it. Following the completion of the third stage, the results are kept on a server that is accessible online, and the final decision is made and communicated to the end users, who may be medical professionals.

Figure 3. Proposed KSK approach for BP patient health monitoring

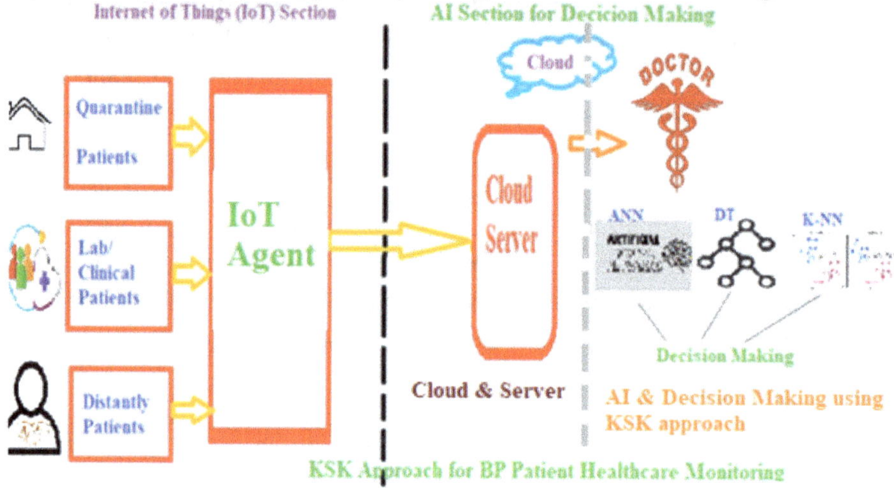

1. Information gathering: A range of techniques are employed to gather patient data, including information gathered from the patient's home, clinic, or laboratory as well as information obtained remotely. A multitude of sensors and IoT devices are needed for the collecting of patient data in real time. For patients who remain in their own homes, sensors within the required range have been placed. The laboratory personnel provide clinical and analytical data to an IoT agent. People who live in really isolated areas have several sensors implanted in them. These sensors collect the data, which is subsequently sent to an IoT agent for additional processing.
2. The pre-processing of the provided data consists of two steps: filtering and looking for missing values. These actions are a part of the data pre-processing and calculation.
3. After pre-processing is finished, the data is moved to a cloud server to begin processing. In this case, three AI classifiers—DT, ANN, and K-NN—employed to compute and classify the data. It is advised to employ these classifiers while using the KSK method of decision making.

DISCUSSION

Among the most innovative developments of the past few years is the AI-Powered-IoT (AIIoT), which combines AI and IoT. There has been a significant expansion in the field of healthcare as a direct result of the development of technology. The marriage of artificial intelligence with the IoT represents a few of the most significant recent developments. Within the realm of patient monitoring, this integration has the potential to bring about a complete transformation in the manner in which healthcare is delivered. This article will discuss the KSK technique, which is a decision-making system that is based on the IoT and is used to monitor the medical care of individuals who have high blood pressure.

The condition known as hypertension, which is also referred to as high blood pressure (BP) in some circles, is a significant health risk that affects billions of people all over the Globe. Due to the fact that the condition is chronic, continuous care and monitoring are required in order to prevent complications that will persist over time. When utilizing the standard monitoring strategy, patients may discover that it is challenging and time-consuming to visit their healthcare practitioner on a consistent basis. This is where the IoT comes into play, providing patients with a technique of monitoring their blood pressure that is both more accurate and more effective.

A decision-making tool that continuously analyzes, evaluates, and renders judgments on the patient's blood pressure levels is the KSK (K S Kazi) Approach. This approach makes use of AI algorithms and IoT sensors. A monitoring platform, a decision-making system, and sensors are the three fundamental elements that make up this strategy.

To collect data on the patient's blood pressure measures in real time, sensors are placed to the patient with the intention of collecting the data. It is possible that these sensors may be incorporated into everyday goods such as clothing or furniture, or they could take the form of a gadget that can be worn comfortably. Following the collection of data by these sensors, the information is then transmitted to the decision-making system, which is the basis of the KSK method.

In order to provide the patient with information about their blood pressure readings in real time, the decision-making system performs an analysis on the data collected by the sensors. Within the realm of artificial intelligence, algorithms are utilized by the system. For the purpose of providing accurate and individualized results, this device is designed to continuously learn from and adapt to the unique blood pressure trends of each individual patient. In addition, it is able to detect any anomalies or sudden changes in the patient's blood pressure, which allows it to alert the physician in the event of an emergency.

The monitoring platform establishes a connection between the patient, the healthcare professional, and the system that ultimately makes decisions. In terms of the KSK strategy, this platform constitutes the third ingredient. Through the platform's intuitive user interface, the patient is able to review their blood pressure data and obtain individualized guidance on how to effectively manage their condition. It also makes it possible for medical professionals to remotely monitor patients and respond quickly to any emergency situations that may arise.

A notable advantage of the KSK technique is that it can anticipate the patient's blood pressure readings in advance, which is one of the most significant advantages of the strategy. Due to the fact that it continuously monitors and evaluates patient data, this decision-making system is able to identify patterns and make predictions regarding blood pressure readings. It is possible that healthcare providers may find this to be useful in order to make proactive decisions and avert any potential harm to the health of their patients.

Additionally, the KSK approach encourages patient participation and empowerment with regard to their care. Patients are given the ability to take charge of their own health care by providing them with access to individualized recommendations and data that is updated in real time through the monitoring platform used. As a consequence of this, individuals might be better competent to take care of their condition on their own, which might consequently lead to better outcomes.

There are, however, some limits associated with the IoT-based decision-making system, just like there are with any other technology. There is a direct correlation between the precision and dependability of artificial intelligence algorithms and sensors and the progression of this technology. In the event that there are any mistakes in the technique that was used to collect or process the data, it is possible that wrong decisions would be made, which could put the patient in risk. Because of this, the system needs to be subjected to routine maintenance and upgrades in order to guarantee that it displays accurate information.

Within the context of the healthcare system, the decision-making system that is based on IoT and is being implemented by KSK has the potential to totally transform the way in which blood pressure patients are monitored. Through the utilization of this technology, it is feasible to monitor, anticipate, and regulate their status in a manner that is both more precise and more economical. As IoT and AI continue to grow, we should anticipate increased inventiveness in the healthcare industry. The outcomes for patients as well as their quality of life will be improved as a result of these solutions.

RESULTS

The tests that were conducted with several classification algorithms, including DT, ANN, and K-NN in the KSK approach, will be examined. The section that follows provided a description of these experiments. Blood pressure-related disease datasets are among the many diverse disease datasets that have been used. The dataset—which comprised several samples—that was actually used is given in Table 1 and Figure 4.

Table 1. Dataset utilized for experimentation

Sr. No.	Dataset	Number of Samples
1	BP	780
2	Training Dataset used	624
3	Testing dataset	156

To make experimental research easier, the dataset is divided into two ratios. 20% and 80% are the ratios. Eighty percent of the data set goes towards developing categorization techniques, with the remaining twenty percent going towards testing. We perform an analysis on each of the three different classifiers to evaluate their sensitivity, specificity, and precision.

Figure 4. Dataset segregation

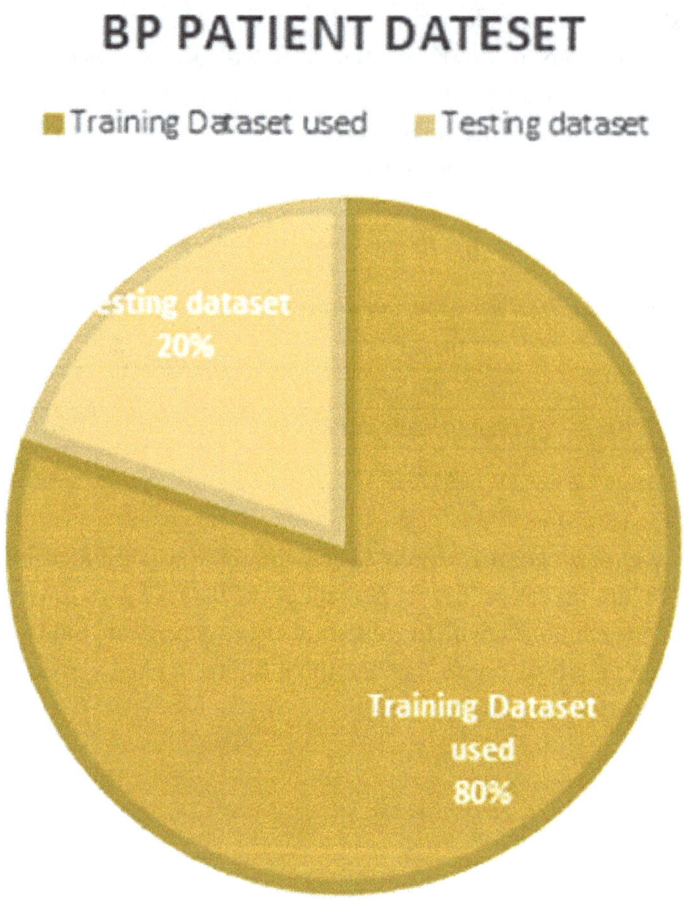

There are three different classifiers used for BP, and each has a unique set of performance metrics. According to Dr. K S Kazi's KSK method, three different classifiers should have been used for the BP dataset. The accuracy, precision, and recall of these classifiers are shown in Figures 5, 6, and 7, respectively.

Figure 5. Accuracy for KSK approach with BP dataset

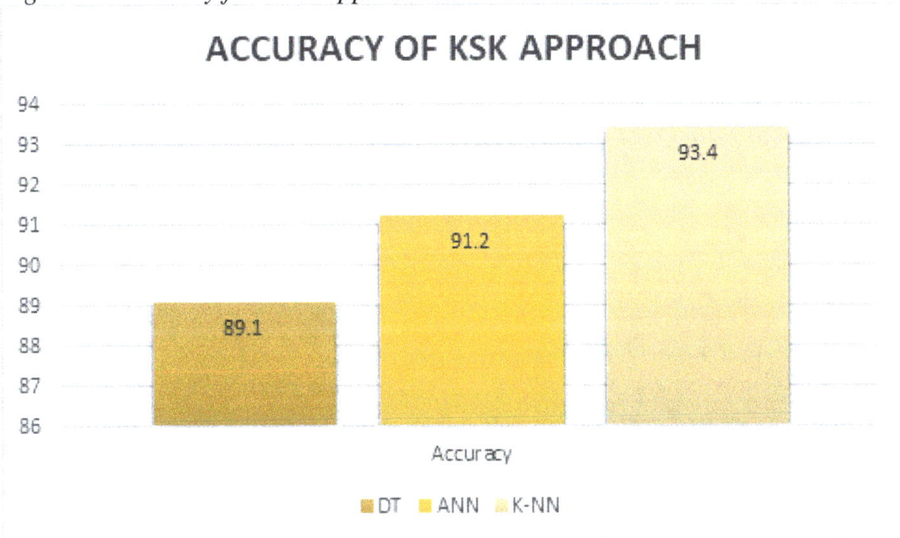

From Figure 5, the accuracy of proposed KSK approach with DT is 89.1%, with ANN is 91.2% and with K-NN is 93.4%. The accuracy for K-NN is higher than other two methods, hence the decision is that the accuracy is 93.4% with KSK approach.

Figure 6. Precision for KSK approach with BP dataset

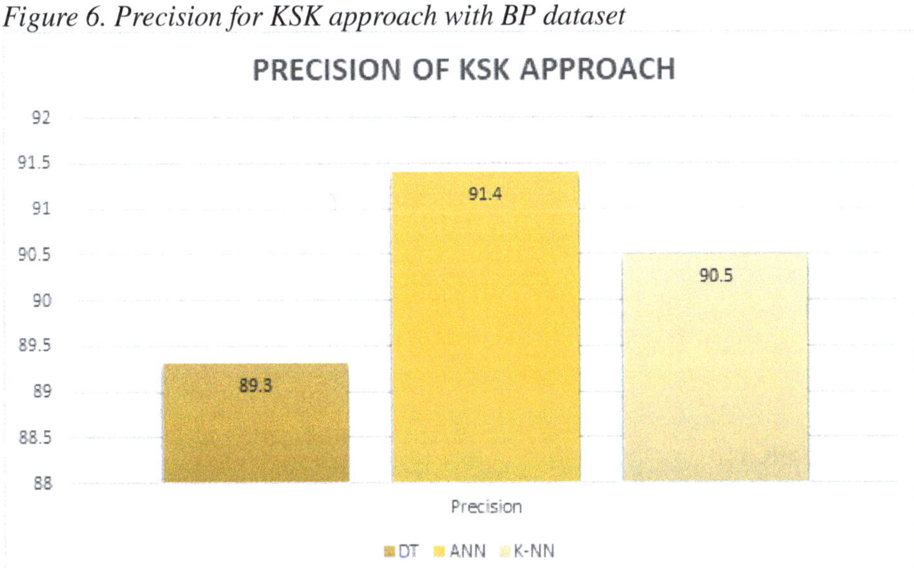

From Figure 6, the precision of proposed KSK approach with DT is 89.3%, with ANN is 91.4% and with K-NN is 90.5%. The precision for ANN is higher than other two methods, hence the decision is that the accuracy is 91.4% with KSK approach.

Figure 7. Recall for KSK approach with BP dataset

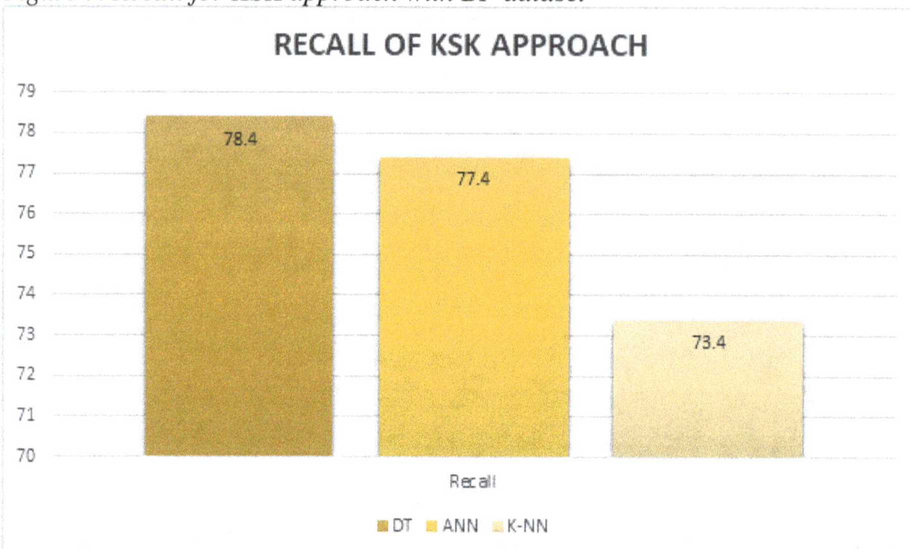

From Figure 7, the recall of proposed KSK approach with DT is 78.4% with ANN is 77.4% and with K-NN is 73.4%. The accuracy for DT is higher than other two methods, hence the decision is that the accuracy is 78.4% with KSK approach.

As can be seen in Figures 5, 6, and 7, recall of DT is higher than ANN and K-NN (78.4%), accuracy of K-NN is higher than ANN and DT (95.4%), and precision of ANN is more than the other two (01.4% and 78.4%). For decision-making, the KSK method therefore recommends DT, ANN, and K-NN. The KSK strategy is the most appropriate method if we wish to base any decision on memory, accuracy, or precision. Thus, at the end, we determined that DT had a higher recall, ANN had a higher precision, and K-NN had a higher accuracy.

CONCLUSION

In a nutshell the application of AI classification algorithms to the prediction and decision-making of diseases and illnesses is still in its infancy. The KSK approach suggests using the k-nearest-neighbors(K-NN) algorithm, decision tree (DT), and artificial neural networks (ANN) for decision making. Using three different AI classification algorithms—Decision Tree (DT), Artificial Neural Network(ANN), and K-Nearest Neighbors (K-NN)—we constructed a healthcare model for the proposed study. This model was created especially for the intended investigation. These classifiers are used on disease datasets, specifically blood pressure datasets. The effectiveness of the KSK method is evaluated using three metrics. Recall, accuracy, and precision are among the metrics. The accuracy rate of the current KSK approach in the healthcare industry ranges from 89% to 93% for each ailment. Therefore, based on Figure 5, Figure 6, and Figure 7, we can ultimately draw the conclusion that K-NN has higher accuracy, ANN has higher precision, and DT has higher recall.

FUTURE SCOPE: In future, we will Implement the Low-BP patient health using KSK1 approach.

REFERENCES

Dhanwe, S. S., (2024). AI-driven IoT in Robotics: A Review. *Journal of Mechanisms and Robotics*, 9(1), 41–48.

Halli, U. M. (2022). Nanotechnology in IoT Security, *Journal of Nanoscience. Nanoengineering & Applications*, 12(3), 11–16.

Kasat, K., Shaikh, N., Rayabharapu, V. K., & Nayak, M. (2023). Implementation and Recognition of Waste Management System with Mobility Solution in Smart Cities using Internet of Things, *2023 Second International Conference on Augmented Intelligence and Sustainable Systems (ICAISS)*, Trichy, India, 2023, pp. 1661-1665, DOI: 10.1109/ICAISS58487.2023.10250690

Kazi, K. (2024). Modelling and Simulation of Electric Vehicle for Performance Analysis: BEV and HEV Electrical Vehicle Implementation Using Simulink for E-Mobility Ecosystems. In L. D., N. Nagpal, N. Kassarwani, V. Varthanan G., & P. Siano (Eds.), E-Mobility in Electrical Energy Systems for Sustainability (pp. 295-320). IGI Global. Available at: https://www.igi-global.com/gateway/chapter/full-text-pdf/341172DOI: 10.4018/979-8-3693-2611-4.ch014

Kazi, K. (2024). AI-Driven IoT (AIIoT) in Healthcare Monitoring. In Nguyen, T., & Vo, N. (Eds.), *Using Traditional Design Methods to Enhance AI-Driven Decision Making* (pp. 77–101). IGI Global., available at https://www.igi-global.com/chapter/ai-driven-iot-aiiot-in-healthcare-monitoring/336693, DOI: 10.4018/979-8-3693-0639-0.ch003

Kazi, K. (2024). Complications with Malware Identification in IoT and an Overview of Artificial Immune Approaches. *Research & Reviews. The Journal of Immunology : Official Journal of the American Association of Immunologists*, 14(01), 54–62.

Kazi, K. (2024a). Machine Learning (ML)-Based Braille Lippi Characters and Numbers Detection and Announcement System for Blind Children in Learning. In Sart, G. (Ed.), *Social Reflections of Human-Computer Interaction in Education, Management, and Economics*. IGI Global., DOI: 10.4018/979-8-3693-3033-3.ch002

Kazi, K. (2024a). IoT Technologies for the Intelligent Dairy Industry: A New Challenge. In Thandekkattu, S. G., & Vajjhala, N. R. (Eds.), *Designing Sustainable Internet of Things Solutions for Smart Industries*. IGI Global. DOI: 10.4018/979-8-3693-5498-8.ch012

Kazi, K. (2024b). Machine Learning-Driven-Internet of Things(MLIoT) Based Healthcare Monitoring System. In Wickramasinghe, N. (Ed.), *Impact of Digital Solutions for Improved Healthcare Delivery*. IGI Global.

Kazi, K. (2024c). Moonlighting in Carrier. In Tunio, M. N. (Ed.), *Applications of Career Transitions and Entrepreneurship*. IGI Global.

Kazi, K. (2024d). Heart Health Monitoring Using IoT and Machine Learning Methods. In Shaik, A. (Ed.), *AI-Powered Advances in Pharmacology*. IGI Global.

Kazi, K. S. (2017). Significance And Usage Of Face Recognition System. *Scholarly Journal For Humanity Science and English Language*, 4(20), 4764–4772.

Kazi, K. S. (2024). Computer-Aided Diagnosis in Ophthalmology: A Technical Review of Deep Learning Applications. In Garcia, M., & de Almeida, R. (Eds.), *Transformative Approaches to Patient Literacy and Healthcare Innovation* (pp. 112–135). IGI Global., Available at https://www.igi-global.com/chapter/computer-aided-diagnosis-in-ophthalmology/342823, DOI: 10.4018/979-8-3693-3661-8.ch006

Kazi, K. S. (2024). Artificial Intelligence (AI)-Driven IoT (AIIoT)-Based Agriculture Automation. In Satapathy, S., & Muduli, K. (Eds.), *Advanced Computational Methods for Agri-Business Sustainability* (pp. 72–94). IGI Global., DOI: 10.4018/979-8-3693-3583-3.ch005

Kazi, K. S. (2024). Machine Learning-Based Pomegranate Disease Detection and Treatment. In Zia Ul Haq, M., & Ali, I. (Eds.), *Revolutionizing Pest Management for Sustainable Agriculture* (pp. 469–498). IGI Global., DOI: 10.4018/979-8-3693-3061-6.ch019

Kazi, K. S. (2024b). IoT Driven by Machine Learning (MLIoT) for the Retail Apparel Sector. In Tarnanidis, T., Papachristou, E., Karypidis, M., & Ismyrlis, V. (Eds.), *Driving Green Marketing in Fashion and Retail* (pp. 63–81). IGI Global., DOI: 10.4018/979-8-3693-3049-4.ch004

Kazi, K. S. L. (2018). Significance of Projection and Rotation of Image in Color Matching for High-Quality Panoramic Images used for Aquatic study. *International Journal of Aquatic Science*, 09(02), 130–145.

Kazi, K. S. L. (2024). IoT and Sensor-based Smart Agriculturing Driven by NodeMCU. *Research & Review: Electronics and Communication Engineering*, 1(2), 25–33.

Kazi, K. S. L. (2024). Smart Agriculture based on AI-Driven-IoT(AIIoT): A KSK Approach, *Advance Research in Communication Engineering and its. Innovations*, 1(2), 23–32.

Kazi, K. S. L. (2024). Nanotechnology in BattleField: A Study. *Journal of Nanoscience. Nanoengineering & Applications.*, 14(2), 18–30p.

Kazi, K., & Sayyad, L., (2024). Explainable AI in Healthcare. In Anitha Kamaraj, A. (Ed.), *Explainable Artificial Intelligence in healthcare System.* Debi Prasanna Acharjya., DOI: 10.52305/GOMR8163

Kazi, K., Sayyad L., (2024). Nanotechnology in Medical Applications: A Study. *Nano Trends: A Journal of Nanotechnology and Its Applications.* 2024; 26(2): 1–11p. DOI: 10.52305/GOMR8163

Kutubuddin, K. (2024c). Vehicle Health Monitoring System (VHMS) by Employing IoT and Sensors, *Grenze International Journal of Engineering and Technology,* Vol 10, Issue 2, pp- 5367-5374. Available at: https://thegrenze.com/index.php?display=page&view=journalabstract&absid=3371&id=8

Kutubuddin, K. (2024e). A Novel Approach on ML based Palmistry, *Grenze International Journal of Engineering and Technology,* Vol 10, Issue 2, pp- 5186-5193. Available at: https://thegrenze.com/index.php?display=page&view=journalabstract&absid=3344&id=8

Kutubuddin, K. (2024e). IoT based Boiler Health Monitoring for Sugar Industries, *Grenze. IACSIT International Journal of Engineering and Technology*, 10(2), 5178–5185. https://thegrenze.com/index.php?display=page&view=journalabstract&absid=3343&id=8

Liyakat, K. K. S. (2023).Detecting Malicious Nodes in IoT Networks Using Machine Learning and Artificial Neural Networks, *2023 International Conference on Emerging Smart Computing and Informatics (ESCI)*, Pune, India, 2023, pp. 1-5, DOI: 10.1109/ESCI56872.2023.10099544

Liyakat, K. K. S. (2023). Machine Learning Approach Using Artificial Neural Networks to Detect Malicious Nodes in IoT Networks. In Shukla, P. K., Mittal, H., & Engelbrecht, A. (Eds.), *Computer Vision and Robotics. CVR 2023. Algorithms for Intelligent Systems.* Springer., DOI: 10.1007/978-981-99-4577-1_3

Liyakat, K. K. S. (2024). Machine Learning Approach Using Artificial Neural Networks to Detect Malicious Nodes in IoT Networks. In Udgata, S. K., Sethi, S., & Gao, X. Z. (Eds.), *Intelligent Systems. ICMIB 2023. Lecture Notes in Networks and Systems* (Vol. 728). Springer., available at https://link.springer.com/chapter/10.1007/978-981-99-3932-9_12, DOI: 10.1007/978-981-99-3932-9_12

Liyakat, K. K. S. (2024). Explainable AI in healthcare. *Explainable Artificial Intelligence in Healthcare Systems*, 2024, 271–284.

Liyakat, K. S. (2023). Intelligent Watering System (IWS) for Agricultural Land Utilising Raspberry Pi. *Recent Trends in Fluid Mechanics.*, 10(2), 26–31.

Liyakat, S. S. (2023a). Nanomedicine as a Potential Therapeutic Approach to COVID-19. *International Journal of Applied Nanotechnology*, 9(2), 27–35p.

Liyakat, S. S. (2023b). IoT Changing the Electronics Manufacturing Industry. *Journal of Analog and Digital Communications*, 8(3), 13–17. DOI: 10.46610/JoADC.2023.v08i03.003

Liyakat, S. S. (2023c). IoT in the Electric Power Industry. *Journal of Controller and Converters*, 8(3), 1–7.

Liyakat, S. S. (2024). IoT-based Alcohol Detector using Blynk. *Journal of Electronics Design and Technology*, 1(1), 10–15.

Liyakat Kazi, K. S. (2024). ChatGPT: An Automated Teacher's Guide to Learning. In Bansal, R., Chakir, A., Hafaz Ngah, A., Rabby, F., & Jain, A. (Eds.), *AI Algorithms and ChatGPT for Student Engagement in Online Learning* (pp. 1–20). IGI Global., DOI: 10.4018/979-8-3693-4268-8.ch001

Mishra Sunil, B.. (2024). AI-Driven IoT (AI IoT) in Thermodynamic Engineering. *Journal of Modern Thermodynamics in Mechanical System*, 6(1), 1–8.

Nagrale, M., Pol, R. S., Birajadar, G. B., & Mulani, A. O. (2024). Internet of Robotic Things in Cardiac Surgery: An Innovative Approach. *African Journal of Biological Sciences*, 6(6), 709–725. DOI: 10.33472/AFJBS.6.6.2024.709-725

Neeraja, P., Kumar, R. G., Kumar, M. S., Liyakat, K. K. S., & Vani, M. S. (2024, February). DL-based somnolence detection for improved driver safety and alertness monitoring. In 2024 IEEE International Conference on Computing, Power and Communication Technologies (IC2PCT) (Vol. 5, pp. 589-594). IEEE.

Nerkar, P. M., & Dhaware, B. U. (2023). Predictive Data Analytics Framework Based on Heart Healthcare System (HHS) Using Machine Learning, Journal of Advanced Zoology, 2023, Volume 44, Special Issue -2. *Page*, 3673, 3686.

Pradeepa, M., ... (2022). Student Health Detection using a Machine Learning Approach and IoT, 2022 IEEE 2nd Mysore sub section International Conference (MysuruCon), 2022.

Prasad, K. R., Karanam, S. R., Ganesh, D., Liyakat, K. K. S., Talasila, V., & Purushotham, P. (2024, May). AI in public-private partnership for IT infrastructure development. *The Journal of High Technology Management Research*, 35(1), 100496. DOI: 10.1016/j.hitech.2024.100496

Kutubuddin, K. (2022). Business Mode and Product Life Cycle to Improve Marketing in Healthcare Units, *E-Commerce for Future & Trends*, 2022, vol 9, issue 3, pp. 1-9. DOI: 10.1016/j.hitech.2024.100496

Kumar, M. S., Ganesh, D., Turukmane, A. V., Batta, U., & Sayyadliyakat, K. K. (2022). Deep convolution neural network based solution for detecting plant diseases. *Journal of Pharmaceutical Negative Results*, 13, 464–471.

Veena, C., Sridevi, M., Liyakat, K. K. S., Saha, B., Reddy, S. R., & Shirisha, N. (2023). *"HEECCNB: An Efficient IoT-Cloud Architecture for Secure Patient Data Transmission and Accurate Disease Prediction in Healthcare Systems," 2023 Seventh International Conference on Image Information Processing*. ICIIP., Available at https://ieeexplore.ieee.org/document/10537627, DOI: 10.1109/ICIIP61524.2023.10537627

Wale, A. D., & Dipali, R.. (2019). Smart Agriculture System using IoT. *International Journal of Innovative Research In Technology*, 5(10), 493–497.

Chapter 8
Mechanism-Based PKPD Models for Rifampicin Evaluation:
Quantitative Systems Pharmacology Through Pharmacometrics

Zuber Peermohammed Shaikh
Savitribai Phule Pune University, India

ABSTRACT

This research paper demonstrates role of QSP modeling efforts in Rifampicin development program via empirical pharmaceutical research, which were selected to cover a wide range of mathematical modeling methods including agent-based modeling, partial differential equation modeling, and ordinary differential equation modeling. Other applications of systems modeling include evaluation of new target pathways; optimization of compound physicochemical properties; characterization of efficacy and toxicity mechanisms of action; recommendation of treatment posology of monotherapies and combination therapies by balancing efficacy and toxicity; and guidance of study subject stratification strategies based on clinical responder features. Particularly, quantitative systems modeling plays a critical role in predicting clinical hematological toxicity risks by translating preclinical data obtained from micro-physiological systems (MPS). The analysis of Rifampicin as personalized medicine in MPS data is routinely performed to simulate clinical outcomes under various dosage regimens.

DOI: 10.4018/979-8-3693-6270-9.ch008

INTRODUCTION

Quantitative Systems Pharmacology through Pharmacometrics: Since its advent as an approach described in the NIH white paper from 2011, quantitative systems pharmacology (QSP) modeling has gained popularity in Rifampicin development. While the scope of QSP modeling needs further clarification, it includes an attempt to quantitatively unravel the complex mechanisms and interactions between physiology and Rifampicins (including investigational Rifampicins) to predict responses given a Rifampicin intervention. *Systems biology-based models* describe biological pathways and their regulatory networks at molecular, cellular, tissue, and organ system levels to further the understanding of biological processes. *Pharmacokinetic-pharmacodynamic (PKPD) modeling* aims towards understanding pharmacological responses by quantifying the relationship between observed Rifampicin exposure and its observed non-clinical or clinical endpoints, often linking exposure to one endpoint whilst QSP models are used to capture multiple longitudinal biomarker measurements simultaneously in disease platform models. PKPD modeling is considered a top-down approach such that it is driven by already-observed data, whereas *systems biology-based modeling* is a bottom-up approach in that it starts from the fundamental understanding of biological knowledge such as molecular or cellular signaling pathways to predict the behavior of biological systems. In this context, *quantitative systems pharmacology modeling* can be considered as a balanced platform of bottom-up and top-down modeling approaches, which allows integration of biological knowledge available *a priori* and observed data obtained posteriori to help Rifampicin development decisions in a science-informed and practical way. *(Asad M.,2020)*

Figure 1. Quantitative systems pharmacology models balance the models

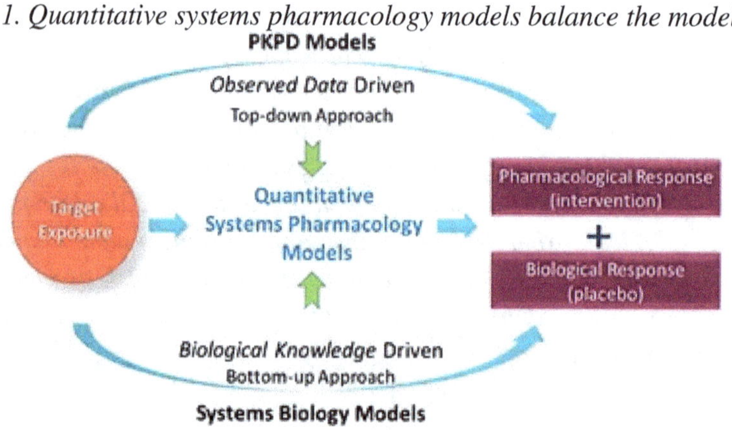

The availability of quantitative longitudinal data from non-clinical research has led to the increased use of these models in the internal decision-making process in pharmaceutical companies. QSP models are developed at various biological scales ranging from cellular, molecular, tissue, organ, patient, and/or population levels, thereby highlighting the use of these models in delineating various multiscale mechanisms of pharmacological responses. These models have been used to determine the affinity required to engage a target; aid the target validation and lead discovery stage; predict and monitor Rifampicin response by identifying appropriate biomarkers; and predict toxicity effects in various organs. QSP models are frequently used for dosage regimen decisions for first-in-human studies by utilizing a wide range of non-clinical data and publishing competitor's clinical data. In addition, the models allow cost-effective assessment to help understand target engagement for efficacy and safety risks for optimization of clinical study designs. Furthermore, the QSP modeling approach can be also taken to efficiently expedite development for an alternate Rifampicin indication during life cycle management process wherein the Rifampicin targets different diseases or patient populations *via* the same or similar mechanism of action. There are several publications that emphasize the emerging potential of QSP applications for pharmaceutical research in improving Rifampicin development decision-making.

The availability of biological knowledge and data from the preclinical stage allows development of QSP models, but the sparsity and limited granularity of observed data still constrains their predictive capability. Nevertheless, employment of these models at the stage, where clinical data is yet to be collected, has the potential to predict clinical responses to make an impact in the decisions of dosage regimen, subject enrollment criteria, sampling/monitoring times, biomarker-adaptive clinical trial design, rescue Rifampicin intervention strategy, *etc.* (*Asare P., 2020)*

QSP model applications in the clinical stage include further addressing the biological mechanism of action of a therapeutic agent; identifying biomarkers to predict clinical success; or understanding disease pathology, which provides a way to address clinical development decisions such as biomarker interpretation, study subject enrollment stratification, or competitive landscape evaluation. An example of a successful application of QSP models from a clinician's point of view may include offering insights on dosage individualization, based on their biomarker levels, to improve the probability of success of the treatment. Precision medicine will be better achieved by providing appropriate diagnostic tools: these technologies can help clinicians quantify multiple relevant biomarkers to subgroup patients in their susceptibility to a disease, prognosis, or likelihood of responding to a Rifampicin, and a QSP approach can guide the decisions on which biomarker(s) is the most informative.

LITERATURE REVIEW

Mechanism Based PKPD Models: These is a schematic showing potential impact of systems modeling in the Rifampicin development pipeline. In this paper, we highlight the impact of QSP modeling *via* three case study applications that answered specific questions in early Rifampicin development. We show how various modeling approaches such as agent-based modeling (ABM); hybrid modeling with ordinary differential equations (ODE), partial differential equations (PDE), and ABM; and non-linear mixed-effects modeling with ODE are routinely used to influence the internal decision-making processes at various Rifampicin development stages at AstraZeneca. *Case 1* shows how an agent-based modeling approach can be used in the context of gastrointestinal safety assessment (predictions of chemotherapy-induced diarrhea); *Case 2* shows a hybrid model in the context of cardiovascular diseases guiding study dosage regimen decisions in human ventricular progenitor therapy development and *Case 3*show how a systems modeling approach was used in oncology for the characterization of the interplay of longitudinal biomarkers given little available data. The mathematical details (code and impact) of these case studies will be discussed in separate stand-alone papers. (*Azad A. K., 2012)*

Computational modeling approach: In pursuit of this dictionary, we developed an agent-based model that simulated the interactions of individual cells (the agents) interacting in the geometry of the crypt. The model incorporates all the major cell types and multiple clinically relevant signaling mechanisms. It replicates the geometry, physical and mechanical forces and cell zonation of *in vivo* crypts and demonstrates many experimentally observed phenotypes. With the assumption that the mechanistic action of a Rifampicin is the same in organoids and real crypts, we used this agent-based model to transfer the experimentally observed effects in human-derived organoids into predictions of chemotherapy-induced diarrhea in real patients. The model can be viewed as an *in silico* organ that, by replicating multiple aspects of human biology, can be used in the Rifampicin-discovery pipeline to make safety and toxicity predictions, circumventing the need for animal studies, and/or test biological hypotheses to gain mechanistic insight.

Figure 2. Applications of quantitative systems models throughout Rifampicin development pipeline

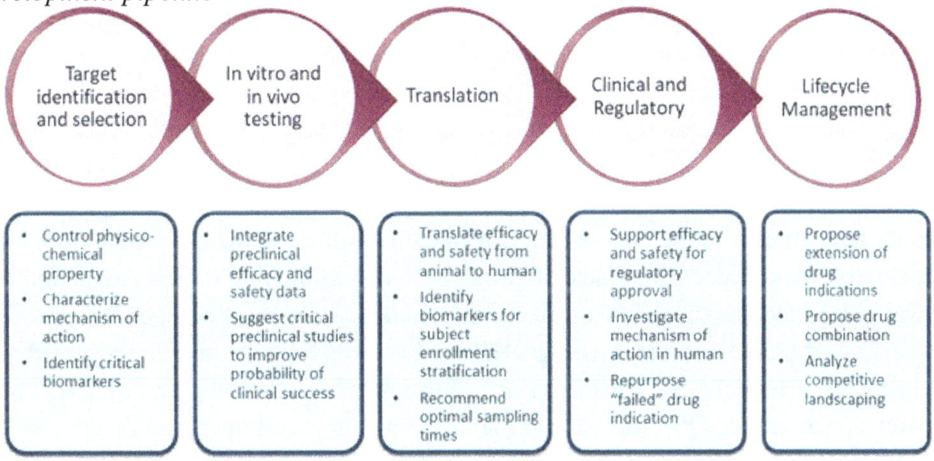

Agent Based Modelling: The intestinal crypt is particularly amenable to an **agent-based modelling approach** for a selection of historic applications of agent-based modelling to the intestinal crypt). The compartmentalization of the cells in the crypt, and the inner workings of signaling mechanisms that cause this, are well studied, with bountiful single-cell data (including signaling knockouts, ablations of single types of cells, and more) with spatial and temporal resolution. Indeed, building an agent-based model of the gastrointestinal crypt is not a new concept, but our new model contains an unprecedented number of sub-systems (internal protein networks and intercellular signaling mechanisms), allowing it to recreate many clinically relevant phenotypes, recovering from a variety of injuries in experimentally verified fashion. For the development of the model, we focused on three key tenets (in roughly ascending order of importance): computational speed/efficiency, modularity, and a focus on emergent behavior. Computational speed has long plagued agent-based modelling and is a topic of great interest. The simulation of all the agents can be computationally intensive and hence time consuming, but in our current model, a full virtual Rifampicin exposure with all analytics obtained from the model can be calculated within minutes on a standard consumer laptop. In a pharmacological setting, this is a vital feature: a quick, efficient model allows many more trial simulations for greater accuracy in results, increasing flexibility in testing hypotheses and vastly improving ease of use.

Biological and Pharmacological systems: Given our understanding of the crucial role that QSP plays, some challenges exist in the path towards achieving the goals set for QSP models. The major challenge is the limitation in data to support complex biological and pharmacological systems. Inconsistent, imbalanced, missing and/or limited data in various datasets can affect the prediction accuracy of these models. Fortunately, project experimentalists are willing to conduct studies to generate essential data if such studies are both feasible to conduct and considered valuable for better clinical prediction *via* modeling. However, complex assay development and inherently complex physiological systems result into scarcity of relevant multi-scale data. These challenges may lead to modeling bias with incorrect assumptions, which requires systems modelers to develop computationally efficient methods to check the model performance (e.g., multi-parameter model diagnostic profiling. Another notable challenge is the accessibility of models with standardized annotation. To meet the accelerated timelines of projects that require model-derived insights, available models in the public domain can be adopted to answer compound-specific questions thereby eliminating the need to build a model from scratch. However, often times, these models can fail to run or fail to reproduce published outcomes. The external sharing of QSP models *via* markup languages and open-source code will help enhance the reusability and collaborative development of these models. This is particularly important if QSP models are to be accepted as a part of regulatory submissions because, from a regulatory perspective, this transparency will improve the admissibility of these models. (*Bakuła Z., 2023)*

There is a steady rise in both ***QSP-related publications and submissions*** to the US Food Rifampicin Administration (FDA), but the inclusion of QSP models in regulatory documents is still at its early stages. In 2014, the US FDA evaluated an alternate dosing regimen in the treatment of hypoparathyroidism, which was possible using an open-source QSP model. Based on the quantitative evaluation of the model, the FDA asked for optimization of the dosing regimen to address safety concerns for hypercalciuria. It is therefore important for QSP models to be transparent, reproducible and be extended beyond the research space to have an impact in Rifampicin development. A consortium-based article by the UK QSP network group (created in 2015) outlined the recommendations and provided a checklist of best practices for QSP models that can enhance the quality, reproducibility, and further applicability of QSP models. Gadkar et al. highlighted the important components of the QSP modeling process crucial for success, which includes the identification of impactful questions, understanding of time constraints and agreement on feasible modeling goals as crucial parts of project initiation. FDA scientists discussed model calibration, validation, and performance of a few published QSP models and proposed a list of questions to be addressed for the QSP model assessment to establish common expectations. (*Bateson A., 2022)*

The systems modeling approaches have been useful for company's discussions thereby facilitating go/no-go decisions or study design decisions. While the potential of QSP modeling approaches needs more clinical verification, the future iterations of these models with clinical data from various stages can especially aid in reducing the Phase I concerns on safety, assisting in repositioning Phase II efficacy 'failures', and/or assisting in patient increase responder rates by proposing study subject stratification strategy. It is important to note that as clinical development is expensive compared to non-clinical and early development, tailoring each step of Rifampicin development with earlier quantitative pharmacological understanding of a Rifampicin candidate can aid overall financial savings. With the recent advancement in biomarker assay methods, novel non-clinical experiment systems, and high computing power, in addition to an interest in model-informed Rifampicin development by academia, regulatory agencies, and pharmaceutical companies, we anticipate more successful use cases of QSP modeling integrated in Rifampicin development and regulatory decisions.

Next-generation sequencing (NGS) has emerged as a powerful tool for understanding the genetic background of various infectious diseases, including TB. In the context of PPPM, NGS can transform and accelerate the delivery of personalized treatment to patients affected by TB, thus revolutionizing the way TB is diagnosed and treated. A more comprehensive Rifampicin susceptibility profile is needed to design an effective treatment plan for patients with Rifampicin-resistant TB. WGS has been identified as a highly promising tool for this particular purpose. Cox et al. recently employed WGS to assess the accuracy of treatment regimens (derived from standard Rifampicin susceptibility testing and clinical information) in individuals with Rifampicin-resistant TB. Overall, 305 (24%) patients had MDR/rifampicin resistant (RR)-TB with second-line TB Rifampicin resistance, where the availability of WGS-derived Rifampicin susceptibility testing (DST) would have enabled more effective treatment personalization for these patients, such as reducing Rifampicin dosages or removing ineffective Rifampicins. Similarly, the results of Korhonen demonstrated that WGS could aid in the selection of optimal treatment regimens in the future, primarily for patients with resistance to ethambutol. The application of WGS in routine clinical practice also enables rapid identification of isoniazid monoresistance, reducing delays in treatment decisions and initiating WHO-recommended treatment for isoniazid-resistant TB. In settings with a low incidence of TB, WGS reduced the time required for appropriate treatment modification, thus decreasing the expenses associated with hospitalization and treatment. (*Berrocal-Almanza L. C., 2022)*

BACKGROUND

As tremendous time and effort is required to develop these complex models, early engagement between modelers and the project team is necessary. Due to the inherent nature of the QSP model framework being multiscale; being computationally complex; and requiring extensive data from non-clinical as well as clinical space, early-stage planning and involvement of QSP modelers in the project team are inevitable. The development and success of these models are dependent on i) the quality, amount, and type of data available from non-clinical to clinical research and ii) the interdisciplinary collaboration among translational scientists, quantitative modelers (who understand pharmacology and systems biology), and clinicians. Especially, rapid advancement in new Rifampicin modalities such as cell therapy, gene therapy, bis-specific engagers, antisense nucleotides to name a few (that accompany a plethora of hypotheses and missing information in addition to observed data) requires input from various expertise to help integrate the available knowledge. This further emphasizes the need for collaboration and makes it inevitable to have continuing conversation, engagement among the modeler, project team, and regulatory agencies regarding model use, model credibility assessment, verification, and risk decision.

Prediction of Toxicity: AI systems that examine the properties and chemical structures of molecules can forecast the toxicity of Rifampicins. Trained in toxicology databases, machine learning algorithms are able to recognize potentially dangerous structural features or predict deleterious consequences. In clinical studies, this helps researchers minimize potential negative reactions and prioritize safer Rifampicins. All things considered, the identification, optimization, and creation of innovative therapeutic candidates may be sped up and streamlined with the use of AI in Rifampicin research and development, ultimately producing more effective and efficient Rifampicins. *(Bonnet I., 2022)*

Two key facets of research using nucleic acids are ***pharmacokinetic modulation and molecular stabilization.*** These molecular forms' pharmacokinetic exposure and improvement are essential objectives. In order to address these problems and find solutions, new technological advances may be useful.

However, because of the grey area in the results, human interpretation is necessary to arrive at the correct conclusion. Algorithm bias can cause problems for AI when it comes to analyzing data for predictions and evaluating theories. Furthermore, it frequently happens that molecules that are inactive are found by docking simulations.

Clinical Trial Predictive Modelling: Clinical trial results can be predicted through the application of supervised learning. The model can learn to predict patient response, treatment efficacy, or safety outcomes by training on historical clinical trial data, which includes patient characteristics, treatment interventions, and trial outcomes. Optimizing patient selection and trial design can be achieved with the help of this information. *(Botha, G. H. R., 2018)*

AI in Treatment of Tuberculosis: The development of novel molecular diagnostic methods has also made a huge contribution to the personalization of therapy and the prevention of TB transmission. Utilizing the full potential of NGS, comprehensive insights into the phylogenetic lineage of infecting strains can provide clinicians with valuable information regarding the likelihood of the strain developing additional Rifampicin resistance. These innovative approaches in TB treatment signify a new era in the management of MDR-TB that will aid in mitigating treatment failure and ongoing transmission. (*Cabibbe A. M., 2020)*

In contrast to the aforementioned advantages, there are several potential knowledge gaps and areas for future research regarding the management of TB and the roles of AI, genetic screening, and WGS. The successful integration of AI into clinical practice for TB management requires a holistic approach that addresses technical, regulatory, educational, and usability aspects. Research in these areas can pave the way for more effective and widespread use of AI to combat TB and improve patient outcomes. In the realm of genetic screening for TB management, research should focus on understanding population-specific variations and assessing the cost-effectiveness of these screening methods. It's essential to determine the accuracy of genetic markers, integrate them effectively into clinical decision-making, and provide ethical patient counseling. Additionally, research should explore the impact on healthcare systems and potential contributions to Rifampicin development. Global collaboration and data sharing are also vital for advancing this field. In summary, addressing these knowledge gaps and conducting research in these areas can contribute to more effective TB control and management strategies, ultimately reducing the global burden of this disease.

METHODOLOGY

Pharmacokinetic/pharmacodynamic (PK/PD) modeling connects PK and PD to facilitate the prediction of the time course of Rifampicin effects that result from a specific dosing regimen. Systems pharmacology is already widely used in the pharmaceutical industry, focusing on PK/PD modeling, predicting dose-exposure responses, and evaluating market potential. This modeling assists in gaining mechanistic insights and facilitates early dose selection. In addition, population PK/PD modeling can help understand the critical PK characteristics and population-level covariates. Physiologically-based pharmacokinetic (PBPK) modeling presents the pharmacokinetic behavior of a compound in the body and predicts the ADME of natural or synthetic substances in humans and other species. Physiologically based pharmacokinetic/pharmacodynamic (PBPK/PD) models connect Rifampicin information with prior knowledge of physiology and biology at the organism level to provide a mechanistic representation of the Rifampicin in biological systems. PBPK models consider different organs and tissues and assist in obtaining quantitative characterizations of concentration–time profiles in the individual compartments. This modeling approach can be utilized to understand tissue-specific PK and PD and estimate Rifampicin interaction risks. According to a survey across 50 pharmaceutical companies, the industry has a vague definition of QSP. Although this survey showed that most pharmaceutical companies used the QSP term to describe their modeling approaches, a significant number of companies used other terms for mentioning their modeling activities. Therefore, to accelerate improvements in Rifampicin discoveries, one suggestion can be to use fixed terminologies that assist in studying and investigating QSP models. The aforementioned study also showed that the most common applications in this field are related to generating and testing hypotheses, optimizing doses or regimens, predicting clinical efficacy, and identifying biomarkers suggesting that future opportunities in the industry can be related to the usage of QSP modeling for evaluating safety and decision-making. *(Cavaco M. J., 2022)*

Target fishing (TF) in silico technique, for instance, is used in medicines to predict biological targets based on chemical structure. The information shown here is based on the biologically annotated data that is accessible in the chemical database. To further explore the mechanism of action and provide the target class information needed for efficient planning, a number of additional techniques were employed, including data mining and chemical structure docking. Combining ***cheminformatics*** tools with machine learning enabled the application of the target fishing technique in Rifampicin discovery. These two are utilized to gather in depth information about how to properly analyze complex structures and create unique therapeutic ingredients that will effectively cure complex disorders. The standard Rifampicin discovery procedures used by various companies are highly expensive since they entail a number of intricate steps that must be correctly completed, such as the identification and selection of the target proteins and a thorough understanding of the small molecules' mechanisms of action. TF was used to expedite this procedure, which helped lower the overall cost of experiments during the Rifampicin development processes. With the aid of 3D descriptors, reference molecules are utilized to predict the target ligand.

This method was employed to determine diethylstilbestrol's strong binding ability, whereas the TF technique is frequently utilized to analyze monthly similarity scores and investigate the Rifampicin's phytopharmacology. This method is computational, and proteomics based, with data points ranked according to how similar their data fusion is to therapeutic targets. It is also applied in the forecasting of possible toxicities for the ligand-based Rifampicin development methodology. With the help of TF, some crucial elements of the Rifampicin development and Rifampicin discovery phases are investigated. These elements include the identification and selection of novel targets, the prediction of phytopharmacological profiles, and the prediction of side effects related to novel therapeutic indications. In order to identify the target for these occurrences, the bioactive compound similarity to the unidentified molecule is applied. A number of medications, including methadone and loperamide, have been effectively characterized by the use of this technique; muscarinic, adrenergic, and neurokinin receptors have been identified as the Rifampicins' respective targets]. With the application of AI models and tools, the field of Rifampicin development has made considerable strides. *(Chen X., 2020)*

Unsupervised AI Learning: Unsupervised learning is a kind of machine learning in which labelled data is not given to the algorithm. Rather, it has to work on its own to find patterns and connections in the data. This method can be helpful in identifying hidden structures or clusters within a dataset and is frequently applied in exploration data analysis. The methodology being discussed is referred to as a "data-driven methodology," and its goal is to identify patterns, structures, or insights in unannotated data. Finding association rules, visualizing data, dimensionality reduction, grouping, and anomaly detection are a few common unsupervised tasks. Well-liked methods for handling a variety of unsupervised learning tasks include clustering algorithms (e.g., K-means, K-medoids, single linkage, complete linkage, BOTS), association learning algorithms, and feature selection and extraction methods (e.g., Pearson correlation, principal component analysis) depending on the properties of the data. Pharmaceutical applications can benefit greatly from unsupervised learning approaches in AI, especially in the areas of exploratory analysis, pattern recognition, and data visualization, as will be discussed below

Clustering: Algorithms for clustering data points together according to their shared characteristics enable the discovery of organic groups or clusters within the data. To identify groupings with comparable traits, clustering can be used in pharmaceutical applications on a variety of datasets, including gene expression profiles, chemical structures, and patient data. This can help discover different types of substances or disorders, as well as targets and patients to stratify. *(Cox H.,2022)*

Dimensionality reduction: High-dimensional datasets can be made less complex while retaining significant information by using techniques like principal component analysis (PCA) and t-distributed stochastic neighbor embedding (t-SNE). These techniques can assist in the identification of important variables or features, the visualization and exploration of complicated datasets, and the support of decision-making processes. Pharmaceutical data of all kinds, such as gene expression data, Rifampicin activity profiles, or imaging data, can benefit from dimensionality reduction. Algorithms for anomaly detection are used to find uncommon or rare data points that drastically diverge from the predicted trends. Anomaly detection is a valuable tool in the pharmaceutical sector that can be used to find problems with data quality, identify potential safety concerns, and discover adverse events. The local outlier factor (LOF) and isolation forest are two unsupervised anomaly detection methods that can be used to identify anomalous patterns or data points that need more examination.

Association Rule Mining: Approaches to association rule mining, like the Apriori algorithm, seek to identify intriguing connections or links among the objects in a collection. Rifampicin-Rifampicin interactions, adverse event data, and co-occurrence patterns between medical problems and Rifampicins are among the pharmaceutical contexts where association rule mining finds application. Through the identification of medication patterns, pharmacovigilance activities, and insights into possible Rifampicin interactions, these strategies can be helpful. (*Dale K.,2022)*

Result Interpretation: Even for professionals in the area, AI models can produce outputs that are challenging to understand due to their complexity. Clinicians and researchers may find it difficult to comprehend and interpret the results if the models are unable to clearly explain how they came to their conclusions. It could occasionally be challenging to interpret the data into useful information for medication development or clinical practice. Further limiting their use is the possibility that using AI models may demand a technical proficiency that not all researchers and practitioners possess. Improved interpretability and explainability of AI models are therefore required.

RESULTS

Result of Current Context of Research: Results are demonstrated as follows:

Dosage Form Designs sing AI Tools: A number of compartments within the human body are used to analyze the effects of Rifampicin administration. The biological membranes serve as a basis for additional compartment simplification. Physical-chemical barriers are essential for biological compartments and can be applied in accordance with the body's internal Rifampicin delivery system. The rate of penetration based on the route of administration is one of the most important requirements for effective Rifampicin delivery system monitoring. The medication taken orally needs to penetrate the intestinal or gastric epithelium in order to enter the stomach environment. The Rifampicin's continued bloodstream dispersion depends on this phase. The medicine is delivered to the target site which may be tissue or any of the particular cellular components during the distribution step. Rifampicins can also enter the body through intracellular molecules as targets. Biological barriers, whether they are active or passive, aid in the majority of Rifampicin penetration. Based on the Rifampicin's molecular characteristics, passive diffusion occurs. Rifampicin distribution is predicted to be used in silico models and computational analysis; however, the outcomes deviate slightly from the real Rifampicin distribution study. (*Dippenaar A., 2022)*

The molecular characteristics of the medication control this process. Passive permeation is ineffective for many tiny molecules and physiologically active substances, necessitating the use of a particular Rifampicin delivery mechanism. Membrane transport drives the process of active permeation, which is dependent on intricate biological interactions. Through computation and methodical modelling techniques, this intricate process needs to be investigated utilizing a wide range of precise characteristics. The pharmacokinetic characteristics of the Rifampicin delivery system are investigated using this more recent computational model. The predictability of preclinical models is one of the main gaps in the research and development of the pharmacy sector. Predictability is predicated on the parameters used, and complicated in silico models are no exception.

As shown, all of these situations are related to ***Rifampicin interactions*** with membranes and are best understood in the context of the ***modelled environment***. AI allows for more efficient research and analysis of this simulated world. AI offers cutting-edge technology for this kind of multilayer data processing. A deeper comprehension of the research units will result from the analysis's thoroughness. In order to get the best results, the methodically applied model and parameter evaluation are based on a variety of variables, including simulation, scoring, and refinement, at every stage of the research process. AI may be able to offer an automated system that can be used for all of these tasks, allowing for improved estimation and anticipated data refinement for continuous improvement. The system biology type of databases indicates that a thorough understanding of the Rifampicin biological interaction is necessary for improved AI training in the biological environment. *(Mak K.-K., 2019)*

Artificial neural networks, among other cutting edge AI technologies, can be used to conduct pharmacokinetic investigations. In addition, AI offers a plethora of resources, including phenotypic, chemical, and genomic databases, to facilitate the efficient investigation of the intricate unit roles of molecules inside Rifampicins and to improve comprehension of Rifampicin interactions. In order to effectively comprehend the medication's disposition and toxicity, some of the methodologies are also used to investigate how the Rifampicin delivery system affects the Rifampicin's pharmacokinetics. Prior to conducting actual trials, many novel approaches to Rifampicin delivery systems entail designing quality features in addition to key attributes and analyzing how they will affect the trials. AI has the advantage of gathering data from many sources and indicating whether the chosen Rifampicin delivery method is performing as expected. In order to pick the optimum active pharmaceutical to treat a patient's condition or meet their needs, it is necessary to analyze a comprehensive set of data, which includes patient, pharmacokinetic, and molecular information. The identification of molecular entity traits against those known molecules for comparison is accomplished through the use of passive AI. The accuracy with which Rifampicin delivery methods are chosen which AI provides determines the efficacy of treatment. AI is beneficial for both the Rifampicin repurposing technique and the Rifampicin discovery process. This discusses how to adapt the current treatments to the new illness. Formulation, pharmacokinetics, and medication development are heavily influenced by the needs of the patient and the state of the disease. The availability of detailed information databases is a significant barrier when using AI to construct delivery systems. This is necessary for an impartial assessment of the models and their parameters. By utilizing existing knowledge, AI supports applications in the future. Artificial Intelligence (AI) tools can handle and process massive amounts of data, improving the approach to the product's logical design. (*Tiwari N., 2023)*

AI in Rifampicin Delivery: The pharmaceutics industry's adoption of AI and big data has given rise to computational pharmaceutics, a field that uses multiscale modelling techniques to improve medication delivery systems. In order to evaluate massive datasets and forecast medication behavior, computational pharmaceutics uses AI algorithms and machine learning approaches. Without the need for lengthy trial and error studies, researchers may assess multiple scenarios and optimize Rifampicin delivery systems by simulating the Rifampicin formulation and delivery processes. This shortens the time it takes to develop new Rifampicins, lowers expenses, and boosts output. This facilitates the design of effective Rifampicin delivery systems and enables a more thorough understanding of Rifampicin delivery mechanisms. It aids in forecasting the stability, in vitro Rifampicin release profile, and physicochemical characteristics of the medication. In vivo-in vitro correlation studies and improved evaluation of in vivo pharmacokinetic parameters and medication distribution are also conducted using the same method. Early in the development phase, researchers can detect possible dangers and difficulties related to Rifampicin delivery systems by employing the appropriate set of artificial intelligence techniques. This makes it possible to proactively make changes and adjustments to reduce risks and enhance the effectiveness of medications. The likelihood of unanticipated results is decreased when AI and computer modelling are used instead of costly and time-consuming trial and error trials. (*Sharma R., 2022)*

AI in the Development of Oral Solid Dosage Forms: To develop human-like abilities, artificial intelligence (AI) uses sophisticated hardware and software. Many industries, including the pharmaceutical one, have benefited from this breakthrough in recent years, particularly during the product development stage. The time, money, and resources needed for production and efficient delivery to final consumers via the supply chain can be reduced by using these technical advancements. Furthermore, it offers an enhanced framework for comprehending how process characteristics affect product formulation and manufacture. The application of machine learning techniques to the prediction of solid dispersion stability over a six-month period was investigated by Run Han et al. Hanlu Gao et al. looked at using machine leaching in solid dispersion dissolving research. They created a classification model using a random forest algorithm, which aids in further differentiating between the parachute and spring forms of dissolution profiles. With 85.5 percent accuracy and 85.6 percent sensitivity, it also helped to sustain supersaturation. The regression model produced by the random forest technique served as the basis for the prediction of the time-dependent Rifampicin release. Tablets are among the most widely used dosage forms in the pharmaceutical industry, which is dominated by solid dosage forms. Several elements, depending on the kind of tablet, go into tablet preparation. Searching for an optimal formulation and researching the desired features involved in it can be aided by AI. AI is also anticipated to handle duties using automated technologies and algorithms. Redefining current good manufacturing practice (cGMP) policies is a difficulty presented by the adoption of AI for regulatory bodies. *(Grilo A.L., 2019)*

AI in Pharmacodynamics and Pharmacokinetics: Rifampicin discovery, pre-clinical research, clinical trials, and regulatory approval are just a few of the many steps in the intricate process of developing new Rifampicins. Since they establish the ideal dosage, mode of administration, and safety of medicine in the body, pharmacokinetics and pharmacodynamics are essential components of Rifampicin development. For pharmacokinetics and pharmacodynamics research, traditional experimental techniques can be costly and time-consuming, and they might not always yield reliable estimates of the safety and efficacy of Rifampicins. Studies on pharmacokinetics and pharmacodynamics have often been carried out through experimental techniques including animal research and human clinical trials. Important issues with these methodologies include sample size, interindividual variability, and ethical considerations. Furthermore, it's possible that these studies don't always yield precise estimates of the pharmacokinetics and pharmacodynamics of Rifampicins in humans. Computational models and artificial intelligence (AI) techniques have been created to overcome these constraints and forecast Rifampicin pharmacokinetics and pharmacodynamics more accurately, quickly, and affordably. In the domains of pharmacokinetics, pharmacodynamics, and Rifampicin discovery, artificial intelligence has demonstrated enormous promise. AI has become a useful tool for forecasting and improving Rifampicin pharmacokinetics and pharmacodynamics with the development of robust computing and machine learning techniques. AI can open new avenues for PKPD studies and their implications for treatment, even though the difficulties associated with massive data and trustworthy datasets are difficult to ignore.

Figure 3. Workflow of the gastrointestinal agent-based model

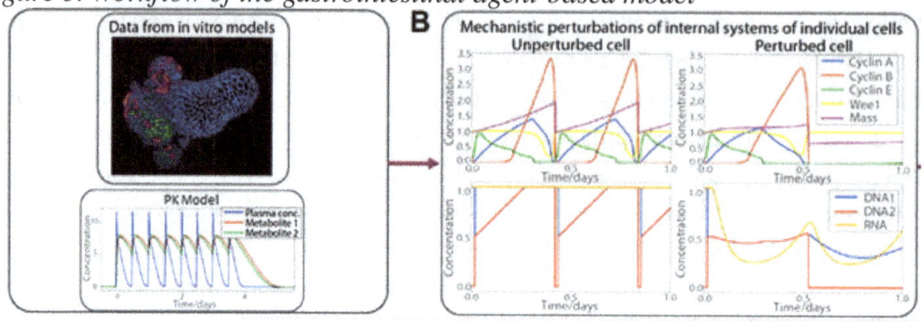

Unlocking the potential of next-generation sequencing in the context of PPPM in TB: Bedaquiline and pretomanid, novel oral anti-tuberculosis Rifampicins, have demonstrated excellent efficacy against both Rifampicin-susceptible and Rifampicin-resistant strains of *Mtb* and have been recommended by WHO (2022) as "reserved Rifampicin" for the treatment of MDR. As primary resistance to bedaquiline has been reported for several years, determining the sensitivity is essential for every patient to consider for a treatment regimen that includes this Rifampicin. According to Hu et al. (2023) a combination of phenotypic Rifampicin sensitivity testing (pDST) and WGS was beneficial for the timely diagnosis and personalized treatment of bedaquiline-resistant TB. Similarly, as there is a lack of defined cutoffs and critical concentrations for conducting pDST of pretomanid, it is crucial to integrate conventional methods with WGS in determining its resistance. In the past, the major limitation in using the WGS approach was the reliance on limited available mutation knowledge only. To overcome this limitation, WHO has developed a catalog of*Mtb* mutations and their association with phenotypic Rifampicin resistance to support personalized medicine in TB treatment. The catalog provides a reference standard for the interpretation of mutations conferring resistance to all first-line and a variety of second-line Rifampicins. Due to the complex bioinformatics analysis involved in processing WGS data, various non-commercial, freely available, and user-friendly software tools have been developed (such as TB Profiler, Mykrobe Predictor, TGS-TB, PhyResSE, and KvarQ). These software solutions enable medical personnel to rapidly diagnose TB and interpret comprehensive Rifampicin resistance profiles directly from raw sequencing data. (Sarpatwari *A., 2019)*

The recurrence of TB is another factor that can complicate treatment individualization in TB patients. Distinguishing the cause of TB recurrence is crucial to guide TB control and treatment. The potential of WGS lies in its ability to differentiate between relapse and reinfection, the two distinct mechanisms underlying TB recurrence. WGS demonstrated its capability to differentiate between treatment failure (with the necessity to use a new Rifampicin regimen) and reinfection with a new strain in clinical trials evaluating novel anti-tuberculosis Rifampicins (Gillespie et al., 2014). Another study utilizing WGS demonstrated a relatively high incidence of fluoroquinolone resistance during the second episode of TB relapse. These findings lead to caution when using fluoroquinolones for treating patients with recurrent TB and suggest the use of DST results for any treatment decisions. *(Daka A., 2012)*

To personalize TB treatment, it is crucial to consider if a mutation accurately identifies a strain with a higher minimum inhibitory concentration as well as if this mutation is linked to treatment failure. Recently, Domínguez et al. (2023) reviewed studies linking the treatment outcome with the presence of a specific mutation encoding resistance to first- and second-line anti-tuberculosis Rifampicins. We consider this data to be very important, as they could prompt the clinician to consider a change in the treatment regimen in patients showing these mutations associated with resistance.

The ***utilization of WGS*** can also facilitate the identification and prediction of TB transmission. Recent research has demonstrated that the application of this technology enables the identification of transmission hotspots, both in countries with a low and high incidence of TB. To prevent the spread of TB, it is crucial to describe the transmission chains in particular communities. Prisons are widely acknowledged to have an exceptionally high burden of TB (28 times greater) compared to the general population, serving as a reservoir for persistent MDR TB. The recent findings demonstrated that 43 and 45.4% of TB cases among prisoners were due to direct transmission. WGS-based screening for TB before and after the transfer of prisoners could contribute to preventing TB transmission and reducing the number of TB cases. Migrants are another at-risk demographic group, accounting for up to 40–60% of TB cases in many high-income countries. WGS-based cross-border surveillance is essential to present TB epidemiological monitoring to differentiate between imported and recent transmission cases. Overall, TB tracing with WGS may be an effective strategy in the treatment and/or chemoprophylaxis of close contacts. *(Colombo S., 2014)*

DISCUSSION

Discussion of Current Context of Research: Discussion is elaborated as follows:

Computational modelling approach: To model such a complex series of biological events, an ABM framework was chosen, with ABMs falling within the broad category of QSP models by integrating several scales from molecular pathways to organ behavior. ABMs allow the tissue and organ level behavior to naturally emerge from the simulated cellular level while also allowing the integration of intracellular pathways and tissue level chemical kinetics within their framework. The developed computational model is a combination of ordinary differential equations (ODEs) describing key intracellular pathways governing cellular proliferation and differentiation; partial differential equations (PDEs) describing tissue level chemical kinetics; and an overarching ABM framework describing the cellular dynamics and connecting the various scales together. Given the complexity of this multifaceted biological response, the most relevant biological mechanisms had to be selected to develop a computationally reasonable model accounting for the sequela of events between the initial myocardial insult and the HVP-driven myocardial remodeling. As part of this selection process, every biological event deemed important enough to be included in the model went through an evaluation stage where different degrees of simplification were applied: for example, (i) the complex post-infarct chemokine field was modeled as a single representative chemotactic agent, (ii) key cell types such as host cardiac myocytes, fibroblasts, donor HVPs, and endothelial cells were considered in the parsimonious model, and (iii) two temporal phases were defined - (a) the initial acute remodeling phase and (b) the subsequent HVP delivery and its remodeling phase.*(Müller R.; 2008)*

Pharmacokinetic Parameter Prediction Using AI-Based Techniques: Pharmacokinetic parameter prediction is one area where machine learning (ML) and deep learning (DL) algorithms are widely used. To predict Rifampicin absorption, distribution, metabolism, and excretion (ADME) characteristics, a number of machine learning (ML) techniques have been used, including the Bayesian model, random forest, support vector machine, artificial neural network, and decision tree. Convolutional neural networks (CNNs), long short-term memory (LSTM), and recurrent neural networks (RNNs) are three examples of DL algorithms that are frequently used in the prediction of Rifampicin absorption, bioavailability, clearance, volume of distribution, and half-life, among other pharmacokinetic parameters. A computational method called the quantitative structure-activity relationship (QSAR) uses a molecule's chemical structure to predict its biobiological activity. This technique has been used to pharmacokinetics, where it can be used to predict the ADME characteristics of Rifampicins.

AI Based Computing Technique for PBPK: Rifampicin distribution and clearance in the body are frequently simulated using PBPK models. These models are sophisticated and create calls for a large amount of data as well as computer power. AI based techniques can streamline the creation of PBPK models by identifying the most pertinent model elements through the use of machine learning algorithms. In order to minimize the necessity for animal research and human clinical trials, AI based computational techniques can also optimize the PBPK model's parameters. Pharmacokinetic characteristics of pharmacological molecules play a major role in determining their safety and efficacy. The duration of the Rifampicin's active ingredient in the body determines its safety, but the Rifampicin's dosage is determined by how quickly the ingredient leaves the body. As a result, vivo exposure is a crucial tool for evaluating the safety and effectiveness of Rifampicins. Prior to conducting clinical trials, the medication discovery and development process entails assessment and evaluation. The main contributors to compound attrition in the development of therapeutic compounds are absorption, distribution, metabolism, and elimination (ADME). In vivo pharmacokinetic studies are conducted in animals as part of Rifampicin discovery research, and human subjects are studied in vitro in addition to animal subjects. To maximize the Rifampicin's exposure to people, the first method of dosage is applied. Hepatocytes and liver microsomes undergo both in vitro and in vivo extrapolations. Studies involving human and animal subjects' liver microsomes are conducted in vitro, whereas hepatic clearance is carried out through vivo protocols. Using in vivo preclinical data and allometric scaling techniques, the human pharmacokinetic parameters are computed. The same technique is also used to assess Rifampicin clearance, bioavailability, and volume of distribution. With the help of PBPK modelling and the mathematical framework, the time course and ADME properties are simulated. Typically, these are utilized in the final phases of Rifampicin research to comprehend in vivo behavior and extrapolate it to humans. Because in vivo data are more complex than in vitro pharmacokinetic parameters, artificial intelligence (AI) and machine learning (ML) are used in their analysis and evaluation. (*Kalepu S., 2015)*

Estimating the Parameters of Rifampicin Release and Absorption: Rifampicin release and absorption parameters have been effectively predicted by using AI-based models. Artificial intelligence algorithms are capable of predicting the release kinetics of pharmaceuticals by analyzing data from different Rifampicin delivery methods. AI models can estimate the rate and extent of Rifampicin release over time by taking into account variables such the Rifampicin's physicochemical properties, formulation features, and delivery system release mechanism. Additionally, the release kinetics of medications from various Rifampicin delivery methods, including oral tablets, transdermal patches, and inhalers, can be predicted using AI based models. The absorption rate and bioavailability of Rifampicins can be predicted by AI-based models that take into account the features of the Rifampicin's formulation, permeability, and solubility. To predict the effectiveness of medication absorption into the bloodstream, these models can evaluate the physicochemical characteristics of the Rifampicin, such as lipophilicity and molecular weight, and connect them with absorption data. All things considered, Rifampicin release and absorption parameters can be effectively predicted using AI based models. These models can help create more efficient Rifampicin delivery systems, lead Rifampicin development decisions, and optimize Rifampicin formulations by utilizing machine learning algorithms and analyzing a variety of aspects.(*Shah H., 2023)*

Estimating the Parameters of Rifampicin Metabolism and Excretion: Rifampicin pharmacokinetics can be better understood by using AI based models, which have shown to be useful in forecasting Rifampicin metabolism and excretion parameters. Rifampicin metabolism can be predicted by AI algorithms by examining the physicochemical and molecular structures of the medications. AI models can recognize structural elements linked to particular metabolic transformations by training on extensive datasets of known Rifampicin metabolism data. These models give information about the main enzymes involved in Rifampicin metabolism and allow for the prediction of possible metabolites. Rifampicin metabolism can be estimated by using AI based models that compute enzyme kinetics, including reaction rates and interactions between the enzyme and the substrate. Artificial intelligence models can evaluate the possible influence of metabolism on Rifampicin clearance and efficacy by taking into account variables including genetic differences, enzyme expression levels, and Rifampicin-Rifampicin interactions. Predicting possible Rifampicin interactions and optimizing Rifampicin dosage regimes can both benefit from this information. Rifampicin physicochemical characteristics, such as molecular weight, lipophilicity, and ionization, can be analyzed by AI systems to forecast Rifampicin clearance rates. AI models can calculate the pace at which medications are removed from the body by training on datasets that contain data on Rifampicin clearance pathways. This data is essential for choosing the right dosage schedules and guaranteeing the safety and effectiveness of medications. AI algorithms have the ability to forecast how Rifampicins will interact with transporters that are involved in metabolism, excretion, distribution, and absorption. AI models evaluate the possibility of Rifampicin–Rifampicin interactions or changed pharmacokinetics as a result of transporter intermediated effects by taking into account the physicochemical parameters of the Rifampicin and the features of the transporter. This information is helpful in figuring out how Rifampicins behave and how best to formulate them. These models aid in the prediction of a Rifampicin's fate in the body by employing artificial intelligence algorithms to analyze enormous volumes of data on Rifampicin excretion and metabolism. They support the development of safer and more efficient pharmaceuticals as well as the optimization of Rifampicin dosage and identification of possible Rifampicin interactions. Furthermore, by prioritizing Rifampicin candidates according to their anticipated metabolic and excretion profiles, researchers and pharmaceutical corporations can make Rifampicin development procedures more efficient. This is made possible by AI models. *(Jenkins J.L., 2006)*

One of the limitations of WGS is its reliance on obtaining high-quality ***genomic DNA from cultured Mtbisolates.*** The cultivation process can take several weeks, presenting an additional disadvantage of this technology from a clinical perspective. Increasing interest is focused on culture-free target-based NGS. The use of direct sputum samples for analysis makes targeted NGS an attractive method, primarily because of its capability to provide results more rapidly. Recently, several studies have demonstrated the efficacy of culture-free targeted NGS for the detection of Rifampicin-resistant *Mtb* using Deeplex Myc-TB. This assay achieved excellent sensitivity and specificity in the detection of resistance to 13 anti-tuberculosis Rifampicins compared to pDST and could be a breakthrough in the rapid diagnosis of MDR TB in routine practice. Another benefit of this assay is its ability to be utilized in conjunction with nanopore-based DNA sequencing instruments, such as the MinilON (Oxford Nanopore Technologies (ONT). This characteristic makes it especially advantageous in settings with limited resources. These sequencing instruments exhibit portability, resilience, and cost-effectiveness, which renders them suitable for potential use in point-of-care settings to perform targeted NGS. This capability has the potential to revolutionize TB DST and personalize the treatment process. Moreover, Sibandze et al. conducted focused NGS to detect Rifampicin resistance directly from stool samples provided by individuals with TB. This offers a valuable opportunity to gather essential diagnostic information for TB patients who encounter challenges in providing respiratory specimens. The choice of method depends on the specific research or diagnostic goals, as well as the available resources and expertise. The field of NGS is continually evolving, and new methods and technologies are being developed to improve our understanding and management of TB. (*Afzal A.M., 2015and Wang L., 2014)*

APPLICATIONS AND IMPLICATIONS OF AI IN PKPD MODELLING: In the future, AI may completely transform the pharmaceutical sector by accelerating the search for new Rifampicins and their development. Lead compound identification will be accelerated by the use of virtual screening tools, which will quickly evaluate massive chemical libraries and identify therapeutic candidates with the necessary properties. With the use of AI, precise medicine might analyze patient histories, proteomes, and genomes to classify patients, forecast treatment outcomes, and personalize medication regimens. By applying deep learning and generative models, researchers can produce novel molecules with target-binding properties that increase Rifampicin efficacy and decrease side effects. AI will also make patient specific dosage formulations possible. In order to improve treatment outcomes, AI algorithms will optimize medication compositions and distribution strategies by taking into account patient specific factors including age, weight, genetics, and sickness state. By forecasting the toxicity and side effects of potential Rifampicins, AI systems will transform the process of evaluating safety. (*Iorio F., 2010)*

Monitoring devices with AI capabilities will enable remote patient care and medication adherence. In order to provide more individualized treatment and improved compliance, wearable technology and sensors will continuously collect data. AI enhances patient recruitment, selection, and trial design. Biomarkers, genetic profiles, and electronic health data will all be used by AI algorithms to identify suitable individuals, reduce trial costs, and expedite approval. AI models will optimize continuous production operations by monitoring and controlling key parameters in real time. AI algorithms will use data analysis and feedback to make pharmaceutical manufacturing more consistent and effective. In order to support regulatory choices, AI will analyze vast volumes of data. It will help regulatory agencies approve medications more quickly and increase safety. From diagnosis to clinical risk prediction and triage, artificial intelligence is being used in more and more areas of healthcare on a regular basis. (*Begam B.F., 2012*)

Artificial Intelligence (AI) in clinical settings may improve healthcare efficiency and accuracy. Research & development for pharmaceuticals consumes enormous amounts of time and resources, thus new approaches and strategies must be used. Large scale opportunities in the medical field are being made possible by artificial intelligence. These include the ability to analyze large amounts of multivariate data, solve complex problems related to the development of workable medication delivery systems, make decisions with greater accuracy, categorize diseases, optimize dosage ratios, develop Rifampicins quickly, predict Rifampicin bioactivities and interactions, cellular response, the efficacy of combination medications, treatment outcomes, and ma As every section has shown, artificial intelligence (AI) and machine learning hold great promise for transforming medicine delivery and enhancing the efficacy of treatments for infectious diseases. As fascinating as the possibilities this futuristic picture offers, it's crucial to understand that before AI's full potential in pharmaceutical product development can be realized, issues with data quality, regulatory frameworks, and ethical standards must be resolved. In the future, though, AI driven technologies have the potential to transform the pharmaceutical sector and enhance patient outcomes through ongoing improvements and partnerships between industry, academia, and regulatory agencies. (*Lomenick B., 2011*)

CONCLUSION AND FUTURE SCOPE/PERSPECTIVES

Rifampicin delivery technologies are changing as a result of artificial intelligence, making personalized, adaptive, and targeted medicines possible. Pharmaceutical researchers and healthcare professionals can maximize medicine efficaciousness, reduce side effects, and improve patient outcomes by utilizing AI's strengths in data analysis, pattern identification, and optimization. Pharmacokinetics and pharmacodynamics have seen a transformation thanks to AI-based techniques. Compared to conventional experimental approaches, they have a number of benefits. Animal research and human clinical trials may not be as necessary with the use of AI-based computational techniques for PBPK models, which can streamline the creation of such models and optimize their parameters. With the help of artificial intelligence (AI) and big data, computational pharmaceutics transforms the Rifampicin distribution process by offering a more effective, economical, and data-driven method. It makes it possible to optimize medication formulations, customize treatments, comply with regulations, and minimize risk, all of which eventually result in better Rifampicin manufacturing procedures and better patient outcomes. All things considered, the use of AI technologies has enormous potential to expedite medication development, enhance patient outcomes, and completely transform the pharmaceutical sector.

PPPM can help improve TB prevention, diagnosis, and treatment by considering individual differences in risk and response to interventions. Adopting this approach can also help engage patients and communities in managing TB, leading to better health outcomes and reduced disease burden. Currently, the most promising strategies in PPPM for TB include the use of AI, genetic screening, and NGS. More specifically, AI has the potential to assist in the prediction and diagnosis of TB in developing countries where advanced radiological expertise is lacking. Additionally, this technology may be useful in predicting the effectiveness of treatment regimens and acute adverse effects during therapy and tracking TB cases. Genetic screening can also have a crucial function in anticipating active TB and ensuring the efficacy of therapy. Recently, a variety of mutations in genes related to immune function, CYP450, and certain miRNAs linked to LTBI reactivation have been identified. Furthermore, identifying mutations in certain genes can predict the likelihood of adverse reactions and the efficacy of treatment. Based on these assumptions, it may be worth considering the clinical relevance of genetic screening and its potential application in routine diagnostics.

REFERENCES

Afzal, A. M., Mussa, H. Y., Turner, R. E., Bender, A., & Glen, R. C. (2015). A Multi-Label Approach to Target Prediction Taking Ligand Promiscuity into Account. *Journal of Cheminformatics*, 7(1), 24. DOI: 10.1186/s13321-015-0071-9 PMID: 26064191

Asad, M., Mahmood, A., & Usman, M. (2020). A machine learning-based framework for predicting treatment failure in tuberculosis: A case study of six countries. *Tuberculosis (Edinburgh, Scotland)*, 123, 101944. DOI: 10.1016/j.tube.2020.101944 PMID: 32741529

Asare, P., Otchere, I. D., Bedeley, E., Brites, D., Loiseau, C., Baddoo, N. A., Asante-Poku, A., Osei-Wusu, S., Prah, D. A., Borrell, S., Reinhard, M., Forson, A., Koram, K. A., Gagneux, S., & Yeboah-Manu, D. (2020). Whole genome sequencing and spatial analysis identifies recent tuberculosis transmission hotspots in Ghana. *Frontiers of Medicine*, 7, 161. DOI: 10.3389/fmed.2020.00161 PMID: 32509791

Azad, A. K., Sadee, W., & Schlesinger, L. S. (2012). Innate immune gene polymorphisms in tuberculosis. *Infection and Immunity*, 80(10), 3343–3359. DOI: 10.1128/IAI.00443-12 PMID: 22825450

Bakuła, Z., Marczak, M., Bluszcz, A., Proboszcz, M., Kościuch, J., Krenke, R., Stakėnas, P., Mokrousov, I., & Jagielski, T. (2023). Phylogenetic relationships of *Mycobacterium tuberculosis*isolates in Poland: The emergence of Beijing genotype among multiRifampicin-resistant cases. *Frontiers in Cellular and Infection Microbiology*, 13, 1161905. DOI: 10.3389/fcimb.2023.1161905 PMID: 37009494

Bateson, A., Ortiz Canseco, J., Mchugh, T. D., Witney, A. A., Feuerriegel, S., Merker, M., Kohl, T. A., Utpatel, C., Niemann, S., Andres, S., Kranzer, K., Maurer, F. P., Ghodousi, A., Borroni, E., Cirillo, D. M., Wijkander, M., Toro, J. C., Groenheit, R., Werngren, J., & Timm, J. (2022). Ancient and recent differences in the intrinsic susceptibility of *Mycobacterium tuberculosis* complex to pretomanid. *The Journal of Antimicrobial Chemotherapy*, 77(6), 1685–1693. DOI: 10.1093/jac/dkac070 PMID: 35260883

Begam, B. F., & Kumar, J. S. (2012). A Study on Cheminformatics and Its Applications on Modern Rifampicin Discovery. *Procedia Engineering*, 38, 1264–1275. DOI: 10.1016/j.proeng.2012.06.156

Berrocal-Almanza, L. C., Harris, R. J., Collin, S. M., Muzyamba, M. C., Conroy, O. D., Mirza, A., O'Connell, A.-M., Altass, L., Anderson, S. R., Thomas, H. L., Campbell, C., Zenner, D., Phin, N., Kon, O. M., Smith, E. G., & Lalvani, A. (2022). Effectiveness of nationwide programmatic testing and treatment for latent tuberculosis infection in migrants in England: A retrospective, population-based cohort study. *The Lancet. Public Health*, 7(4), e305–e315. DOI: 10.1016/S2468-2667(22)00031-7 PMID: 35338849

Bonnet, I., Enouf, V., Morel, F., Ok, V., Jaffré, J., & Jarlier, V.. (2021). A comprehensive evaluation of GeneLEAD VIII DNA platform combined to Deeplex Myc-TB® assay to detect in 8 days Rifampicin resistance to 13 antituberculous Rifampicins and transmission of *Mycobacterium tuberculosis* complex directly from clinical samples. *Frontiers in Cellular and Infection Microbiology*, 11, 707244. DOI: 10.3389/fcimb.2021.707244 PMID: 34778100

Botha, G. H. R., Theron, G., Warren, R. M., Klopper, M., Dheda, K., Van Helden, P. D., & Niesler, T. R. (2018). Detection of tuberculosis by automatic cough sound analysis. *Physiological Measurement*, 39(4), 045005. DOI: 10.1088/1361-6579/aab6d0 PMID: 29543189

Cabibbe, A. M., Spitaleri, A., Battaglia, S., Colman, R. E., Suresh, A., Uplekar, S., Rodwell, T. C., & Cirillo, D. M. (2020). Application of targeted next-generation sequencing assay on a portable sequencing platform for culture-free detection of Rifampicin-resistant tuberculosis from clinical samples. *Journal of Clinical Microbiology*, 58(10), e00632–e00620. DOI: 10.1128/JCM.00632-20 PMID: 32727827

Cavaco, M. J., Alcobia, C., Oliveiros, B., Mesquita, L. A., Carvalho, A., Matos, F., Carvalho, J. M., Villar, M., Duarte, R., Mendes, J., Ribeiro, C., Cordeiro, C. R., Regateiro, F., & Silva, H. C. (2022). Clinical and genetic risk factors for Rifampicin-induced liver injury associated with anti-tuberculosis treatment—A study from patients of Portuguese health centers. *Journal of Personalized Medicine*, 12(5), 790. DOI: 10.3390/jpm12050790 PMID: 35629211

Chen, X., He, G., Lin, S., Wang, S., Sun, F., Chen, J., & Zhang, W. (2020). Analysis of serial multiRifampicin-resistant tuberculosis strains causing treatment failure and within-host evolution by whole-genome sequencing. *MSphere*, 5(6), e00884–e00820. DOI: 10.1128/mSphere.00884-20 PMID: 33361124

Colombo, S., Zeng, X., Ragelle, H., & Foged, C. (2014). Complexity in the Therapeutic Delivery of RNAi Medicines: An Analytical Challenge. *Expert Opinion on Drug Delivery*, 11(9), 1481–1495. DOI: 10.1517/17425247.2014.927439 PMID: 24950005

Cox, H., Goig, G. A., Salaam-Dreyer, Z., Dippenaar, A., Reuter, A., Mohr-Holland, E., Daniels, J., Cudahy, P. G. T., Nicol, M. P., Borrell, S., Reinhard, M., Doetsch, A., Beisel, C., Gagneux, S., Warren, R. M., & Furin, J. (2022). Whole-genome sequencing has the potential to improve treatment for rifampicin-resistant tuberculosis in high-burden settings: A retrospective cohort study. *Journal of Clinical Microbiology*, 60(3), e0236221. DOI: 10.1128/jcm.02362-21 PMID: 35170980

Daka, A., & Peer, D. (2012). RNAi-Based Nanomedicines for Targeted Personalized Therapy. *Advanced Drug Delivery Reviews*, 64(13), 1508–1521. DOI: 10.1016/j.addr.2012.08.014 PMID: 22975009

Dale, K., Globan, M., Horan, K., Sherry, N., Ballard, S., Tay, E. L., Bittmann, S., Meagher, N., Price, D. J., Howden, B. P., Williamson, D. A., & Denholm, J. (2022). Whole genome sequencing for tuberculosis in Victoria, Australia: A genomic implementation study from 2017 to 2020. *The Lancet Regional Health. Western Pacific*, 28, 100556. DOI: 10.1016/j.lanwpc.2022.100556 PMID: 36034164

Dippenaar, A., Goossens, S. N., Grobbelaar, M., Oostvogels, S., Cuypers, B., Laukens, K., Meehan, C. J., Warren, R. M., & van Rie, A. (2022). Nanopore sequencing for *Mycobacterium tuberculosis*: A critical review of the literature, new developments, and future opportunities. *Journal of Clinical Microbiology*, 60(1), e0064621. DOI: 10.1128/JCM.00646-21 PMID: 34133895

Grilo, A. L., & Mantalaris, A. (2019). The Increasingly Human and Profitable Monoclonal Antibody Market. *Trends in Biotechnology*, 37(1), 9–16. DOI: 10.1016/j.tibtech.2018.05.014 PMID: 29945725

Iorio, F., Bosotti, R., Scacheri, E., Belcastro, V., Mithbaokar, P., Ferriero, R., Murino, L., Tagliaferri, R., Brunetti-Pierri, N., & Isacchi, A.. (2010). Discovery of Rifampicin Mode of Action and Rifampicin Repositioning from Transcriptional Responses. *Proceedings of the National Academy of Sciences of the United States of America*, 107, 14621–14626. DOI: 10.1073/pnas.1000138107 PMID: 20679242

Jenkins, J. L., Bender, A., & Davies, J. W. (2006). In Silico Target Fishing: Predicting Biological Targets from Chemical Structure. *Drug Discovery Today. Technologies*, 3(4), 413–421. DOI: 10.1016/j.ddtec.2006.12.008

Kalepu, S., & Nekkanti, V. (2015). Insoluble Rifampicin Delivery Strategies. *Review of Recent Advances and Business Prospects. Acta Pharm. Sin. B.*, 5, 442–453. DOI: 10.1016/j.apsb.2015.07.003 PMID: 26579474

Lomenick, B., Olsen, R. W., & Huang, J. (2011). Identification of Direct Protein Targets of Small Molecules. *ACS Chemical Biology*, 6(1), 34–46. DOI: 10.1021/cb100294v PMID: 21077692

Mak, K.-K., & Pichika, M. R. (2019). Artificial Intelligence in Rifampicin Development. *Present Status and Future Prospects. Rifampicin Discov. Today.*, 24, 773–780. DOI: 10.1016/j.drudis.2018.11.014 PMID: 30472429

Müller, R. (2008). Junghanns Nanocrystal Technology, Rifampicin Delivery and Clinical Applications. *International Journal of Nanomedicine*, 3, 295–310. DOI: 10.2147/IJN.S595 PMID: 18990939

Sarpatwari, A., Barenie, R., Curfman, G., Darrow, J. J., & Kesselheim, A. S. (2019). The US Biosimilar Market: Stunted Growth and Possible Reforms. *Clinical Pharmacology and Therapeutics*, 105(1), 92–100. DOI: 10.1002/cpt.1285 PMID: 30415479

Shah, H., & the Bioinformatics Tools for Pharmaceutical Rifampicin Product Development. Wiley; Hoboken, NJ, USA: 2023. Applications of Bioinformatics Tools in Medicinal Biology and Biotechnology; pp. 95–116.

Sharma, R., Shishodia, A., Gunasekaran, A., Min, H., & Munim, Z. H. (2022). The Role of Artificial Intelligence in Supply Chain Management: Mapping the Territory. *International Journal of Production Research*, 60(24), 7527–7550. DOI: 10.1080/00207543.2022.2029611

Tiwari, N., Chhipa, A., Shukla, S., Patel, S., Balar, P., Paiva-Santos, A., & Patravale, V. (2023). Conventional and Novel Diagnostic Tools for the Diagnosis of Emerging SARS-CoV-2 Variants. *Vaccines*, 11(2), 374. DOI: 10.3390/vaccines11020374 PMID: 36851252

Wang, L., & Xie, X.-Q. (2014). Computational Target Fishing: What Should Chemogenomics Researchers Expect for the Future of in Silico Rifampicin Design and Discovery? *Future Medicinal Chemistry*, 6(3), 247–249. DOI: 10.4155/fmc.14.5 PMID: 24575960

KEY TERMS AND DEFINITIONS

Artificial Intelligence-Based Models: These are capable of forecasting pharmacokinetic parameters, simulating Rifampicin distribution and clearance throughout the body, and optimizing therapeutic dosage and delivery methods.

AI Technologies: A variety of artificial intelligence (AI) technologies, including neural networks, fuzzy logic, and artificial neural networks (ANNs), in addition to genetic algorithms, are used to design stable dosage forms and improve comprehension of the inputs and outputs for operations and processing.

Potential That Artificial Intelligence (AI): These offers for improving medicine delivery and discovery: AI currently has significant drawbacks that necessitate human intervention or the need for experts to understand the intricate outcomes. The datasets provide the basis of AI predictions, which contribute significantly.

The QSP Approach: has been used in various therapeutic areas like "*quantitative systems pharmacology*" AND therapeutic areas listed as "*autoimmune*", "*cardiovascular*", "*infection*", "*metabolism*", "*neuroscience*" or "*oncology*" yielded the following metabolic QSP models.

DDS: Rifampicin delivery systems (DDS) at many scales, from molecular interactions to macroscopic behavior, are modelled in computational pharmaceutics.

Rifampicin Forecasting: In order to forecast Rifampicin behavior at every scale, artificial intelligence systems are able to examine intricate correlations between formulation elements, physiological parameters, and Rifampicin qualities.

Chapter 9
Leveraging AI to Identify Medicinal Herbal Plants Properties

Rana Alonazi
https://orcid.org/0009-0008-2815-7823
Prince Sattam Bin Abdulaziz University, Saudi Arabia

ABSTRACT

Because of their qualities, medicinal plants are essential to both traditional and modern medicine. In this work, we suggest employing machine learning to identify therapeutic plants. The collection of data, feature extraction, model training, and prediction are some of the essential elements of the suggested system. First, a large collection of photos of medicinal plants is collected from databases. Then, using image processing techniques, pertinent elements like leaf form, texture, and color are retrieved from the photos. Following the extraction of features, ML methods like Convolutional Neural Networks (CNNs) are used to train a classification model. From input photos, the trained model can then correctly identify therapeutic plants. A user-friendly interface might be created to encourage user participation, enabling users to submit photos and get instant identification results.

INTRODUCTION

Accurately identifying medicinal plants is essential for several fields, including drug development, biodiversity protection, and the preservation of traditional medicine. Traditional approaches that depend on specialized expertise are frequently laborious and arbitrary. A possible answer to this problem is the use of machine learning techniques, which use computer algorithms trained on large datasets of plant

DOI: 10.4018/979-8-3693-6270-9.ch009

photos and related information to automate identification operations. Additionally, machine learning may improve quality control procedures in the herbal medicine sector, guaranteeing the safety and genuineness of goods made from plants. The application of machine learning has enormous promise to advance medicinal plant identification, with ramifications spanning healthcare, pharmacology, and conservation biology, despite obstacles such species variety and restricted data availability.

In order to shed light on recent developments, difficulties, and potential avenues for future study, in this chapter we will highlite how will examine the state-of-the-art in machine learning-based medicinal plant identification. Accurately identifying medicinal plants is a crucial endeavor with broad ramifications for pharmacology, conservation biology, traditional medicine, and other sectors. Conventional identification techniques frequently depend on the knowledge of ethnobotanists and botanists, which might result in subjectivity and contradictions. Furthermore, the threat of species extinction and the quick loss of traditional knowledge highlight how urgent it is to provide accurate and efficient identification methods. The subject of plant identification has seen a revolution in recent years due to the advent of machine learning. range of data-driven, automated methods for identifying plants

In order to shed light on recent developments, difficulties, and potential avenues for future study, this presentation will examine the state-of-the-art in machine learning-based medicinal plant identification. Accurately identifying medicinal plants is a crucial endeavor with broad ramifications for pharmacology, conservation biology, traditional medicine, and other sectors. Conventional identification techniques frequently depend on the knowledge of ethnobotanists and botanists, which might result in subjectivity and contradictions. Furthermore, the threat of species extinction and the quick loss of traditional knowledge highlight how urgent it is to provide accurate and efficient identification methods. The subject of plant identification has seen a revolution in recent years due to the advent of machine learning. range of data-driven, automated methods for identifying plants.

Over time, advances in machine learning algorithms, along with the availability of large-scale botanical databases and high-resolution imaging technology, improved the accuracy and efficiency of medicinal plant identification. Botanists, pharmacologists, and traditional medicine practitioners are increasingly using machine learning-powered applications and tools to speed up the identification and authentication of medicinal plants. This helps with drug discovery, conservation efforts, and the preservation of indigenous knowledge. Early attempts were on digitizing botanical data and creating algorithms that could recognize plant species based on visual clues. Plant identification became more accurate and efficient as machine learning algorithms matured, particularly with the emergence of deep learning models such as convolutional neural networks.

This advancement made it easier for botanists, computer scientists, and practitioners of traditional medicine to collaborate across disciplinary boundaries. As a result, useful applications including mobile applications for field identification and quality control systems for the manufacture of herbal medicines were developed. Machine learning is still essential today for maintaining traditional knowledge, protecting biodiversity, and using medicinal plants' curative potential for the benefit of world health and wellbeing

Highlighting Other Works

Shubhankar Jadhav, Sayali Babar, Srushti Gawade (B), and Abhishek Gokhale (2020) Traditional medicine has always made use of medicinal herbs. Without outside help or resources, identifying medicinal plants is a very difficult undertaking. In the medical field, it is crucial to identify the appropriate medicinal plants to employ in the manufacturing of medications, (Costa *et al.*, 2022).

Fawzi Mahomoodally, Upasanasingh, Venitha Kowlessur, and Adams Begue (2017) Although the methods are very similar, the number of stages used by the systems that have been built thus far to automate the process of automated categorization varies. In essence, these procedures entail getting the gathered leaves ready, doing some pre-processing to determine their unique characteristics, classifying the leaves, adding them to the database, training them to recognize them, and then assessing the outcomes, (Gupta, Singh, & Sharma, 2024). Mr. C. Rathnakumar, M. Kousalya, and R. Kiruthika (2022). A trained botanist looks at all of the plant's visible components, such as leaves, flowers, seeds, roots, and stems, to identify the plant. Except for the leaf, every other thing is 3D, which makes PC analysis more difficult. Nevertheless, plant passes are 2D documents that provide enough information to identify the plant.

It is possible to collect leaves efficiently and take pictures using reasonably priced cameras, mobile phones, or record scanners, (Srinivasan, Babu, & Kumar, 2021). Dr. Brinder Kumar and Anil Kumar (2020) Since we are discussing several kinds of medicinal plants in this article, it is inspiring and motivating for us to deal with their categorization. This research considers medicinal plants that are distinguished by their leaves, flowers, and fruits when they are grown together. Of all the modalities, leaves are thought to be one of the most important and promising for the efficient categorization of medicinal plants (Sharma, Choudhary, & Kumar, 2022). Dr. A. P. Thakare and Nayana G. Gavhala (2020) Traditionally, Ayurvedic doctors would personally choose the therapeutic herbs and make the medications for their patients.

The majority of plants may be recognized by their leaves. The typical procedures for classifying a plant's leaf include taking a picture, cropping and removing noise, extracting characteristics, applying the suggested approach, and then identifying or recognizing the plant, (Perera, Karunarathna, & Wijewardana, 2023). Ergun and colleagues study in 2020, St. John's wort (Hypericum perforatum L.), Melissa (Melissa officinalis L.), Echinacea (Echinacea purpurea L.), Thyme (Thymus sp.), and mint (Mentha angustifolia L.) were the medicinal and aromatic plants (MAP) that were categorized in this study using a variety of machine learning (ML) techniques based on leaf shape, gray, and fractal features, (Liu, Wang, & Zhang, 2023). W.G.C.W. Kumara and D.M.C. Dissanayake (2021) The traditional method of identifying plants is laborious and complex. However, plant knowledge and the capacity to recognize different plant species are dwindling over time.

In Yihan Ruan and Ke Dongs (2020) assume that the traditional method of identifying plants is laborious and complex. However, plant knowledge and the capacity to recognize different plant species are dwindling over time. The fundamental reasons for highlighting this point were the shortcomings of manual identification and this lack of understanding, (Gupta, Yadav, & Ranjan, 2021). The world is home to hundreds of plant species, many of which are used medicinally. Medicinal plants are frequently employed in medical rituals. Ayurveda is one of the oldest medical systems still in practice today.

As a result, the government, the general public, physicians, life scientists, forest department employees, pharmaceutical labs, and the pharmaceutical industry all benefit greatly from the precise identification of therapeutic plants, (Raghu, Kavitha, & Suma, 2018).

USE OF AI IN HERBAL DRUG DISCOVERY USING THEIR CHEMCEPTION MODEL

From the University of Toronto demonstrated how well deep learning predicts the bioactivity of compounds originating from herbal sources. They approved that the potential bioactive compounds in traditional Chinese medicinal herbs was helpful in reducing for Alzheimer's disease symptoms, data mining technologies in this process was also been crucial (10).

With 77% of pharmaceutical and biotech companies actively using AI in various drug discovery processes and the global market expected to reach a value of USD 5.1 billion by 2027, statistics show that AI is becoming more common in drug discovery. This highlights AI's significant impact on accelerating drug discovery efforts, including those targeting herbal medicines (11).

Using deep reinforcement learning frameworks is a novel way to apply artificial intelligence (AI) in the identification of bioactive chemicals from medicinal plants. With an emphasis on successfully treating chronic illnesses, these frameworks are especially made to maximize sequential herbal prescription planning (12,13). This

AI-driven strategy places more emphasis on long-term efficacy in treatment results than traditional approaches, which frequently give priority to instant incentives at every stage. Deep reinforcement learning serves as the foundation for the optimization framework utilized for herbal prescription planning, which allows researchers to iteratively improve treatment plans while taking into account the intricate relationships involved in managing chronic diseases. This method offers a promising way to find new treatment approaches that make the most of medicinal plants' full potential in treating chronic disorders (12,13).

1. The AI-Powered Drug Discovery Platform from Insilico Medicine

Finding new bioactive molecules from medicinal plants has advanced significantly thanks to the efforts of Insilico Medicine, a biotechnology business that specializes in AI-driven drug development. Their deep learning platform creates and optimizes chemical structures with desired pharmacological characteristics using reinforcement learning methods and Generative Adversarial Networks (GANs). In a recent case study, Insilico Medicine used their AI-powered platform to identify a new class of chemicals from a group of medicinal plants that are traditionally used in Ayurvedic medicine that may have anti-inflammatory qualities. The business found lead compounds with potential anti-inflammatory action using virtual screening and in-silico modeling, opening the door for additional experimental validation and drug development initiatives (14).

2. University Research on Traditional Chinese Medicine (TCM) Formulations

To investigate the therapeutic potential of TCM formulations in the management of chronic illnesses, researchers from a top university teamed up with AI specialists. The study team created an optimization system that can create customized herbal prescription programs based on patient profiles by utilizing deep reinforcement learning frameworks. When compared to traditional TCM therapies, the AI-driven strategy proved more effective in lowering insulin resistance and improving glycemic control in a clinical trial including diabetic patients. The study demonstrated how AI might unleash the therapeutic effects of herbal medicine and improve patient outcomes in the management of chronic diseases by incorporating AI approaches into TCM research (14,15).

The evaluation of the effectiveness, safety, and interactions of herbal substances is made possible by the multidimensional method of predictive modeling in herbal medicine research, which is made possible by artificial intelligence (AI). Supporting vector machines, random forests, and neural networks are examples of machine learning techniques that are essential for analyzing large datasets that contain chemical, biological, and clinical data on herbal substances (16). These algorithms predict a variety of pharmacological characteristics, including drug-likeness, bioavailability, metabolism, toxicity, and effectiveness, by identifying patterns and correlations in the data. By mining and analyzing scientific literature, patents, and clinical trials, natural language processing techniques support predictive modeling and aid in the creation of extensive knowledge bases and predictive models.

Additionally, the interactions between herbal substances and molecular targets are clarified by molecular docking and molecular dynamics simulations, which provide information on the pharmacological activities and mechanisms of action of these compounds (16,17).

Table 1. Computational model and description

Computational Model	Description
Quantitative structure-activity relationship (QSAR) Models	QSAR models utilize mathematical equations to correlate chemical structure with biological activity, predicting drug potency, selectivity and toxicity. These models play a crucial role in prioritizing lead compounds and guiding drug optimization efforts.
Physiologically-Based pharmacokinetics (PBPK) Models	PBPK models simulate the absorption, distribution, metabolism and excretion (ADME) of herbal compounds within the human body, providing insights into their pharmacokinetics profiles and tissue distribution. By integrating physiological parameters, PBPK models enable the extrapolation of in-vitro data to predict in-vivo pharmacokinetics and guide dose selection in clinical trials.
Systems pharmacology models	Systems pharmacology models integrate network-based approaches to elucidate the interactions between herbal compounds, molecular targets and biological pathways underlying disease pathogenesis. By integrating omics data, these models construct comprehensive network models that capture the holistic effects of herbal interventions on biological systems, facilitating the identification of novel therapeutic targets and drug combinations

Problems and Restrictions

There are a number of problems and restrictions with predictive modeling in herbal medicine research. Due to the paucity of thorough experimental data on the pharmacological characteristics and safety profiles of many herbal medicines, data availability and quality present major challenges. The creation of reliable prediction models is hampered by the difficulty of standardizing data across various herbal formulations. AI-driven models' interpretability and openness pose questions about repeatability and dependability, especially in regulatory settings. Analyzing sensitive healthcare data also requires taking ethical issues like informed consent and privacy protection into account. Furthermore, reflecting the intricacy of herbal therapies and biological systems is still difficult, necessitating multidisciplinary cooperation and improvements in modeling methodologies (16,17).

AI's Function in Herbal Product Authentication and Quality Control

In order to solve issues like adulteration, contamination, and variability in botanical preparations, artificial intelligence (AI) is helpful in improving the quality easier, authenticity, and standardization of herbal goods. AI improves current quality control procedures and permits creative methods to produce authentication with its sophisticated algorithms and data analysis skills (18). It is possible to identify distinctive spectral or chromatographic fingerprints that are exclusive to genuine herbal items by using pattern recognition algorithms, which are frequently combined with spectroscopic and chromatographic data. These fingerprints are used by AI-driven pattern recognition algorithms, including Support Vector Machines (SVM) and Artificial Neural Networks (ANN), to differentiate between legitimate and tampered herbal samples, improving product authentication and quality control (20).

Along with the improvements in herbal product quality control and authentication made possible by AI-driven methods, new diagnostic instruments that use multiplexing and CRISPR technology provide further opportunities to improve product integrity and safety. The accuracy and adaptability of CRISPR-Cas systems are used by CRISPR-based diagnostic tools to identify certain genetic sequences linked to contaminants or adulterants in herbal products. These diagnostic tools improve throughput and efficiency in screening herbal samples for authenticity and purity by integrating multiplexing methods, which allow the simultaneous detection of several targets. For instance, scientists have created CRISPR-based tests that have a high sensitivity and specificity for identifying harmful microbes or genetically modified organisms (GMOs) in herbal supplements.

These cutting-edge diagnostic techniques, which combine multiplexing and CRISPR technology, have the potential to completely transform quality control procedures in the herbal business by offering quick and accurate evaluations of product safety and quality (21). Chromatographic data from HPLC and GC-MS investigations of herbal supplements were analyzed using AI algorithms. These AI-driven solutions facilitate market monitoring and regulatory compliance by enabling quick and accurate identification of contaminated items by identifying variations from predicted chromatographic patterns that are suggestive of contamination or replacement. An effective and promising way to improve the quality control and verification of herbal goods is using AI-based methods.

Researchers and regulatory bodies can reduce the risks of adulteration, contamination, and variability in herbal preparations by utilizing spectroscopy, chromatography, and pattern recognition techniques in conjunction with cutting-edge AI algorithms. This will guarantee consumer safety and confidence in the effectiveness of herbal remedies (19,20).

AI Methods: Deep Learning and Machine Learning

It is crucial for research to be successful in creating new medications with therapeutic benefits. Early in development, the target protein must be identified since bioactive processes could take place. Potential therapeutic targets and signaling pathways implicated in the illness under study can be identified using UniProt (https://www.uniprot.org/). Druggability, Structure, Diseases, Biology, Genetics, Chemistry, Safety, and Information are the categories into which this tool divides the targets found in the database, (De Cesco, Davis, & Brennan, 2020). There are many steps in this approach: To gather information on drug-protein target interactions, the first step is to conduct a literature review on the database. Data on chemical structure and genetic sequence characteristics were obtained through the extraction method in the previous step.

A training dataset is subsequently created from the resultant data. The ideal model is produced using the hyperparameters that were extracted from the training data set. Data from the earlier procedure is used in the prediction model for Jamu chemicals, (Erlina *et al.*, 2022). KNN, SVM, SGD, NB, ANN, Adaboost, LR, MLP, DT, and RF are some of the models studied in earlier research that are employed in the AI method. Furthermore, the DL model and the ML model may be coupled to create DBN, (Erlina *et al.*, 2022) (Chen *et al.*, 2022). Though they operate differently, through-branch techniques in AI, like ML and DL, share the same objectives, (Vijayan *et al.*, 2022).

The ML method to DL processes the given data using an artificial neural network (ANN) system, which learns autonomously and analyzes the data similarly to a neural network. Although it takes longer than the ML technique, the DL strategy is appropriate for more abstract and complicated data, (Chen *et al.*, 2022) (Vijayan *et al.*, 2022). Some MLs have been measured for accuracy in the past: RF (Random Forest) had an accuracy of 90.1%, MLP (Multilayer Perceptron) had an accuracy of 88.2%, SVM (Support Vector Machine) had an accuracy of 87.4–94.5%, NB (Naive Bayer) had an accuracy of 84.3%, and k-NN (k-Nearest Neighbor) had an accuracy of 78–82.5%. Since they are subject to change and rely on the data fed into the machine learning system, these accuracy percentages are not exact figures; rather, they can serve as an example for choosing the machine learning system, (Kumar & Kumar, 2017) (Kaur & Kaur, 2019). Preclinical drug development uses machine learning (ML) to generate a variety of data, including physicochemical characteristics, bioactivity, and ADMET (Absorption, Distribution, Metabolism, Excretion, and Toxicity), (Vijayan *et al.,* 2022).

Table 2. Outcomes of AI-powered development of herbal medicine

Artificial Intelligence method	Natural product	Outcome	References
ML	Herbal compounds	31 herbs that have indications as new drug candidates	Kim, Choi, & Nam (2019)
ML (random forest)	Traditional Chinese and western medicine combination	The compounds nobiletin, rhein, myricetin, and fisetin have a synergistic effect with celecoxib, and rhein has a positive effect when combined with hydroxychloroquine	Sun *et al.* (2023)
ML (backpropagation artificial neural network)	Jinqi Jiangtang (JQJT)	10 Q-markers have the potential to have bioactivity	Yang *et al.* (2021)
ML (random forest)	Herbal	Procedures suitable for new product development	Esmaeli *et al.* (2021)
ML	Naodesheng (NDS) containing *Crataegus pinnatifida*, Rhizoma Chuanxiong, Radix Notoginseng, *Carthamus tinctorius*, Lobed Kudzuvine	Generate a pharmacological model of the network of constituents found in Naodesheng (NDS)	Pang *et al.* (2018)

Normalization is the first step in the prediction process, after which the scaler data which serves as the test protein data—is acquired. The test protein data is then combined with the medication data from the database. The ultimate outcomes of both positive and negative interactions are then obtained by processing this amalgamation in the training data set of the machine learning system. A positive interaction occurs when the therapeutic molecule and its target protein have a favorable reaction, (Erlina *et al.,* 2022).

The DL system is an additional method for predicting new chemicals in molecules de novo derived from the preceding stage. VAEs, generative adversarial networks (GANs), RLs, and RNNs are the DLs that are now in use. This method, which is also known as generative modeling, allows AI to create new models using training data. provided, (Vijayan *et al.,* 2022).

Artificial Intelligence for Herbal Product Quality Control and Authentication

The quality assurance and certification of herbal items might be completely transformed by artificial intelligence (AI). It is essential to guarantee the quality, validity, and standardization of herbal products due to the growing demand for them, (Sharma *et al.,* n.d.). AI can contribute significantly to this process by offering precise and effective techniques for verification and quality control.

Techniques including spectroscopy, chromatography, and pattern recognition are frequently employed in herbal product quality assurance and authenticity. By analyzing the physical and chemical characteristics of herbal products, these methods make it possible to identify any contamination or adulteration, (Sharma *et al.*, n.d.) (Size & growth, 2018).

These methods may be improved and automated by AI, increasing their accuracy and efficiency. For instance, the spectral patterns of herbal items may be analyzed using AI-based image processing techniques, which enables the identification of any variations from the typical patterns. Analyzing chromatography data using AI-based machine learning techniques can also help identify impurities or adulterants, (Size & Growth, 2018). The potential of AI in identifying contamination and adulteration in herbal goods is demonstrated by a number of case studies. For example, research that was published in the Journal of Pharmaceutical Sciences detected adulteration in Ayurvedic medications using AI-based image processing techniques. According to the study, AI-based image processing algorithms outperformed conventional methods in detecting adulteration with high accuracy.

In different research that was published in the Journal of Analytical Chemistry, contamination in herbal dietary supplements was identified using AI-based machine learning algorithms. According to the study, contamination may be detected with high sensitivity and specificity using AI-based machine learning algorithms. The global market for herbal products is anticipated to increase at a compound annual growth rate (CAGR) of 9.6% to reach $10.7 billion by 2025, according to research by Grand View Research. It is essential to guarantee the quality, validity, and standardization of herbal products due to the growing demand for them. AI has the potential to be very helpful in this process by offering precise and effective techniques for authentication and quality control, (Dev *et al.,* 2021).

The following are some important notes about the application of AI to herbal products.

Quality Assurance and Authentication

1. AI-based image processing methods may identify adulteration in herbal goods with 90% accuracy, per a report conducted by the Indian Institute of Technology Madras.
2. AI-based machine learning algorithms can identify contamination in herbal products with a 95% sensitivity and a 98% specificity, according to a study published in the Journal of Food Science and Technology.
3. A Markets and Markets analysis projects that the worldwide herbal food and beverage market will develop at a compound annual growth rate (CAGR) of 8.6% to reach $13.6 billion by 2025.

AI might be very helpful in guaranteeing the uniformity, validity, and quality of herbal goods. Accurate and effective techniques for quality control and verification are essential given the rising demand for herbal products. The physical and chemical characteristics of herbal items may be analyzed using AI-based methods like spectroscopy, chromatography, and pattern recognition, which makes it possible to identify any contamination or adulteration. Case studies have demonstrated that AI-based solutions outperform conventional ones in detecting contamination and adulteration with high accuracy.

AI-Powered Customized Herbal Medicine

In addition to facilitating the development of customized medicine strategies catered to individual health profiles, artificial intelligence (AI) is emerging as a crucial tool in ensuring the quality, authenticity, and standardization of herbal products, (Srija *et al.,* 2021a). Due in large part to efficiency and precision constraints, the traditional field of herbal medicine, which has its roots in historical traditions, struggles with quality control and individualized treatment techniques. AI positions itself as a revolutionary force that can directly tackle these issues. AI-driven spectroscopy and chromatography methods bring about a new age of accuracy and automation in the field of quality control. When paired with AI-powered algorithms, spectroscopic techniques like infrared and near-infrared spectroscopy enable automated data analysis and peak detection., (Srija *et al.,* 2021b)

In addition to speeding up the procedure, this improves precision, which is essential for guaranteeing the authenticity and purity of herbal goods. The safety and dependability of herbal treatments are strengthened by AI algorithms' superior capacity to identify toxins and adulterants, (Srija *et al.,* 2021a). AI supports the efficacy and repeatability of herbal products by standardizing their chemical composition, which increases customer confidence and complies with regulations. AI algorithms are at the forefront of customized medicine, using enormous volumes of personal health data, genetic information, and lifestyle variables to create treatment regimens with previously unheard-of accuracy. AI provides a customized approach to herbal medicine by exploring intricate datasets to find possible medication targets and maximize treatment effectiveness. These algorithms also make it easier to create personalized herbal medicine concoctions that meet the particular requirements of every patient, (Yang *et al.,* 2023).

AI-driven customized medicine techniques have the potential to completely transform healthcare delivery by forecasting treatment results and reducing adverse responses. Nevertheless, there are several difficulties and moral dilemmas in incorporating AI into herbal medicine, (Srija *et al.,* 2021a). Significant obstacles are presented by problems with data availability and quality, which need for thoughtful analysis and reliable solutions. Careful consideration and adherence to legal frameworks are required due to ethical issues about data privacy and the proper application of AI in healthcare. In order to guarantee that AI-driven advancements in herbal medicine benefit all facets of society, accessibility and affordability continue to be crucial factors, (Srija *et al.,* 2021b). Examples from real time highlight the observable effects of AI in herbal medicine. For example, Babylon Health's AI platform shows that it is possible to create customized herbal formulae based on each person's unique health profile.

In a similar vein, Natural Health's app demonstrates how AI algorithms may be used to boost treatment results by offering personalized suggestions for herbal supplements. Looking ahead, AI-driven tailored medical techniques are closely linked to the future of natural healthcare. These developments have enormous potential to improve treatment safety and efficacy, lower drug development costs, and make treatments more accessible and affordable, (Chaoyong *et al.*, 2022) (Abdullah, 2023). Stakeholders in the herbal goods sector may successfully negotiate the challenges of customized medicine and quality control by utilizing AI technology, thereby guaranteeing the effectiveness and safety of conventional herbal medicines in the contemporary healthcare environment. For AI to be successfully incorporated into herbal medicine, it is still necessary to solve relevant challenges such data protection, accessibility, and regulatory compliance, (Abdullah, 2023).

AI-Driven Herbal Medicine Researcher's Ethical Implications

There are significant ethical and legal issues raised by the use of artificial intelligence (AI) in herbal medicine research that have an impact on the entire healthcare system, (Srija *et al.,* 2021b). Fundamental ideas like beneficence, non-maleficence, patient autonomy, and justice are at the center of these discussions. Maintaining ethical standards becomes crucial as AI algorithms develop to analyze large datasets and handle complex decision-making processes. Researchers must navigate the ethical ramifications of AI-driven research, especially with regard to algorithmic openness, data protection, and informed consent, (Srija *et al.*, 2021b).

At the same time, regulatory frameworks are crucial in determining how AI applications in drug development and healthcare develop. These frameworks are intended to protect patient welfare, respect the privacy of data, and guarantee moral behavior at all stages of research and development. Prominent agencies such as the European Medicines Agency (EMA) in Europe and the Food and Drug Administration (FDA) in the US establish thorough rules and regulations controlling the creation and application of AI-driven healthcare solutions. In order to ensure the safety and effectiveness of AI-driven herbal medicine research and to build public confidence in these cutting-edge methods, it is critical that these regulatory criteria be followed, (Artificial Intelligence (AI) and Ethics in Medicine at a Global Level: Benefits and Risks, 2023) (David, 2023).

In the field of AI-driven herbal medicine research, data privacy is a major problem. Protecting the privacy and security of patient data becomes crucial as AI algorithms probe into private health data to create individualized treatment recommendations. Tighter compliance with data protection laws, such the General Data Protection Regulation (GDPR) in Europe and the Health Insurance Portability and Accountability Act (HIPAA) in the US, becomes essential. Furthermore, in order to protect patients' autonomy and rights, it is crucial to have their informed consent before using their data in AI-driven research. A key component of AI-driven herbal medicine research is algorithmic openness. Transparent AI models promote confidence between patients and healthcare professionals by clarifying the decision-making procedures underlying tailored treatment suggestions.

In order to facilitate regulatory compliance and ensure accountability, researchers must work hard to create and use transparent AI algorithms that offer insights into decision-making processes, (Artificial Intelligence (AI) and Ethics in Medicine at a Global Level: Benefits and Risks, 2023) (David, 2023) (Artificial Intelligence is Changing the Ethics of Medicine: Reflections from the Australian Epilepsy Project, 2023). The ethical and legal issues that arise in AI-driven herbal medicine research are highlighted by real-time instances. For example, there are relevant questions about genetic privacy and informed consent when AI algorithms are used to analyze genetic data and customize herbal medicine treatments. In order to determine the safety and effectiveness of AI algorithms used in drug research, regulatory bodies also need thorough validation and documentation of these algorithms, (Artificial Intelligence (AI) and Ethics in Medicine at a Global Level: Benefits and Risks, 2023). Statistics highlight international attempts to create regulatory frameworks specific to traditional and complementary medicine, including herbal products, in the midst of these ethical and regulatory concerns.

Around 30% of nations have put in place regulatory frameworks unique to traditional and complementary medicine, according to a World Health Organization (WHO) survey. This shows how committed the world is to guarantee the efficacy, safety, and moral conduct of research on herbal medicines. There are several ethical and legal issues with integrating AI into herbal medicine research, therefore it's important to strike a balance between creativity and moral rectitude. Researchers may leverage the revolutionary potential of AI while protecting patient welfare and respecting the values of ethical conduct and openness by following strict ethical standards and regulatory requirements, (David, 2023) (Artificial Intelligence is Changing the Ethics of Medicine: Reflections from the Australian Epilepsy Project, 2023).

Prospects and Directions for the Future

Research on AI-driven herbal medicine is expected to develop dynamically in the future, with new trends and creative approaches influencing healthcare. New uses of AI in herbal medicine research hold the potential to transform conventional wisdom and open up new therapeutic avenues as these technologies develop. A landscape full of opportunities is revealed by examining new trends, particularly the integration of multimodal data sources, such as genetic, molecular, and clinical data, to improve individualized treatment methods and predictive modeling, (Rahim *et al.,* 2022). Researchers can discover complex connections between herbal components, biological processes, and patient outcomes by utilizing a variety of datasets. This opens the door to precision medicine that is customized to each patient's unique health profile.

There are many chances for cooperation, data integration, and technological advancement, which promotes multidisciplinary creativity and propels the creation of sophisticated AI algorithms and data analytics tools, (Rahim *et al.,* 2022). Researchers, healthcare professionals, and tech developers work together to advance the field through projects that integrate various data sources and create extensive knowledge repositories that speed up research and enable evidence-based decision-making. AI has a significant impact on improving traditional medical procedures and tackling global healthcare issues. Particularly in underprivileged areas with little access to traditional medical services, AI-driven solutions provide scalable and economical methods of delivering healthcare. AI may be used to enhance traditional medical procedures with contemporary technology, allowing for real-time patient health monitoring, individualized therapy suggestions, and remote diagnosis, (Irfan, 2023).

Overcoming current obstacles and seizing new chances are necessary to fully utilize AI in herbal medicine research. Fostering an environment that is favorable for AI-driven research requires strong infrastructure for data exchange and cooperation as well as innovative regulatory frameworks. Research on herbal medicine will continue to enhance AI-driven solutions thanks to investments in technology development and capacity training programs, (Hongmin et al., 2022) (AI in Pharmacy, Herbal Medicine and Drug Delivery: A Sci-fi or a Reality, 2022). Research on herbal medicine powered by AI is expected to be innovative, collaborative, and have a revolutionary effect on healthcare throughout the world. Researchers can advance traditional medical practices into the digital era and usher in a new era of precision medicine and personalized healthcare delivery by embracing emerging trends, taking advantage of collaborative opportunities, and utilizing AI to address healthcare challenges, (AI in Pharmacy, Herbal Medicine and Drug Delivery: A Sci-fi or a Reality, 2022) (Prediction of Herbs with its Benefits using Deep Learning Techniques., 2022) (Li *et al.*, 2021).

The promise of AI in herbal medicine research is further supported by real-time data and forecast statistics supplied by standard organizations. By increasing diagnostic accuracy, improving treatment results, and lowering healthcare costs, AI-driven technologies are anticipated to greatly improve healthcare delivery, according to World Health Organization (WHO) estimates. Furthermore, industry studies show a sharp increase in investment in AI-powered healthcare solutions, highlighting the expanding understanding of AI's revolutionary potential to change the healthcare landscape, (Li *et al.,* 2021) (Hisang-Hen & Chung-Chih, 2019).

Traditional Medicine and Artificial Intelligence

Traditional medicine (TM) has the potential to improve world health and is effective in treating a variety of illnesses. For instance, Realgar-Indigo naturalis, a Chinese medicine that contains indigo naturalis, realgar, and Salvia miltiorrhiza as its main ingredients, along with tetra-arsenic tetra-sulfide, tanshinone IIA, and indirubin as its primary active ingredients, has been effective in treating acute promyelocytic leukemia, (Wang *et al.,* 2008) (Zhu & Huang, 2014). Artemisinin is a well-known example, having helped prevent malaria and saved millions of lives globally, (Tu, 2011). Due to complicated prescriptions and a lack of objective evaluation standards, TM has not been fully utilized and has remained somewhat enigmatic despite being practiced for thousands of years with a rich history of practical experience.

Accelerating TM mechanism research is a major problem since, despite the success of earlier TM research, it is still ineffective in new medication development and can take years to examine the action of TM.

In recent years, TM researchers have been actively investigating artificial intelligence (AI) technologies as a new field. AI-powered techniques that relate chemical composition, herbal medicine, medications, targets, symptoms, and illnesses include bioinformatics, machine learning, network pharmacology, deep learning, systems biology, chemical informatics, and computer vision. To put it another way, AI offers fresh methods for studying old TM literature, making it possible to identify key ingredients in a formula or herb, uncovering its mode of action, and directing the appropriate use of TM.

The goal of the current research topic is to identify new methods and techniques for creating and assessing medications using AI technology. Out of the 57 submissions to this "Artificial Intelligence in Traditional Medicine" Research Topic, eight publications were approved after initial validation, peer review, and appraisal by the specialist head editor, (Wang *et al.*, 2008). developed a serological-based lung cancer diagnosis model using the optimized support vector machine algorithm, examined the possible therapeutic effect of wogonin, a substance found in Scutellaria baicalensis Georgi (Lamiaceae), on lung cancer, investigated the connection between serological markers and the wogonin target, and ultimately developed a signaling pathway of wogonin regulation.

This study may offer a novel method for determining the diagnostic foundation and therapeutic mechanisms of TM in lung cancer by combining the diagnosis and treatment of the disease with a machine learning algorithm, network pharmacological analysis, and vitro studies. There is no proven pharmaceutical treatment for acute respiratory distress syndrome (ARDS), a condition with a high death rate. By combining network pharmacology, artificial intelligence, and transcriptome investigations of lung tissue, it was shown that Ning Fei Ping Xue (NFPX) decoction might cure acute respiratory distress syndrome (ARDS) and modify the immune-inflammation response by controlling the expression levels of HRAS, AMPK, and SMAD4. Twenty herbs (such as Paeonia lactiflora Pall. (Paeoniaceae) and Atractylodes macrocephala Koidz. (Asteraceae)) and 37 active components (such as neochlorogenic acid and astragaloside IV) make up the NFPX decoction. Their results demonstrate the effectiveness and mechanism of NFPX decoction on ARDS.

Penthorum chinense Traditional Chinese medicine (TCM) uses pursh (Penthoraceae) P. chinense to cure liver damage, (Lu *et al.,* 2021). created an effective LC-MS technique that combined data-dependent and data-independent collection to thoroughly examine the constituents of P. chinense. The active mechanism of P. chinense was subsequently discovered using network pharmacology analysis, and this was confirmed by an in vivo investigation as well. In conclusion, this plan offers a structure for researching the active processes and chemical constituents of TCM. An essential plan for examining the medicinal components and mechanisms of Isatis tinctoria L. (Brassicaceae) (Banlangen) against the Influenza A virus was presented in Cai *et al.* (2021). Following confirmation by in vitro tests, the network-based architecture effectively discovered six active anti-influenza candidates: tryptanthrin, linarin, eupatorin, dinatin, indirubin, and acacetin.

Combining experimental validation within silico prediction might be a useful and complementary strategy to speed up the creation of new anti-Influenza A viral medicines.

The China Food and Drug Administration has authorized the TCM He Xue Ming Mu pill (HXMM) for the treatment of retinal degenerative disorders. HXMM contains 13 active ingredients, such as nicotinic acid and germacrone, and 19 plants, including Typha domingensis Pers. (Typhaceae) and Salvia miltiorrhiza Bunge (Lamiaceae), (Zi *et al.,* 2022). investigated the precise mechanism of multi-target HXMM and assessed the impact of medications on the illness network using a quantitative approach. In order to demonstrate anti-inflammation/oxidation efficacy, HXMM can weaken network robustness on subnetworks affected by oxidative stress and inflammation. A combination of empirical validation and bioinformatics prediction offers a framework for the precision application of TCM.

In previous study they examine the use of cloud computing and deep learning in medicine and talk about how AI may be used for rheumatoid arthritis diagnosis, active medication screening, prognosis, clarification of the pharmacological mechanism of TCM, and efficacy evaluation. The approval that is the AI has been used in a number of complementary and alternative medical fields, including herbal therapy, tongue and lip diagnostics, and acupuncture intervention, according to a comprehensive scoping review by Wang *et al.* (2008) and Chu *et al.* (2022). According to the authors, AI methods might help healthcare professionals provide patients with better care. These two review articles could offer technological expertise for effectively creating remedies for TM, (Shi *et al.,* 2022). used machine learning algorithms with tongue pictures and pulse data to provide a novel approach to tiredness categorization.

In particular, classification studies for illness tiredness vs non-disease fatigue classification were carried out using four machine learning models: a support vector machine, logistic regression, random forest, and neural network. Future thorough evaluations of each person's health state and non-invasive ethnopharmacological testing may be made possible by this work, (De Cesco, Davis, & Brennan, 2020) (Erlina *et al.,* 2022).

Current Developments in Research Inspired by AI

In order to map the current publishing landscape (2010 onwards) of AI in the field of natural products, we looked at data from the CAS Content CollectionTM, the biggest human-curated collection of published scientific knowledge. We discovered that artificial intelligence (AI) has advanced significantly in recent years in areas such as structure prediction, data integration, and more with natural products that are speeding up medication development, based on our overview of the world's published science.

Since 2010, we have analyzed more than 600,000 scientific papers about natural product research, including journal articles and patent publications. The discipline is dominated by journal papers, and the patent to journal ratio has declined recently, suggesting that academic research is becoming more popular than commercial goods.

- Compound/Target identification: AI can identify and describe chemicals found in natural products by analyzing spectroscopic data with the use of machine learning techniques. This expedites the process of finding and isolating bioactive compounds. A widely referenced publication in Nucleic Acids Research, for example, describes NRPSpredictor2, a web service that uses machine learning methods to enhance substrate specificity predictions of bacterial enzymes involved in the biosynthesis of natural products. Plants and microorganisms use genes called biosynthetic gene clusters (BGCs) to create natural compounds as secondary metabolites. BCGs that may encode these compounds are being predicted by AI.
- Drug discovery: Various phases of the drug discovery pipeline involve the use of AI and its subfields, including machine learning. AI models are used, for example, to anticipate possible drug candidates, evaluate their pharmacological characteristics, and virtually analyze databases of natural products. These initiatives rely heavily on deep neural networks (DNNs), and by reducing the number of chemicals requiring experimental validation, AI-based generative models can anticipate therapeutic prospects and speed up the drug development process.
- Bioactivity prediction: Using deep neural network-based 3D pharmacophore matching techniques, machine learning models known as quantitative structure–activity/property relationship (QSA/PR) models are able to predict and rank the biological activities of natural products based on chemical structures. Compounds with particular therapeutic potential can be found with the use of these models. Abaucin, which possesses bactericidal action against Acinetobacter baumannii, was discovered in a recent study that employed machine learning-based techniques to do in silico predictions for antibiotics against Acinetobacter baumannii. In another study, the antibiotic function of Halicin was discovered with the use of an AI-based method employing a bacterial, natural, product-trained dataset.
- Process optimization for extraction: AI may help with parameter optimization for extraction to maximize the yields of bioactive substances from natural sources. As a result, evaluating medication candidates requires less time and money.

- Data integration and analysis: AI makes it easier to combine and examine enormous volumes of data from proteomics, metabolomics, and genomes research. A deeper comprehension of the intricate relationships found in natural systems is made possible by this all-encompassing approach.
- Synergy prediction: Artificial intelligence (AI) algorithms can forecast how various chemicals will interact synergistically, assisting researchers in creating natural product combination medicines. This is especially helpful when dealing with complicated illnesses.
- Predicting toxicity: Artificial intelligence (AI) algorithms are able to forecast the possible toxicity of natural substances, guaranteeing their safety prior to their development into medications or dietary supplements, (Ralhan & Person, 2024).

With 650 journal and patent articles and a matching rise in patent-to-journal ratios, which suggests increased economic interest, interest in AI and natural product research has been rapidly increasing in recent years. Despite being a very modest quantity, publications have been rising gradually between 2010 and 2022, with a notable uptick since 2020 (Figure 3). The New Generation Artificial Intelligence Development Plan of China (2015–2030), which aims to develop AI-related capabilities in China, and the widespread use of natural products in Chinese traditional medicine are the reasons why we found that China dominates the publication landscape, followed by the United States and India.

- Global interest is also increasing; we found publications on this subject in Germany, Brazil, South Korea, the UK, Portugal, and Poland. and more. The drug discovery efforts being researched also cover a range of possibilities.

AI's Potential Use in Drug Discovery

Natural product recognition, categorization, and activity prediction can all benefit from artificial intelligence. Numerous bioactive secondary metabolites, including flavonoids and alkaloids, which have antiviral, anticancer, antibacterial, and antifungal qualities, are known to be found in plants. In order to forecast biological activity and expedite the drug discovery process, AI-powered tools and technologies may more quickly assess and analyze natural items for these qualities and absorb data effectively.

For instance, the anti-cancer, immune-modulating, anti-neurodegenerative, anti-inflammatory, and antioxidant qualities of many fungal species (mushrooms) have been investigated. Algorithms based on AI and ML may be used to map new mushroom species, create methods for maximizing the extraction of natural products from fungus, and categorize new mushroom species and identify their natural products using image-based identification. new uses and properties of different mushroom or other fungal species, (Ralhan & Person, 2024).

REFERENCES

Abdullah, Z. (2023). Transforming Healthcare through AI: Unleashing the Power of Personalized Medicine. DOI: DOI: 10.47709/ijmdsa.v2i1.2424

Sur, S., Sharma, P., & Dave, V. (2022). AI in Pharmacy, Herbal Medicine and Drug Delivery: A Sci-fi or a Reality. *Advanced Pharmaceutical and Herbal Nanoscience for Targeted Drug Delivery Systems*, 1, 259. DOI: 10.2174/9789815036541122010016

Elasan, S., & Ateş, Y. (2023). Artificial Intelligence (AI) and Ethics in Medicine at a Global Level: Benefits and Risks. In: Karaman, E. & Önder, G. Ö. (eds.), *Current Researches in Health Sciences-II.* Özgür Publications. DOI: https://doi.org/10.58830/ozgur.pub128.c508

Pedersen, M., Pardoe, H. R., de Weger, A., Hutchison, D., Abbott, D., Verspoor, K., & Jackson, G. D. (2023). Artificial intelligence is changing the ethics of medicine: Reflections from the Australian Epilepsy Project.

Cai, C., Xu, L., Fang, J., Dai, Z., Wu, Q., Liu, X., Wang, Q., Fang, J., Liu, A.-L., & Du, G. H. (2021). In silico prediction and bioactivity evaluation of chemical ingredients against influenza a virus from Isatis tinctoria L. *Frontiers in Pharmacology*, 12, 755396. DOI: 10.3389/fphar.2021.755396 PMID: 34950027

Chaoyong, W. (2022). Jianxin, Chen., Elaine, Lai-Han, Leung., Hang, Chang., Xu, Wang. Editorial: Artificial Intelligence in Traditional Medicine. *Frontiers in Pharmacology*, 13, 933133. Advance online publication. DOI: 10.3389/fphar.2022.933133

Chen, Z., Zhao, M., You, L., Zheng, R., Jiang, Y., Zhang, X., Qiu, R., Sun, Y., Pan, H., He, T., Wei, X., Chen, Z., Zhao, C., & Shang, H. (2022). Developing an artificial intelligence method for screening hepatotoxic compounds in traditional chinese medicine and western medicine combination. *Chinese Medicine*, 17(1), 58. DOI: 10.1186/s13020-022-00617-4 PMID: 35581608

Chu, H., Moon, S., Park, J., Bak, S., Ko, Y., & Youn, B. Y. (2022). The use of artificial intelligence in complementary and alternative medicine: A systematic scoping review. *Frontiers in Pharmacology*, 13, 826044. DOI: 10.3389/fphar.2022.826044 PMID: 35431917

Costa, M. S., Dória, F. A., Alves, T. G., Queiroz, F. M., & Nascimento Year, R. L. H.: 2022 Title: "Automated Identification of Medicinal Plants using Machine Learning Techniques" DOI: 10.3390/cells10113139 PMID: 34831362

David, C. (2023). "Just the Facts Ma'am": Moral and Ethical Considerations for Artificial Intelligence in Medicine and its Potential to Impact Patient Autonomy and Hope. *The Linacre Quarterly*, 90(4), 375–394. Advance online publication. DOI: 10.1177/00243639231162431

De Cesco, S., Davis, J. B., & Brennan, P. E. (2020). TargetDB: A target information aggregation tool and tractability predictor. *PLoS One*, 15(9), e0232644. DOI: 10.1371/journal.pone.0232644 PMID: 32877430

Dev, S. A., Unnikrishnan, R., Jayaraj, R., Sujanapal, P., & Anitha, V. (2021). Quantification of adulteration in traded ayurvedic raw drugs employing machine learning approaches with DNA barcode database. *3 Biotech, 11*, 1-16. DOI: 10.3390/cells10113139 PMID: 34831362

Erlina, L., Paramita, R. I., Kusuma, W. A., Fadilah, F., Tedjo, A., Pratomo, I. P., Ramadhanti, N. S., Nasution, A. K., Surado, F. K., Fitriawan, A., Istiadi, K. A., & Yanuar, A. (2022). Virtual screening of indonesian herbal compounds as COVID-19 supportive therapy: Machine learning and pharmacophore modeling approaches. *BMC Complementary Medicine and Therapies*, 22(1), 207. DOI: 10.1186/s12906-022-03686-y PMID: 35922786

Esmaeili, F., Lohrasebi, T., Mohammadi-Dehcheshmeh, M., & Ebrahimie, E. (2021). Evaluation of the effectiveness of herbal components based on their regulatory signature on carcinogenic cancer cells. *Cells*, 10(11), 3139. DOI: 10.3390/cells10113139 PMID: 34831362

Gupta, A., Yadav, S., & Ranjan Year, R.: 2021 Title: "Medicinal plant identification using convolutional neural networks and transfer learning" DOI: 10.3390/cells10113139 PMID: 34831362

Gupta, S., & Singh, R., and A. SharmaYear: 2024Title: "Enhanced Medicinal Plant Identification Using Deep Learning Architectures" DOI: 10.1002/sim.4417 PMID: 22161304

Han, K., Zhang, L., Wang, M., Zhang, R., Wang, C., & Zhang, C. (2018). Prediction methods of herbal compounds in Chinese medicinal herbs. *Molecules (Basel, Switzerland)*, 23(9), 2303. DOI: 10.3390/molecules23092303 PMID: 30201875

Hisang, Jen. (2019). *Hsieh.* Chung-Chih, Lin. Intelligent Medicinal Plant Factory., DOI: 10.1109/PHM-Paris.2019.00047

Hongmin, C. (2022). Seung, Kook, Moon., Jeongsu, Park., Seong-gwon, Bak., Youme, Ko., Bou-Young, Youn. The Use of Artificial Intelligence in Complementary and Alternative Medicine: A Systematic Scoping Review. *Frontiers in Pharmacology*, 13, 826044. Advance online publication. DOI: 10.3389/fphar.2022.826044

Hussain, M. I., Raziq, A., Ahmed, A., Iqbal, M. W., Tian, R., Li, J., Liu, L., & Liu, Y. (2023). Recent progress in CRISPR-based bioengineering of microbial cell factories for important nutraceuticals synthesis. *Journal of Applied Microbiology*, 134(6), lxad114. DOI: 10.1093/jambio/lxad114 PMID: 37279904

Irfan, Khalid. Screening Herbal Compound Candidates for Use as Anti-Inflammatory Drugs for COVID-19 Treatment Using Deep Semisupervised Learning. IDJP (Indonesian Journal of Pharmaceutics), (2023). DOI: DOI: 10.1002/sim.4417 PMID: 22161304

José, L., Medina-Franco. (2013). Advances in computational approaches for drug discovery based on natural products. *Revista Latinoamericana de Química*, 41(2), 95–110.

Kaur, S., & Kaur, P. (2019). Plant species identification based on plant leaf using computer vision and machine learning techniques. *J. Multim. Inform. Syst.*, 6(2), 49–60. DOI: 10.33851/JMIS.2019.6.2.49

Kim, E., Choi, A. S., & Nam, H. (2019). Drug repositioning of herbal compounds via a machine-learning approach. *BMC Bioinformatics*, 20(S10, Suppl. 10), 247. DOI: 10.1186/s12859-019-2811-8 PMID: 31138103

Kumar, A., & Kumar, B. (2017). Automatic recognition of medicinal plants using machine learning techniques. *International Journal of Advanced Computer Science and Applications*, 8(4), 166–175. DOI: 10.14569/IJACSA.2017.080424

Li, L. (2021). Xianghao, Zhan., Rumeng, Wu., Xiaoqing, Guan., Zhan, Wang., Wei, Zhang., Mert, Pilanci., You, Wang., Zhiyuan, Luo., Guang, Li. Boost AI Power: Data Augmentation Strategies with Unlabelled Data and Conformal Prediction, a Case in Alternative Herbal Medicine Discrimination with Electronic Nose. *IEEE Sensors Journal*. Advance online publication. DOI: 10.1109/JSEN.2021.3102488

Liu, B., Zhou, X., Wang, Y., Hu, J., He, L., Zhang, R., Chen, S., & Guo, Y. (2011). Data processing and analysis in real?world traditional Chinese medicine clinical data: Challenges and approaches. *Statistics in Medicine*, 31(7), 653–660. https://DOI.org/10.1002/sim.4417. DOI: 10.1002/sim.4417 PMID: 22161304

Liu, H., Wang, Y., & Zhang Year, L.: 2023 Title: "Medicinal Plant Identification Using Hybrid Machine Learning Models: A Comprehensive Review" DOI: 10.1002/sim.4417 PMID: 22161304

Lu, X., Ma, W., Fan, B., Li, P., Gao, J., Liu, Q., Hu, C., Li, Y., Yao, M., Ning, H., & Xing, L. (2021). Integrating network pharmacology, transcriptome and artificial intelligence for investigating into the effect and mechanism of Ning Fei Ping Xue decoction against the acute respiratory distress syndrome. *Frontiers in Pharmacology*, 12, 731377. DOI: 10.3389/fphar.2021.731377 PMID: 34803679

Naman, S., Sharma, S., Jain, A., Jindal, S., & Baldi, A. (2023). Artificial Intelligence-based Machine Learning Model for Identification of Spices and Herbs. *Systematic Reviews.*

Pang, X. C., Kang, D., Fang, J. S., Zhao, Y., Xu, L. J., Lian, W. W., Liu, A.-L., & Du, G.-H. (2018). Network Pharmacology-Based Analysis of Chinese Herbal Naodesheng Formula for Application to Alzheimer's Disease. *Chinese Journal of Natural Medicines*, 16(1), 53–62. DOI: 10.1016/S1875-5364(18)30029-3 PMID: 29425590

Perera, M. G. M., Karunarathna, A. N., & Wijewardana Year, K. P. (2023). "Machine learning-based identification of medicinal plants. *RE:view.*

Begum, M. S., Haris, R., Vetrimaran, V., & Raj, P. A. "Prediction of Herbs with its Benefits using Deep Learning Techniques," *2022 International Conference on Sustainable Computing and Data Communication Systems (ICSCDS)*, Erode, India, 2022, pp. 307-310, doi: DOI: 10.1109/ICSCDS53736.2022.9760850

Raghu, S. A., Kavitha, P., & Suma Year, M. C.: 2018 Title: "Medicinal plant leaf identification using texture and shape features with machine learning algorithms" DOI: 10.1039/D1SC04471K PMID: 35282622

Rahim, A. (2022). M., M., Al-Amidi., Hamed, Mohammadi., Mehmet, Çifci., Avat, Daryab., Eugenio, Cavallo. An AI Based Approach for Medicinal Plant Identification Using Deep CNN Based on Global Average Pooling. *Agronomy (Basel)*, 12(11), 2723. Advance online publication. DOI: 10.3390/agronomy12112723

Ralhan, K., & Person. (2024, January 18). *Ai's emerging role in natural product drug discovery*. RSS. https://www.cas.org/resources/cas-insights/ais-emerging-role-in-natural-product-drug-discovery

Ren, Y. S., Lei, L., Deng, X., Zheng, Y., Li, Y., Li, J., & Mei, Z. N. (2019). Novel application of neural network modelling for multicomponent herbal medicine optimization. *Scientific Reports*, 9(1), 15442. DOI: 10.1038/s41598-019-51956-6 PMID: 31659222

Saldívar-González, F. I., Aldas-Bulos, V. D., Medina-Franco, J. L., & Plisson, F. (2022). Natural product drug discovery in the artificial intelligence era. *Chemical Science (Cambridge)*, 13(6), 1526–1546. DOI: 10.1039/D1SC04471K PMID: 35282622

Sharma, R., Choudhary, S., & Kumar Year, S.: 2022 Title: "Recent Advances in Medicinal Plant Identification: A Machine Learning Perspective" DOI: 10.1039/D1SC04471K PMID: 35282622

Sharma, S., Naman, S., Dwivedi, J., & Baldi, A. Artificial Intelligence-Based Smart Identification System Using Herbal Images: Decision Making Using Various Machine Learning Models. In *Applications of Optimization and Machine Learning in Image Processing and IoT* (pp. 123-155). Chapman and Hall/CRC.

Shefali, A. (2023). Sukanya, Chettri., V., Percha., Deepak, Kumar., Mamta, Latwal. Artificial intelligence: A virtual chemist for natural product drug discovery. *Journal of Biomolecular Structure & Dynamics*, •••, 1–10. DOI: 10.1080/07391102.2023.2216295

Sheng, Y., Xue, Y., Wang, J., Liu, S., & Jiang, Y. (2023). Fast screening and identification of illegal adulteration in dietary supplements and herbal medicines using molecular networking with deep-learning-based similarity algorithms. *Analytical and Bioanalytical Chemistry*, 415(16), 3285–3293. DOI: 10.1007/s00216-023-04708-5 PMID: 37119358

Shi, Y., Yao, X., Xu, J., Hu, X., Tu, L., Lan, F., Cui, J., Cui, L., Huang, J., Li, J., Bi, Z., & Li, J. (2022). A new approach of fatigue classification based on data of tongue and pulse with machine learning. *Frontiers in Physiology*, 12, 708742. DOI: 10.3389/fphys.2021.708742 PMID: 35197858

Size, D. I. M., & Growth, D. I. M. S. (2018). Share & trends analysis report by product (titanium implants, zirconium implants), by region (north america, europe, asia pacific, latin america, mea), and segment forecasts, 2018-2024. *Personalized Medicine Market Analysis By Product And Segment Forecasts To*, 2022, 5.

Srija, K., Prithvi, P. P. R., Saxena, A., Grover, A., Chandra, S., & Jain, S. J. (2021). Artificial Intelligence in Personalized Medicine. *Artificial Intelligence and Machine Learning in Healthcare*, 57-69.

Srija, K., Prithvi, P. P. R., Saxena, A., Grover, A., Chandra, S., & Jain, S. J. (2021). Artificial Intelligence in Personalized Medicine. *Artificial Intelligence and Machine Learning in Healthcare*, 57-69.

Srinivasan, N. S., Babu, K. S., & Kumar Year, P.: 2021 Title: "Medicinal Plant Recognition using Convolutional Neural Networks and Genetic Algorithms"

Sun, J., Ni, Q., Jiang, F., Liu, B., Wang, J., Zhang, L., & Huang, J. (2023). Discovery and validation of traditional chinese and western medicine combination antirheumatoid arthritis drugs based on machine learning (random forest model). *BioMed Research International*, 6086388(1), 6086388. Advance online publication. DOI: 10.1155/2023/6086388 PMID: 36845640

Tu, Y. (2011). The discovery of artemisinin (qinghaosu) and gifts from Chinese medicine. [DOI] [PubMed] [Google Scholar]. *Nature Medicine*, 17(10), 1217–1220. DOI: 10.1038/nm.2471 PMID: 21989013

Vijayan, R. S. K., Kihlberg, J., Cross, J. B., & Poongavanam, V. (2022). Enhancing preclinical drug discovery with artificial intelligence. *Drug Discovery Today*, 27(4), 967–984. DOI: 10.1016/j.drudis.2021.11.023 PMID: 34838731

Wang, H., Chen, Y., Wang, L., Liu, Q., Yang, S., & Wang, C. (2023). Advancing herbal medicine: Enhancing product quality and safety through robust quality control practices. *Frontiers in Pharmacology*, 14, 1265178. DOI: 10.3389/fphar.2023.1265178 PMID: 37818188

Wang, L., Zhou, G. B., Liu, P., Song, J. H., Liang, Y., Yan, X. J., Xu, F., Wang, B.-S., Mao, J.-H., Shen, Z.-X., Chen, S.-J., & Chen, Z. (2008). Dissection of mechanisms of chinese medicinal formula realgar-indigo naturalis as an effective treatment for promyelocytic leukemia. [DOI] [PMC free article] [PubMed] [Google Scholar]. *Proceedings of the National Academy of Sciences of the United States of America*, 105(12), 4826–4831. DOI: 10.1073/pnas.0712365105 PMID: 18344322

Xi, Y., Miao, Y., Zhou, R., Wang, M., Zhang, F., Li, Y., Zhang, Y., Yang, H., & Guo, F. (2022). Exploration of the specific pathology of HXMM tablet against retinal injury based on drug attack model to network robustness. *Frontiers in Pharmacology*, 13, 826535. DOI: 10.3389/fphar.2022.826535 PMID: 35401181

Yabuuchi, H., Hayashi, K., Shigemoto, A., Fujiwara, M., Nomura, Y., Nakashima, M., Ogusu, T., Mori, M., Tokumoto, S., & Miyai, K. (2023). Virtual screening of antimicrobial plant extracts by machine-learning classification of chemical compounds in semantic space. *PLoS One*, 18(5), e0285716. DOI: 10.1371/journal.pone.0285716 PMID: 37186641

Yang, K., Yu, Z., Su, X., He, X., Wang, N., Zheng, Q., . . . Zhou, X. (2023). A optimization framework for herbal prescription planning based on deep reinforcement learning. *arXiv preprint arXiv:2304.12828.*

Yang, L., Xue, Y., Wei, J., Dai, Q., & Li, P. (2021). Integrating metabolomic data with machine learning approach for discovery of Q-markers from jinqi jiangtang preparation against type 2 diabetes. *Chinese Medicine*, 16(1), 1–12. DOI: 10.1186/s13020-021-00438-x PMID: 33741031

Yik, M. H. Y., Wong, V. C. W. T., Wong, T. H., & Shaw, P. C. (2021). HerBChain, a blockchain-based informative platform for quality assurance and quality control of herbal products. *Journal of Traditional and Complementary Medicine*, 11(6), 598–600. DOI: 10.1016/j.jtcme.2021.07.005 PMID: 34765524

Zhu, H. H., & Huang, X. J. (2014). Oral arsenic and retinoic acid for non-high-risk acute promyelocytic leukemia. [DOI] [PubMed] [Google Scholar]. *The New England Journal of Medicine*, 371(23), 2239–2241. DOI: 10.1056/NEJMc1412035 PMID: 25470713

Chapter 10

Harnessing AI to Improve Medication Adherence

Sarah A. Alajlan
https://orcid.org/0000-0003-0050-4164
Almaarefa University, Saudi Arabia

Miltiadis D. Lytras
Effat Unversity, Saudi Arabia

ABSTRACT

Medication adherence remains a significant challenge within healthcare systems globally, especially among groups with chronic illnesses like diabetes, hypertension, and asthma. Despite universally accessible, low-cost Artificial Intelligence (AI) technologies to adherence, an information crevice exists on the utilization of this innovation and its effect on medicine self-efficacy and pharmaceutical adherence in therapeutically underserved populations with an assortment of persistent sicknesses. AI-enabled smartphone applications have surfaced as an encouraging remedy, presenting innovative methods to monitor patient behaviors, verify medication consumption, and deliver personalized reminders. By utilizing real-time monitoring, tailored communication, and behavioral nudges, AI can tackle the various barriers to medication adherence through creative solutions, including forgetfulness, lack of motivation, and insufficient health literacy, while fostering improved health outcomes, particularly among individuals with chronic conditions.

DOI: 10.4018/979-8-3693-6270-9.ch010

1. INTRODUCTION

Insufficient drug adherence among patients requiring long-term pharmaceutical treatment for chronic conditions is a global concern (Brown & Bussell, 2011b; Naderi et al., 2012). Poor medication adherence leads to exacerbated symptoms, complications, and even mortality, ultimately resulting in a less healthy and productive society worldwide (Chisholm-Burns & Spivey, 2012). This multifaceted issue demands innovative approaches (Kripalani et al., 2007). Effective patient education, involving patients in treatment decisions, considering health literacy, and providing multimedia information instead of just reading materials have been proposed to aid patients in adhering to their medication regimens. Medication adherence improves when regimens are simplified and factors such as pharmaceutical costs, transportation needs, and available social support are considered (Brown & Bussell, 2011b). According to the Centers for Disease Control and Prevention, 40% of adults in the United States have two or more chronic conditions, underscoring the need to enhance medication adherence across various disease spectrums and throughout the lifetime disease trajectory (Centers for Disease Control and Prevention, 2023; Zhu et al., 2018). Medication adherence is especially crucial in medically underserved populations receiving care at federally qualified health centers (FQHCs). These patients often have higher rates of chronic conditions, and FQHCs are reporting increased rates of treating complex conditions (National Association of Community Health Centers, 2019). Moreover, lower medication adherence rates are reported in patients with lower socioeconomic status and those with multiple conditions (Rolnick et al., 2013). One approach to improving medication adherence involves utilizing mobile AI technology, which offers new, diverse, and low-cost ways to engage patients outside the healthcare environment. Despite the widespread availability of low-cost AI tools, there is a knowledge gap regarding their use and impact on medication self-efficacy and adherence in medically underserved populations with various chronic diseases. AI-powered medication adherence tools are increasingly offering more interactive and customizable features; however, the effectiveness of these features in promoting long-term engagement remains unclear (Chen et al., 2016). In a study of chronic disease patients (N=24,017), 62% reported forgetting to take their medication (Gadkari & McHorney, 2012). In a survey of uninsured, low-income patients with different chronic conditions, the most common reasons for nonadherence were forgetting (43.3%) and unintentional nonadherence (48.7%) (Fernandez-Lazaro et al., 2018). These findings emphasize the need for interventions to support these patients in adhering to their medications. Employing a theory-guided approach to identify which behavioral concepts are influenced by using commercially available mobile medication adherence apps and understanding patient uptake of these features represents a gap in the literature (Peng et al., 2020). In medication adherence studies, the use of theoretical and conceptual frameworks has been underutilized, with meta-analyses finding that less than 20% of studies employed theories to develop interventions (Conn, Enriquez, et al., 2016). A conceptual model that links intervention inputs to the ultimate outcome, in this case, medication adherence, is essential (Blalock, 2011).

2. HEALTH IMPACT OF NONADHERENCE

Adherence can be defined as 'the degree to which the patient's actions align with established recommendations from the prescriber (Horne, Weinman, Barber, Elliott, & Morgan, 2005). The term adherence has typically superseded compliance, which can be defined as the degree to which the patient's behavior aligns with the prescriber's suggestions (Haynes, Taylor, & Sackett, 1979). However, this term has faced criticism because it appears to imply a relationship in which the clinician's role is to determine the suitable treatment and provide the pertinent instructions, while the patient's role is to passively 'follow the doctor's orders.' In contrast, adherence acknowledges the significance of patient autonomy and that an 'agreement' is inherent. The term concordance has also been used to describe medication-taking behavior, indicating the interaction between the patient and prescriber and the degree to which their views on the prescription coincide. However, the term does not characterize patient behavior and cannot be a synonym for adherence (Horne, Weinman, Barber, Elliott, & Morgan, 2005).

Beyond terminology, the meaning of adherence becomes even more contentious. This is straightforward if adherence is viewed as an 'all or nothing' reaction in which the patient either strictly complies with the prescriber's instructions (adherence) or departs from them in some manner (nonadherence). However, such a rigid definition is of minimal utility in practice. The degree of adherence required to attain the desired outcome differs among medications, across individuals, and within individual cases. A threshold of 80% is frequently employed to classify patients into adherent versus nonadherent categories (Nieuwlaat et al., 2014). Such classifications rely on approximations of the extent of nonadherence that is expected to be clinically important. Nonetheless, this differs among patients and medications, and thresholds can solely offer rough measures of clinical significance.

The underlying assumption of adherence interventions is that adherence enhances patient outcomes. This assumption was not, however, rigorously examined (DiMatteo et al., 2002). DiMatteo and colleagues reviewed 63 studies examining the connection between adherence to medical guidance (including prescribed medications, dietary changes, physical exercise, and eye patch usage) and outcomes (including survival rates, reported pain levels, blood pressure management, visual clarity, cholesterol levels, and organ rejection). Generally, the probability of achieving a favorable treatment outcome was three times greater among high and low adherers. Additionally, the increased risk of individuals dying due to 'poor' adherence in contrast to those with 'good adherence' is 2–3 times higher (Simpson et al., 2006). It has been proposed that enhancing medication adherence might have a more significant effect on the population's health than advancements in any medical treatment (Haynes et al., 2002). Not adhering to a prescribed medication is likely to indicate that the patient is not obtaining the complete therapeutic advantage of the medication. Depending on the role and outcome of a given medicine, the impact of non-adherence is likely to be more problematic for some health conditions than others. Nonadherence and non-initiation are arguably most important in those health conditions in which nonadherence has been demonstrated to have an impact on clinical outcomes (e.g., increase in severity of symptoms, morbidity, and mortality) such as HIV, cancer, diabetes, asthma, cardiovascular disease (CVD), mental illness, organ transplant, etc. (Horne, Weinman, Barber, Elliott, & Morgan, 2005). Similarly, low adherence has been linked to an elevated risk of mortality in cardiovascular disease (CVD), diabetes, and end-stage renal disease.

Nevertheless, it is crucial to acknowledge that nonadherence might only sometimes be detrimental to the patient. It might serve a protective role if the prescription is unsuitable and potentially harmful or have a neutral impact if it is less than optimal. In their seminal review of the subject, Sackett et al. regard the prescribing of a medication as a 'therapeutic experiment,' the outcome of which is shaped by the actions of the prescriber in choosing an appropriate diagnosis and treatment, as well as the patient in following the regimen. However, if the prescription was based on evidence and suitable for the patient, we can likely infer that higher adherence correlates with greater therapeutic efficacy.

In a review concerning adherence to long-term therapies, the World Health Organization (WHO) remarked that the effects of nonadherence intensify as the burden of chronic disease escalates globally and that the economically disadvantaged are disproportionately impacted by a 'two-way interdependent relationship between economic poverty and chronic disease.'.

3. PREVALENCE OF NOON ADHERENCE

Although it is widely cited that up to 50% of medications are not taken as prescribed (Sabaté, 2003), these rates vary considerably across different treatments and conditions, and even within conditions based on the definition and measurement of nonadherence, as well as the stage of nonadherence outlined (Vrijens et al., 2012). At initiation, around 20–30% of new prescriptions are estimated not to get filled

(Fischer et al., 2011; OECD, 2018; Sabaté, 2003). A recent systematic review analyzed initiation rates across asthma, chronic obstructive pulmonary disease (COPD), depression, diabetes mellitus, hyperlipidemia, hypertension, and osteoporosis and discovered that rates of non-initiation were highest among those with osteoporosis and hyperlipidemia (25%) and lowest among those with depression (12%) and diabetes (10%) (Cheen et al., 2019).

Most of the research on adherence focuses on implementation, with between 50% and 70% of patients estimated to take their medication as prescribed, although this varies considerably across conditions. Briesacher et al. (2008) compared adherence rates, measured using prescription refill rates, for 706,032 patients with gout, hypercholesteremia, hypertension, hypothyroidism, osteoporosis, seizure disorders, and type 2 diabetes. Adherence rates were highest in hypertension, with 72% of participants having an 80% adherence rate, compared to 55%, 51%, and 36% for those with hypercholesteremia, osteoporosis, and gout, respectively.

Non-persistence with medications prescribed for long-term conditions is often problematic, with non-persistence rates increasing steadily from initiation to two years (OECD, 2018; Yeaw et al., 2009). For example, estimates suggest that 16–50% of patients with hypertension discontinue treatment entirely within the first 12 months of initiation (Brown & Bussell, 2011). Estimates also suggest that 73% of patients with diabetes are persistent six months after initiation, with only 39% persistent at two years (OECD, 2018), and 25–50% of patients with hypercholesterolemia discontinue their statin medication within the first 6–12 months since initiation (Svensson et al., 2015). One study exploring adherence to urate-lowering therapy in a large cohort of 9823 patients with gout found that within 12 months of initiation, non-persistence rates were 56% (Solomon et al., 2008). In a longitudinal database study of 4783 patients with hypertension, approximately only 50% of patients who were prescribed an antihypertensive drug continued taking it 12 months after initiation.

4. AI TECHNOLOGIES TO INCREASE MEDICATION ADHERENCE

4.1 Mobile Phone Applications

Medication compliance guarantees treatments' effectiveness for chronic illnesses and enhances patient outcomes. Noncompliance is prevalent, leading to inadequate treatment results and elevated healthcare expenses. Conventional techniques for monitoring adherence, such as pill counts or self-reported information, are frequently unreliable and susceptible to inaccuracies. To tackle these issues, there has been an increasing interest in applying advanced technologies, especially Artificial Intelligence (AI), to observe and enhance medication adherence in real-time.

AI-based smartphone applications have surfaced as an encouraging remedy, presenting innovative methods to monitor patient behavior, verify medication consumption, and deliver personalized reminders. These applications utilize computer vision, facial recognition, and neural network algorithms to evaluate adherence with high precision. Numerous studies have investigated the implementation of AI-enabled apps to improve medication adherence, demonstrating substantial advancements in patient compliance across various medical conditions, including stroke and schizophrenia, as well as many diseases.

AI smartphone applications ("apps") have been assessed as apparatuses for evaluating and empowering medication adherence in a limited number of studies (Labovitz et al., 2017)—created an AI smartphone app to degree medicine adherence in stroke patients taking coordinated verbal anticoagulant treatment. The AI application utilized neural organized computer vision calculation with the smartphone camera to outwardly distinguish the understanding, the sedate, and the affirmed ingestion. The program's pharmaceutical updates and dosing are enlightening. In this 12-week randomized parallel-group, plasma medication concentration levels showed 100% adherence within the intercession gathers that experienced every day observing through the AI stage, compared with 50% within the control gather who got no day-by-day checking. The outright enhancement of sedate adherence was 67% in patients observed by the AI app; 83. In a post-study survey, 3% of patients respected the stage as "extremely good" when asked to rate the AI stages as a pharmaceutical administration instrument and strategy to progress the doctor-patient relationship.

Nevertheless, the consideration was little (n=28) and ran for a moderately brief period, highlighting the requirement for bigger things to decide whether significant enhancement in medicine adherence can be kept up with such stages over more extended periods. Most clinical trials right now utilize circuitous and possibly wrong measures of adherence, such as pill tallies and self-reported information (Bain et al., 2017) assessed a real-time checking strategy on a smartphone-based AI stage to evaluate adherence in Stage II clinical trial of a 7-nicotinic receptor enemy (ABT-126) in 53 patients with concurrent schizophrenia and cognitive impedance. The AI stage facial acknowledgment, computer vision, and computer program calculations made a difference in recognizing understanding and medication and affirming ingestion in a 24-week trial. Discoveries appeared to have a 179% higher adherence within the AI bunches. The control gathers who got altered straightforwardly watched treatment. The makers concluded that the AI organization may more rapidly recognize non-adherence and expect future non-adherence compared with schedule methodologies.

4.2 Reminder System

AI has Moreover been utilized to convey well-being communication to energize adherence; for case, robotized frameworks have been used to supply updates to required pharmaceuticals (Prayaag et al., 2019) (Prayag et al., 2018b) survey an SMS-based refill update arrangement utilizing conversational AI, the "mPulse-Mobile" in more seasoned patients with NCDs. A higher pharmaceutical refill rate was observed within the mediation group than in the control group (who did not get SMS updates) (Prayag et al., 2018b). So also, the ChronologyMDventure for Crohn's illness utilized a framework of patient-sourced "observations of everyday living" (ODLs) with computer-mediated AI back to empower patients to track their pharmaceutical adherence, movement, and indications on a day-by-day or hourly premise; this data was at that point consequently made accessible to suppliers to move forward choice making (Kreps & Neuhauser, 2013). Patients detailed that the AI components of the framework empower them to track, get, and screen their ODLs more effortlessly and precisely, whereas too making a difference for them to keep in mind requires their drugs.

4.3 AI for Patient Empowerment

AI has moreover appeared to backhanded medicine adherence benefits through quiet back and strengthening. "Vik" may be a chatbot planned to enable patients with breast cancer and their relatives (Chaix et al., 2019). They use personalized content messages. It gives pertinent, quality-checked therapeutic data for breast cancer, the study of disease transmission, medicines, and side impacts, and data on almost all ways of life, richness, repayment, patients' rights, and so on. The ponder appeared that the more the members chatted with Vik, the more attentive they were when employing treatment update work. The standard compliance of patients utilizing the medicine update highlighted more than 20% strides. Then again, automated colleagues may be another strategy to extend quiet strengthening; AI robot assistants have appeared to be supportive of the self-management of diabetes and affront control in children. (Al-Taee et al., 2016) (Cañamero & Lewis, 2016) (Henkemans et al., 2013).

4.4 AI in Integrated Care

Coordinated care programs are, by and large, alluded to as care frameworks that cultivate coordination inside and between healthcare organizations and healthcare experts to move forward clinical results and the involvement of patients. These programs can upgrade the care and treatment of patients NCDs and are moreover prescribed for complex patients, such as those with multimorbidity (characterized as the nearness of more than one concurrent NCD) (Palmer et al., 2017). detailed beneficial impacts of coordinated care for grown-ups with NCDs on a few results, counting decreased mortality, diminished healing center confirmations and re-admissions, and moved forward adherence to treatment rules (counting adherence to medications or diets and/or supplier adherence to regulations). Coordinates care includes a few components that might be bolstered by AI-assisted innovation, counting multidisciplinary systems, sharing data between healthcare suppliers and utilizing electronic quiet records and computerized clinical charts, reinforcing patients' self-management and self-efficacy, shared choice making, and the utilization of individualized care plans, among others (Palmer et al., 2017). Standard dialect handling and cognitive computing AI strategies empower restorative information directors to organize naturally and mine information from unstructured electronic restorative records. AI-assisted innovation can optimize medicines by prioritizing drugs that coordinate the patients' insurance/preferred drug store, drug-drug intuition, etc. AI has appeared to be valuable for pharmaceutical compromise, which may be a method frequently used to decrease pharmaceutical blunders. An AI-assisted instrument was created to progress medicine compromise by locks in the quiet and healthcare suppliers as a group using a tablet-based as well. The AI component assisted the patients in recognizing their claim medicines and reporting inconsistencies for the clinicians to survey, thus moving forward with pharmaceutical precision and decreasing pharmaceutical mistakes (Long et al., 2016).

5. BENEFITS OF AI TO IMPROVE MEDICATION ADHERENCE

5.1 Assessing Adherence Levels

AI has appeared promising in both measuring adherence levels and progressing pharmaceutical adherence. Evaluating pharmaceutical adherence and its essential impacting components can be challenging for doctors and analysts. There are many coordinates and roundabouts, as well as objective and subjective strategies accessible for measuring these; quiet self-report, electronic measures, and drug store refill and claims data are the foremost commonly utilized measures in inquiring about, scheduling hone, and epidemiological and mediation think about. In any case, self-reported measures have, as it were, a weak-to-moderate relationship with, for illustration, medicine refills and electronic measures. A combination of these strategies is expected to be a valuable approach to increment the legitimacy and reliability of adherence estimations. This can be accomplished using AI strategies, particularly machine learning (Lehmann et al., 2013).

5.2 Increasing Adherence

A few trials evaluating AI-assisted advances have illustrated expanded adherence rates in patients utilizing innovation vs. routine care (Labovitz et al., 2017c) (Bain et al., 2017b) (Prayaga et al., 2018c). Expanded pharmaceutical adherence is related to progressive clinical results in NCD patients. For illustration, adherence to cardioprotective drugs in patients with diabetes and ischemic heart illness appeared to be related to lower all-cause mortality (Ho et al., 2006). Adherence to statins and beta-blockers in patients with intense myocardial localized necrosis was linked to a lower hazard of long-term mortality (middle of two. 4 a long time) (Rasmussen et al., 2007). Moreover, an efficient audit concluded that clinic confirmations related to no adherence to medicine are a common issue, particularly in connection to cardiovascular solutions (Mongkhon et al., 2018).illustrated a 21% diminishment in long-term mortality hazard with excellent pharmaceutical adherence in comparison to pharmaceutical no adherence, and a 17% higher risk of all-cause hospitalization related with non-adherence in more seasoned grown-ups (Walsh et al., 2019). Clinical results may be influenced by case; diabetic patients who do not follow their pharmaceutical regimen have poorer clinical results, such as higher glycosylated hemoglobin levels, systolic and diastolic blood weight, and low-density lipoprotein cholesterol levels, as well as a better chance of all-cause mortality and all-cause hospitalization (Ho, Rumsfeld, et al., 2006). Pharmaceutical nonadherence moreover places a critical fetched burden on healthcare frameworks; an orderly audit assessed the yearly balanced disease-specific financial fetched of nonadherence as US$949 toUS$44,190 per individual (in 2015), and the costs credited to all-cause non-adherence extended from US$5,271 to US$52,341(Cutler et al., 2018). Expanding medicine adherence is additionally vital for patient-related results as intercessions have appeared that expanding adherence can lead to better, a much better, higher, stronger, and improved" distant better information of drugs as well as changes in quality of life, physical work, and indications (Conn et al., 2016).

5.3 Time Saving

In clinical hone, patients' subjective gauges of adherence can be wrong, and doctors may not have time to investigate and address the fundamental reasons behind non-adherence, particularly since a complex range of factors can influence it (Brown & Bussell, 2011) (GelLad et al., 2011). Utilizing AI-assisted innovations may help free up the time of healthcare suppliers for fundamental clinical exercises and more in-depth illness- and treatment-related communication with patients. AI may empower a more exact understanding of telemedicine adherence so that doctors can devote more time to judgment and passionate insights for creating personalized methodologies to optimize adherence (Fogel & Kvedar, 2018). Besides, considering the progress of COVID-19, it must be known that AI-assisted intercessions and observation may be essential for NCD administration in periods where face-to-face healthcare is limited. For illustration, the widespread practice has driven a considerable decrease in affirmations for intense cardiovascular infection within the number of methods and longer delays between indication onset and clinic treatment (Kiss et al., 2020). Even though constrained investigations are accessible on how the widespread contamination control measures have mainly influenced medicine adherence in NCD patients, one orderly audit detailed the critical disappointment of provocative bowel illness patients to follow treatments amid the widespread COVID-19 (Jena et al., 2020). Besides, a few, but not all, consider have detailed higher anti-microbial endorsing rates in further essential care interviews compared with face-to-face settings.AI, with the potential to survey adherence through smartphones and tablet-based observing frameworks, as depicted over, may in this way give extra benefits through inaccessible checking of patients and expanding communication with healthcare specialists amid widespread times (Han et al., 2020).

6. OPPORTUNITIES CREATED FOR ADHERENCE OWING TO DIGITIZATION OF THE HEALTH CARE SECTOR

To date, interests include advanced arrangements broadly utilized for exterior well-being care. Still, as it has been as of late, they have been utilized within the pharmaceutical field and offer extraordinary guarantees toward made strides and more effective care. In 2018, the European Commission created an arrangement for the computerized exchange of health and care within the Advanced Single Showcase to speed up this process. The arrangement is based on three columns as follows: (1) securing information to and sharing; (2) interfacing and sharing well-being information for inquiry about, quicker determination, and progressed individualized well-being care administrations and well-being results; and (3) fortifying citizen strengthening and person care through advanced administrations (European This arrange may be a portion of the overarching European Procedure for Information Commission, 2020). Digitization of the well-being care division creates an opportunity for utilizing enormous information analytics instruments and strategies to survey nonadherence, progress clinical hone or well-being care administrations, and advance the utilization of custom-made intercessions. Routinely collected data on endorsing and apportioning, accessible in EHRs, drug store apportioning databases, wellbeing protection claims frameworks, and national well-being frameworks records, empowers a more intensive investigation of the relationship between adherence and well-being results. Patients' rising utilization of mHealth for self-monitoring and infection administration is another potential information source for examination. In this way, huge amounts of information may speak to an effective and generally low-cost asset for exploring imperative open well-being concerns in real-life scenarios, counting the predominance of nonadherence, its drivers, and the results of non-adherence. Huge information can also supply data for planning modern medications and focusing on avoiding and administering non-adherence. Besides, enormous information permits investigation on an exceptional scale, covering expansive populaces (e.g., essential nonadherence, a degree of unfilled medicines, was as of late surveyed in a cohort of 1. 6 million Catalonian essential care patients (Aznar-Lou et al., 2017).and in a national populace-based think about in Poland (Kardas et al., 2020). Unlike restorative trials, huge amounts of information allow for longitudinal surveying adherence (e.g., an Estonian thinks about analyzing a national database for 15 years (Laius et al., 2017). All this is often conceivable without commonplace impediments in fetched, meddling, and inclination, which are characteristic of utilizing other sorts of information for adherence estimation and checking. Nevertheless, at display, uniform and acknowledged measures of adherence estimation for enormous amounts of information are still lacking. Additionally, as of now, huge information collection is not consistently designed or organized for adherence estimation, which implies that nontrivial operations are required to permit this kind of investigation. In this manner, to construct a strong proven base for adherence administration in clinical settings, it is fundamental to standardize adherence estimation and encourage the suitable utilization of these benchmarks (Laius et al., 2017). Adherence inquiries are not the as-it-are zone of investigating confronting issues with standardization regarding advanced well-being. For illustration, there are no worldwide guidelines for EHRs (OECD, 2019). Different authentic, social, financial, and political reasons can be cited as causative variables. This is still the case despite the exercises of a few open and private interoperability activities (Auffray et al., 2016). A few standardization improvement organizations have created exceptionally developed and broadly actualized benchmarks, such as Clinical RecordEngineering (Health Level Seven International, n.d.) and Fast Healthcare Interoperability Resources (HL7, n.d.).by HL7, and CEN-ISO 13606(ISO, 2019). However, their interoperability is restricted. Interests: ISO 10781:2015 gives a reference list of capacities that will be displayed in a framework, and of these, the taking after work handles adherence evaluation: Care Understanding Back CPS 3. 1 Work on "Support for Standard Assessments" (ISO, 2015). A systemic survey of the challenges for the utilization of huge amounts of information in well-being care recognized issues in information structure, security, information standardization, capacity and exchange, and administrative aptitudes, such as information administration, to be the foremost regularly given within the current writing (Kruse et al., 2016). Viable challenges included information preprocessing and curation, show preparation, refinement of frameworks, moral and lawful issues, information security and security, the conclusion of clients understanding acknowledgment, etc. (Ngiam & Khor, 2019) (Shortreed et al., 2019).

7. CHALLENGES OF USING AI IN HEALTHCARE:

7.1 Patient Characteristics

Utilizing AI for measuring or expanding pharmaceutical adherence may lead to imbalances in healthcare between people as the characteristics of clients can affect the adequacy of an AI device. For illustration, a consideration on the viability of an SMS-based refill update arrangement utilizing conversational AI in patients with persistent illness found that race, ethnicity, dialect, age, and social determinants of well-being influenced the level of engagement with the AI arrangement to progress refill adherence (Prayaga et al., 2019b). A consumer survey (Esmaeilzadeh, 2020) proposed that mechanical, moral, and belief components, as well as administrative concerns, essentially contribute to the dangers of utilizing AI applications in healthcare. Mainly, mechanical concerns were the foremost critical, especially execution uneasiness (i.e., the user's discernment that the IT framework will break or not work as aimed) and communication obstructions (i.e., the degree to which the client considers that the AI gadget might diminish human aspects of relations within the treatment prepared). Besides, Ailed chat-box administrations in healthcare can be influenced by the user's reliability and can be seen as having poorer IT abilities and loathe to talk to computers (Nadarzynski et al., 2019). Numerous components influencing a user's capacity and readiness to lock in with AI innovations may be too autonomously related to non-adherence. A precise audit in more seasoned patients recognized three sorts of obstructions to adherence: patient-related variables (sociodemographic, psychosocial profile, comorbidities, cognitive capacity, and wellbeing convictions); drug-related variables (number of drugs taken, unfavorable impacts, and organization regimens); and other variables (patient–prescriber relationship, get to medicine, and social bolster)(Gellad et al., 2011b).In this way, it is fundamental that future inquiries explore whether patients with a high hazard of non-adherence can lock in well with AI-assisted intercessions to extend adherence or whether the utilization of such advances will lead to advanced disparity in healthcare between people.

7.2 Concerns About Depersonalization

Another obstruction to the utilization of AI in healthcare is the potential concern from patients, relatives, and healthcare experts that it may "depersonalize" pharmaceuticals. This may be more articulated in specific statistic bunches; for case, in the field of AI and gerontechnology, some concerns algorithm-based standardization and automatization may lead to the depersonalization of care, that the care relationship may be dehumanized through automatization, which minority bunches may involvement segregation through generalization, thus challenging the "4p medicine" (prescient, personalized, preventive, and participatory) patient-centered show of care (Rubeis, 2020). Moreover, there is skepticism toward mechanization, and the seen hazard stems from appointing control to machines and their particular control instruments. An efficient audit of adherence mediation is too detailed that face-to-face intercessions were more successful than mediation conveyed in other ways, such as using a computer, phone, and/or content message (Conn & Ruppar, 2017). Even though such challenges apply to a run of disarrangements and distinctive regions of healthcare, they are pertinent to pharmaceutical adherence and NCDs. Imperatively, as people age, there is a hazard of having more than one constant condition (moreover known as multimorbidity) increments, and this is frequently related to polypharmacy and related negative results, such as antagonistic sedate responses. AI innovations that screen adherence may give critical openings for NCD patients on polypharmacy. It has been recommended that patients with multimorbidity advantage from coordinated care models with standard observing and appraisal by a group of masters (Palmer et al., 2017b). Hence, the above-mentioned concern of depersonalized care may be particularly significant to complex patients with different comorbid conditions. In any case, if connected, AI-assisted innovation has the potential to improve the 4p show by freeing doctors from time-consuming errands and possibly wrong strategies for measuring subjective reports of adherence, hence giving them more time to form passionate associations with their patients, expanding shared choice making, and empowering them to address person reasons fundamental non-adherence.AI is improbable to supplant doctors at the bedside but can give valuable openings to improve patient-physician communication; for case, the AI-assisted pharmaceutical compromise instrument depicted over (Long et al.) locked in patients and healthcare suppliers as a group by empowering patients to report pharmaceutical inconsistencies for their clinicians to audit(Long et al., 2016b). Innovation has been recommended as an essential component of coordinated care models for NCD patients, particularly those with multimorbidity (Palmer et al., 2017c).

7.3 Infrastructure, Training, and Cost Effectiveness

The victory and broad utilization of AI advances will depend on information capacity, handling control, and other framework capacities inside healthcare frameworks. For illustration, there may be challenges in relocating information over electronic and paper well-being records. Information and acquiring about it must be reasonable by healthcare experts and, in a few cases, patients. Healthcare frameworks ought to moreover back workers and the appropriation of AI arrangements by giving preparation courses to workers. Nevertheless, less than half of healthcare insiders report that AI preparation is given to their representatives (KPMG, 2020), and it was recommended that "Building an AI-ready workforce requires a discount alter within the approach to preparing and how to secure ability. Having individuals who understand how AI can unravel enormous, complex issues is critical". This may offer assistance to diminish the hazard of "AI-washing," that is, where engineers include an "AI" name to program stages with essential calculations to energize and misuse buyers, counting healthcare frameworks and person specialists. Subsequently, preparing workers at numerous levels of the healthcare framework will result in a superior assessment of the viability of an AI arrangement so that healthcare experts can consider the long-term potential to progress persistent results and weigh up the cost-effectiveness. A later orderly survey highlighted the need to investigate altogether tending to the financial effect appraisal of AI in healthcare inside the current writing (Wolff et al., 2019). By the way, the costs of creating and starting AI mediations may be a significant boundary to utilizing these innovations in healthcare inquiry and hone. As said already (Cutler et al., 2018b). Medicine non-adherence is related to significant increments in understanding costs, so it is of most extreme significance to set up whether AI and AI-assisted mediations increment or diminish the costs associated with non-adherence in the future, well-designed cost-effectiveness.

7.4 Ethical Issues

There are a bunch of moral concerns that hinder the utilization of AI in healthcare. Who claims the information that is being mined amid machine learning and colossal information analytics? Have protection issues been addressed, and have satisfactory steps been taken to guarantee the security and secrecy of quiet information? Are all clients mindful of controls and rules for utilizing AI-generated information and comes about? Will using AI encourage disparities in healthcare, for example, concurring with racial or financial components? (Keskinbora, 2019). There may be racial and ethnic contrasts concerning impediments to partaking in the gift of biospecimens for investigation, which may, in turn, have imperative suggestions for machine learning. Within the field of NCDs, there are racial disparities in terms of NCD hazard components as well as treatment issues, including adherence to drugs for common NCDs, for case, antidiabetic, antihypertensive, or antihyperlipidemic drugs (Xie et al., 2019). Moreover, given the profoundly touchy nature of persistent therapeutic records, three-quarters of healthcare insiders are concerned that AI undermines quiet information security (KPMG, 2020). The specific measures sought to be taken to address the morals of gerontechnology, the rate of NCDs, the number and complexity of maladies, and multimorbidity increment with age, and are related to polypharmacy (Rubeis, 2020b) (Ioakeim-Skoufa et al., 2020). Consideration ought to be taken concerning advances with disciplinary components (i.e., coordinate or backhanded teaching by driving patients to adjust to the measures set by the AI). Developments that at first show up enable quiet and make strides in their well-being, which may become an implication to realize objectives that are not in their essential interest. In this way, the improvement and utilization of AI in healthcare investigations require cautious thought of moral standards, dangers, and benefits, security, get to and ease of use, and information administration (Nebeker et al., 2019b).

8. DISCUSSION AND CONCLUSION

Medication adherence remains a notable challenge within healthcare systems globally, especially among groups with chronic illnesses like diabetes, hypertension, and asthma. Failure to follow prescribed medication regimens leads to a variety of detrimental health outcomes, such as disease worsening, hospitalization, and early mortality. Besides the negative health impacts, nonadherence significantly increases healthcare expenses due to the heightened demand for hospital admissions, urgent care, and further treatments. Given these obstacles, there is increasing interest in the ability of artificial intelligence (AI) technologies to improve medication adherence through creative solutions. AI-driven tools, such as mobile apps, medication reminder systems, and patient empowerment resources, can transform how healthcare providers interact with patients and assist them in managing their health challenges. By utilizing real-time monitoring, tailored communication, and behavioral nudges, AI can tackle the various barriers to adherence, including forgetfulness, lack of motivation, and insufficient health literacy, while fostering improved health outcomes, particularly in underserved populations who frequently encounter additional challenges in accessing care. Incorporating AI into medication adherence strategies offers an exhilarating opportunity for enhancing patient engagement and health management. Tools driven by AI allow healthcare providers to observe patient behavior in real time, providing a data-informed approach to medication adherence that conventional methods have been unable to achieve. AI-powered applications can deliver personalized reminders to patients, monitor their adherence behavior, and alert healthcare providers when a patient is in danger of missing a dose. These tools effectively track medication adherence from a distance, eliminating the necessity for frequent in-person visits. Research indicates that AI-enabled apps positively influence adherence rates across different chronic conditions. For instance, studies have shown that AI-powered applications aimed at patients with chronic illnesses like diabetes and hypertension enhance medication adherence, improve disease management, and reduce hospitalizations. These AI systems not only prompt patients to take their medications but also provide customized advice based on real-time data such as blood pressure readings or glucose levels, improving the overall relevance and effectiveness of the intervention. Furthermore, AI systems can be programmed to send encouraging messages, provide positive reinforcement for timely medication intake, and offer information on the long-term health advantages of consistent adherence. These interventions can assist in narrowing the gap between a patient's intent to adhere to their treatment plan and their actual adherence behavior, ultimately resulting in better health outcomes. While the opportunity for AI to enhance medication adherence is evident, numerous challenges must be tackled to ensure the extensive usage and efficacy of AI solutions within healthcare systems. One significant obstacle to AI implementation is patient attributes, particularly their technological literacy. While younger, more tech-savvy individuals might feel at ease using mobile applications and AI tools, older adults and individuals with restricted access to smartphones or internet services may find interacting with digital health solutions challenging. Research indicates that older adults, especially those suffering from chronic ailments, often possess lower levels of technological literacy, hindering their ability to utilize AI-driven tools efficiently. This challenge is especially noticeable in low-income and rural populations, who may lack access to smartphones, dependable internet connections, or training in digital skills. Therefore, when developing AI solutions aimed at medication adherence, it is crucial to consider the technological constraints different patient demographics face. AI systems should be created with accessibility as a priority, ensuring they are user-friendly and intuitive for patients with diverse levels of technological proficiency. Furthermore, healthcare organizations must consider offering education and support for patients, particularly older individuals, to aid them in effectively using AI tools. This may entail training programs or assistance via healthcare providers to ensure that patients are not excluded due to technological obstacles. By enhancing the accessibility of these tools, healthcare providers can guarantee that all patients, irrespective of age or technological skills, can gain from AI-driven solutions. In addition to technological literacy, concerns regarding the depersonalization of care pose another challenge in adopting AI in medication adherence strategies. One potential drawback of AI is that it may diminish the amount of personal interaction between healthcare providers and patients, particularly as AI takes over administrative duties such as reminders, tracking, and follow-ups. Some patients may view this change as a decline in the quality of care since the human aspect is crucial to many patients' trust and satisfaction in healthcare. While AI can improve efficiency and provide valuable insights, it cannot substitute for the empathy, compassion, and nuanced understanding that human healthcare providers deliver. For instance, some patients may experience feelings of alienation if they perceive their healthcare interactions as being excessively automated or impersonal. Therefore, the effective integration of AI into healthcare systems must achieve a delicate balance between employing technology to enhance efficiency and ensuring that the human elements of care remain intact. Healthcare providers must utilize AI to support, rather than supplant, human interaction, which is vital to establishing trust and promoting a positive patient experience. For instance, AI could manage routine tasks, such as sending medication reminders or gathering basic health information, allowing healthcare providers to engage more meaningfully with patients. This balance would guarantee that AI enhances the quality of care without undermining the therapeutic relationships between patients and providers. The extensive adoption of AI in medication adherence necessitates considerable investments in healthcare infrastructure and education. Healthcare systems must possess the required digital infrastructure to facilitate AI technologies, which includes secure data storage options, cloud-based services, and compatibility with current electronic health record (EHR) systems. Without these essential components, AI systems might not reach their full capabilities. Additionally, healthcare professionals need to be sufficiently trained in utilizing AI-powered tools. Although AI can offer meaningful insights and suggestions, healthcare providers must understand how to effectively interpret and utilize these data points to make well-informed clinical choices. This demands adequate training in the technical elements of AI tools and their incorporation into clinical processes. Providers must also be knowledgeable about how to involve patients in conversations regarding AI, as patients might have concerns about data safety, precision, and the place of technology in their treatment. To guarantee the effective implementation of AI solutions, healthcare organizations should emphasize infrastructure investment and training initiatives to prepare patients and providers with the competencies they need to utilize AI-driven tools confidently. Ethical considerations also hold considerable importance in implementing AI for medication adherence. As AI systems gather and evaluate extensive amounts of patient data, including confidential medical information, it is crucial to maintain patient privacy and confirm that data is utilized responsibly. Healthcare providers must comply with stringent data protection regulations, like HIPAA in the United States or GDPR in Europe, to protect patient information and ensure that AI systems operate transparently regarding their data handling processes. Furthermore, AI algorithms must be crafted to prevent bias, as algorithmic bias can result in unequal treatment or missed chances for intervention, especially for underrepresented populations. AI systems learning from non-diverse datasets may generate inaccurate or inadequate recommendations for patients from various ethnic or socioeconomic backgrounds. To mitigate these problems, AI systems ought to be developed using representative datasets and routinely examined for fairness. Additionally, healthcare providers must guarantee that AI-driven tools are available to all patients, regardless of socioeconomic status, geographic location, or technological resources. Ensuring fair access to these technologies is vital for addressing health inequities and fostering inclusivity in healthcare. Governments, policymakers, and healthcare entities need to work together to lower access barriers by offering subsidies for low-income patients or supplying affordable devices and internet services.

In conclusion, AI-powered solutions show considerable potential for enhancing medication adherence, especially among individuals with chronic conditions. AI technologies can empower patients to manage their health and improve their adherence to prescribed medication routines by providing real-time monitoring, tailored reminders, and proactive interventions. Furthermore, AI allows healthcare providers to connect with patients creatively, resulting in improved health outcomes and lower healthcare expenses. However, several obstacles must be overcome to harness the advantages of AI completely in medication adherence. These encompass ensuring that AI solutions are accessible and easy to use for all patient populations, preserving the human aspect of care, investing in infrastructure and training, and addressing ethical issues related to data privacy, algorithmic bias, and equitable access. By addressing these challenges thoughtfully and systematically, AI can be integrated into healthcare systems to boost medication adherence, enhance patient outcomes, and contribute to the overall standard of care.

REFERENCES

Al-Taee, M. A., Kapoor, R., Garrett, C., & Choudhary, P. (2016). Acceptability of Robot Assistant in Management of Type 1 Diabetes in Children. *Diabetes Technology & Therapeutics*, 18(9), 551–554. DOI: 10.1089/dia.2015.0428 PMID: 27479198

Auffray, C., Balling, R., Barroso, I., Bencze, L., Benson, M., Bergeron, J., Bernal-Delgado, E., Blomberg, N., Bock, C., Conesa, A., Del Signore, S., Delogne, C., Devilee, P., Di Meglio, A., Eijkemans, M., Flicek, P., Graf, N., Grimm, V., Guchelaar, H., & Zanetti, G. (2016c). Making sense of big data in health research: Towards an EU action plan. *Genome Medicine*, 8(1), 71. Advance online publication. DOI: 10.1186/s13073-016-0323-y PMID: 27338147

Aznar-Lou, I., Fernández, A., Gil-Girbau, M., Fajó-Pascual, M., Moreno-Peral, P., Peñarrubia-María, M. T., Serrano-Blanco, A., Sánchez-Niubó, A., March-Pujol, M. A., Jové, A. M., & Rubio-Valera, M. (2017). Initial medication non-adherence: Prevalence and predictive factors in a 1.6 million primary care patients cohort. *British Journal of Clinical Pharmacology*, 83(6), 1328–1340. DOI: 10.1111/bcp.13215 PMID: 28229476

Bain, E. E., Shafner, L., Walling, D. P., Othman, A. A., Chuang-Stein, C., Hinkle, J., & Hanina, A. (2017). Use of a Novel Artificial Intelligence Platform on Mobile Devices to Assess Dosing Compliance in a Phase 2 Clinical Trial in Subjects with Schizophrenia. *JMIR mHealth and uHealth*, 5(2), e18. DOI: 10.2196/mhealth.7030 PMID: 28223265

Bain, E. E., Shafner, L., Walling, D. P., Othman, A. A., Chuang-Stein, C., Hinkle, J., & Hanina, A. (2017c). Use of a Novel Artificial Intelligence Platform on Mobile Devices to Assess Dosing Compliance in a Phase 2 Clinical Trial in Subjects with Schizophrenia. *JMIR mHealth and uHealth*, 5(2), e18. DOI: 10.2196/mhealth.7030 PMID: 28223265

Blalock, S. J. (2011). The theoretical basis for practice-relevant medication use research: Patient-centered/behavioral theories. *Research in Social & Administrative Pharmacy*, 7(4), 317–329. DOI: 10.1016/j.sapharm.2010.11.001 PMID: 21272552

Briesacher, B. A., Andrade, S. E., Fouayzi, H., & Chan, K. A. (2008). Comparison of drug adherence rates among patients with seven different medical conditions. *Pharmacotherapy*, 28(4), 437–443. DOI: 10.1592/phco.28.4.437 PMID: 18363527

Brown, M. T., & Bussell, J. K. (2011). Medication adherence: WHO cares? *Mayo Clinic Proceedings*, 86(4), 304–314. DOI: 10.4065/mcp.2010.0575 PMID: 21389250

Brown, M. T., & Bussell, J. K. (2011). Medication Adherence: WHO Cares? *Mayo Clinic Proceedings*, 86(4), 304–314. DOI: 10.4065/mcp.2010.0575 PMID: 21389250

Brown, M. T., & Bussell, J. K. (2011b). Medication Adherence: WHO Cares? *Mayo Clinic Proceedings*, 86(4), 304–314. DOI: 10.4065/mcp.2010.0575 PMID: 21389250

Cañamero, L., & Lewis, M. (2016). Making New "New AI" Friends: Designing a Social Robot for Diabetic Children from an Embodied AI Perspective. *International Journal of Social Robotics*, 8(4), 523–537. DOI: 10.1007/s12369-016-0364-9

Centers for Disease Control and Prevention. (2023). *Chronic diseases in America*. National Center for Chronic Disease Prevention and Health Promotion. https://www.cdc.gov/chronicdisease/pdf/infographics/chronic-disease-in-america-H.pdf

Chaix, B., Bibault, J., Pienkowski, A., Delamon, G., Guillemassé, A., Nectoux, P., & Brouard, B. (2019). When Chatbots Meet Patients: One-Year Prospective Study of Conversations Between Patients with Breast Cancer and a Chatbot. *JMIR Cancer*, 5(1), e12856. DOI: 10.2196/12856 PMID: 31045505

Cheen, M. H., Tan, Y. Z., Ng, S. W., Chan, H. K., & Lim, L. M. (2019). A systematic review of medication adherence and health outcomes in patients with chronic disease. *Journal of Clinical Pharmacy and Therapeutics*, 44(1), 1–10. DOI: 10.1111/jcpt.12768 PMID: 30171815

Chen, S., Gong, E., Kazi, D. S., Gates, A. B., Karate, K. M., Girder, N., Bai, R., Alabi, K. F., Li, C., Sun, K., Hong, L., Fu, H., Peng, W., Liu, X., Chen, L., Schwalm, J., & Yan, L. L. (2016). Development of a mobile phone-based intervention to improve adherence to secondary prevention of coronary heart disease in China. *Journal of Medical Engineering & Technology*, 40(7–8), 372–382. DOI: 10.1080/03091902.2016.1213904 PMID: 27686107

Chisholm-Burns, M. A., & Spivey, C. A. (2012). The "cost" of medication nonadherence: Consequences we cannot afford to accept. *Journal of the American Pharmacists Association*, 52(6), 823–826. DOI: 10.1331/JAPhA.2012.11088 PMID: 23229971

Conn, V. S., Enriquez, M., Ropar, T. M., & Chan, K. C. (2016). Meta-analyses of Theory Use in Medication Adherence Intervention Research. *American Journal of Health Behavior*, 40(2), 155–171. DOI: 10.5993/AJHB.40.2.1 PMID: 26931748

Conn, V. S., & Ruppar, T. M. (2017). Medication adherence outcomes of 771 intervention trials: Systematic review and meta-analysis. *Preventive Medicine*, 99, 269–276. DOI: 10.1016/j.ypmed.2017.03.008 PMID: 28315760

Conn, V. S., Ruppar, T. M., Rn, M. E., & Cooper, P. S. (2016). Patient-Centered Outcomes of Medication Adherence Interventions: Systematic Review and Meta-Analysis. *Value in Health*, 19(2), 277–285. DOI: 10.1016/j.jval.2015.12.001 PMID: 27021763

Cutler, R. L., Fernandez-Llimos, F., Frommer, M., Benrimoj, C., & Garcia-Cardenas, V. (2018). The economic impact of medication non-adherence by disease groups: A systematic review. *BMJ Open*, 8(1), e016982. DOI: 10.1136/bmjopen-2017-016982 PMID: 29358417

Cutler, R. L., Fernandez-Llimos, F., Frommer, M., Benrimoj, C., & Garcia-Cardenas, V. (2018b). The economic impact of medication non-adherence by disease groups: A systematic review. *BMJ Open*, 8(1), e016982. DOI: 10.1136/bmjopen-2017-016982 PMID: 29358417

Dima, A., Allemann, S., & Dediu, D. (2019). AdhereR: An Open Science Approach to Estimating Adherence to Medications Using Electronic Healthcare Databases. *PubMed*, 264, 1451–1452. DOI: 10.3233/shti190479 PMID: 31438176

DiMatteo, M. R., Giordani, P. J., Lepper, H. S., & Croghan, T. W. (2002). Patient Adherence and Medical Treatment Outcomes. *Medical Care*, 40(9), 794–811. DOI: 10.1097/00005650-200209000-00009 PMID: 12218770

Esmaeilzadeh, P. (2020). Use of AI-based tools for healthcare purposes: A consumer survey study. *BMC Medical Informatics and Decision Making*, 20(1). Advance online publication. DOI: 10.1186/s12911-020-01191-1 PMID: 32698869

European Commission. (2020, April 13). *Health: Digital health and care*. European Commission. https://ec.europa.eu/health/ehealth/overview_en

Fernandez-Lazaro, C. I., Adams, D. P., Fernandez-Lazaro, D., Garcia-González, J. M., Caballero-Garcia, A., & Miron-Canelo, J. A. (2018). Medication adherence and barriers among low-income, uninsured patients with multiple chronic conditions. *Research in Social & Administrative Pharmacy*, 15(6), 744–753. DOI: 10.1016/j.sapharm.2018.09.006 PMID: 30241872

Fischer, M. A., Stedman, M. R., Lii, J., Vogeli, C., Shrank, W. H., Brookhart, M. A., & Weissman, J. S. (2011). Primary medication non-adherence: Analysis of 195,930 electronic prescriptions. *Journal of General Internal Medicine*, 25(4), 284–290. DOI: 10.1007/s11606-010-1253-9 PMID: 20131023

Fogel, A. L., & Kvedar, J. C. (2018). Artificial intelligence powers digital medicine. *NPJ Digital Medicine*, 1(1), 5. Advance online publication. DOI: 10.1038/s41746-017-0012-2 PMID: 31304291

Gadkari, A. S., & McHorney, C. A. (2012). Unintentional non-adherence to chronic prescription medications: How unintentional is it? *BMC Health Services Research*, 12(1), 98. Advance online publication. DOI: 10.1186/1472-6963-12-98 PMID: 22510235

Gellad, W. F., Grenard, J. L., & Marcum, Z. A. (2011). A Systematic Review of Barriers to Medication Adherence in the Elderly. *The American Journal of Geriatric Pharmacotherapy*, 9(1), 11–23. DOI: 10.1016/j.amjopharm.2011.02.004 PMID: 21459305

Gellad, W. F., Grenard, J. L., & Marcum, Z. A. (2011b). A Systematic Review of Barriers to Medication Adherence in the Elderly: Looking Beyond Cost and Regimen Complexity. *˜the œAmerican Journal of Geriatric Pharmacotherapy, 9*(1), 11–23. DOI: 10.1016/j.amjopharm.2011.02.004

Han, S. M., Greenfield, G., Majeed, A., & Hayhoe, B. (2020). Impact of Remote Consultations on Antibiotic Prescribing in Primary Health Care: Systematic Review. *Journal of Medical Internet Research*, 22(11), e23482. DOI: 10.2196/23482 PMID: 33031045

Haynes, R., McDonald, H., Garg, A., & Montague, P. (2002). Interventions for helping patients to follow prescriptions for medications. *The Cochrane Library*. Advance online publication. DOI: 10.1002/14651858.CD000011 PMID: 12076376

Haynes, R. B., Taylor, D. W., & Sackett, D. L. (1979). *Compliance in health care* (1st ed.). The John Hopkins University Press.

Henkemans, O. B., Bierman, B. P., Janssen, J., Neerincx, M. A., Looije, R., Van Der Bosch, H., & Van Der Giessen, J. A. (2013). Using a robot to personalize health education for children with diabetes type 1: A pilot study. *Patient Education and Counseling*, 92(2), 174–181. DOI: 10.1016/j.pec.2013.04.012 PMID: 23684366

Ho, P. M., Magid, D. J., Masoudi, F. A., McClure, D. L., & Rumsfeld, J. S. (2006). Adherence to cardioprotective medications and mortality among patients with diabetes and ischemic heart disease. *BMC Cardiovascular Disorders*, 6(1), 48. Advance online publication. DOI: 10.1186/1471-2261-6-48 PMID: 17173679

Ho, P. M., Rumsfeld, J. S., Masoudi, F. A., McClure, D. L., Plomondon, M. E., Steiner, J. F., & Magid, D. J. (2006). Effect of Medication Nonadherence on Hospitalization and Mortality Among Patients with Diabetes Mellitus. *Archives of Internal Medicine*, 166(17), 1836. DOI: 10.1001/archinte.166.17.1836 PMID: 17000939

Horne, R., Weinman, J., Barber, N., Elliott, R., & Morgan, M. (2005). *Concordance, adherence, and compliance in medicine taking*. National Coordinating Centre for NHS Service Delivery and Organisation R&D. https://www.ahpo.net/assets/NCCSDo %20Compliance%202005.pdf

Horne, R., Weinman, J., Barber, N., Elliott, R., & Morgan, M. (2005). *Concordance, adherence, and compliance in medicine taking*. National Coordinating Centre for NHS Service Delivery and Organisation R&D. https://www.ahpo.net/assets/NCCSDO %20Compliance%202005.pdf

Infulata, R., Wilczynski, N., Navarro, T., Hobson, N., Jeffery, R., Keepanasseril, A., Agoritsas, T., Mistry, N., Iorio, A., Jack, S., Sivaramalingam, B., Iserman, E., Mustafa, R. A., Jedraszewski, D., Cotoi, C., & Haynes, R. B. (2014). Interventions for enhancing medication adherence. *Cochrane Database of Systematic Reviews*, 11(11), CD000011. Advance online publication. DOI: 10.1002/14651858.CD000011. pub4 PMID: 25412402

Ioakeim-Skoufa, I., Poblador-Plou, B., Carmona-Pírez, J., Díez-Manglano, J., Navickas, R., Gimeno-Feliu, L. A., González-Rubio, F., Jureviciene, E., Dambrauskas, L., Prados-Torres, A., & Gimeno-Miguel, A. (2020). Multimorbidity Patterns in the General Population: Results from the EpiChron Cohort Study. *International Journal of Environmental Research and Public Health*, 17(12), 4242. DOI: 10.3390/ ijerph17124242 PMID: 32545876

ISO. (2015). *ISO/HL7 10781:2015 Health informatics — HL7 electronic health records-system functional model, Release 2 (EHR FM)*. ISO. https://www.iso.org/ standard/57757.html

ISO. (2019). *ISO 13606-1:2019 Health Informatics Electronic Health Record Communication Part 1: Reference model*. ISO. https://www.iso.org/standard/67868.html

Jena, A., Singh, A. K., Kumar-M, P., Sharma, V., & Sebastian, S. (2020). Systematic review on failure to adhere to IBD therapies during the COVID-19 pandemic: Correct information is crucial. *Digestive and Liver Disease*, 52(11), 1254–1256. DOI: 10.1016/j.dld.2020.09.012 PMID: 33011089

Kardas, P., Cieszyński, J., Czech, M., Banaś, I., & Lewek, P. (2020). Primary nonadherence to medication and its drivers in Poland: The electronic prescription pilot analysis findings. *Polish Archives of Internal Medicine*, 130(1), 8–16. DOI: 10.20452/pamw.14994 PMID: 31559971

Keskinbora, K. H. (2019). Medical ethics considerations on artificial intelligence. *Journal of Clinical Neuroscience*, 64, 277–282. DOI: 10.1016/j.jocn.2019.03.001 PMID: 30878282

Kiss, P., Carcel, C., Hockham, C., & Peters, S. A. E. (2020). The impact of the COVID-19 pandemic on the care and management of patients with acute cardiovascular disease: A systematic review. *European Heart Journal. Quality of Care & Clinical Outcomes*, 7(1), 18–27. DOI: 10.1093/ehjqcco/qcaa084 PMID: 33151274

KPMG. (2020). *Living in an AI world 2020 report: Healthcare insiders: Taking the temperature of artificial intelligence in healthcare*. KPMG. https://advisory.kpmg.us/content/dam/advisory/en/pdfs/2020/healthcare-living-in-an-ai-world.pdf

KPMG. (2020). *Living in an AI world 2020: Healthcare insiders*. KPMG. https://advisory.kpmg.us/content/dam/advisory/en/pdfs/2020/healthcare-living-in-an-ai-world.pdf

Kreps, G. L., & Neuhauser, L. (2013). Artificial intelligence and immediacy: Designing health communication to engage consumers and providers personally. *Patient Education and Counseling*, 92(2), 205–210. DOI: 10.1016/j.pec.2013.04.014 PMID: 23683341

Kripalani, S., Yao, X., & Haynes, R. B. (2007). Interventions to Enhance Medication Adherence in Chronic Medical Conditions. *Archives of Internal Medicine*, 167(6), 540. DOI: 10.1001/archinte.167.6.540 PMID: 17389285

Kruse, C. S., Goswamy, R., Raval, Y., & Marawi, S. (2016). Challenges and Opportunities of Big Data in Health Care: A Systematic Review. *JMIR Medical Informatics*, 4(4), e38. DOI: 10.2196/medinform.5359 PMID: 27872036

Labovitz, D. L., Shafner, L., Gil, M. R., Virmani, D., & Hanina, A. (2017). Using Artificial Intelligence to Reduce the Risk of Nonadherence in Patients on Anticoagulation Therapy. *Stroke*, 48(5), 1416–1419. DOI: 10.1161/STROKEAHA.116.016281 PMID: 28386037

Labovitz, D. L., Shafner, L., Gil, M. R., Virmani, D., & Hanina, A. (2017b). Using Artificial Intelligence to Reduce the Risk of Nonadherence in Patients on Anticoagulation Therapy. *Stroke*, 48(5), 1416–1419. DOI: 10.1161/STROKEAHA.116.016281 PMID: 28386037

Laius, O., Pisarev, H., Maasalu, K., Kõks, S., & Märtson, A. (2017). Adherence to osteoporosis medicines in Estonia—A 15-year retrospective prescriptions database study. *Archives of Osteoporosis*, 12(1), 59. Advance online publication. DOI: 10.1007/s11657-017-0354-z PMID: 28643266

Lehmann, A., Aslani, P., Ahmed, R., Celio, J., Gauchet, A., Bedouch, P., Bugnon, O., Allenet, B., & Schneider, M. P. (2013). Assessing medication adherence: Options to consider. *International Journal of Clinical Pharmacy*, 36(1), 55–69. DOI: 10.1007/s11096-013-9865-x PMID: 24166659

Long, J., Yuan, M. J., & Poonawala, R. (2016). An Observational Study to Evaluate the Usability and Intent to Adopt an Artificial Intelligence–Powered Medication Reconciliation Tool. *Interactive Journal of Medical Research*, 5(2), e14. DOI: 10.2196/ijmr.5462 PMID: 27185210

Long, J., Yuan, M. J., & Poonawala, R. (2016b). An Observational Study to Evaluate the Usability and Intent to Adopt an Artificial Intelligence–Powered Medication Reconciliation Tool. *Interactive Journal of Medical Research*, 5(2), e14. DOI: 10.2196/ijmr.5462 PMID: 27185210

Master Grid of Standards. Health Level Seven International. URL: https://www.hl7.org/implement/standards/product_brief.cfm?product_id=7V [accessed 2020-04-13]

Mongkhon, P., Ashcroft, D. M., Scholfield, C. N., & Kongkaew, C. (2018). Hospital admissions associated with medication non-adherence: A systematic review of prospective observational studies. *BMJ Quality & Safety*, 27(11), 902–914. DOI: 10.1136/bmjqs-2017-007453 PMID: 29666309

Nadarzynski, T., Miles, O., Cowie, A., & Ridge, D. (2019). Acceptability of artificial intelligence (AI)-led chatbot services in healthcare: A mixed-methods study. *Digital Health*, 5, 205520761987180. DOI: 10.1177/2055207619871808 PMID: 31467682

Naderi, S. H., Bestwick, J. P., & Wald, D. S. (2012). Adherence to Drugs That Prevent Cardiovascular Disease: Meta-analysis on 376,162 Patients. *The American Journal of Medicine*, 125(9), 882–887.e1. DOI: 10.1016/j.amjmed.2011.12.013 PMID: 22748400

National Association of Community Health Centers. (2019). *Research fact sheets and infographics*. https://nachc.org/research-and-data/research-fact-sheets-and-infographics/

Nebeker, C., Torous, J., & Ellis, R. J. B. (2019b). Building the case for actionable ethics in digital health research supported by artificial intelligence. *BMC Medicine*, 17(1), 137. Advance online publication. DOI: 10.1186/s12916-019-1377-7 PMID: 31311535

Ngiam, K. Y., & Khor, I. W. (2019). Big data and machine learning algorithms for healthcare delivery. *The Lancet. Oncology*, 20(5), e262–e273. DOI: 10.1016/S1470-2045(19)30149-4 PMID: 31044724

OECD. (2018).. . *Health at a Glance. Europe*, 2018, •••. https://www.oecd.org/health/health-at-a-glance-europe-23056088.htm

OECD. (2019). Health in the 21st Century: Putting Data to Work for Stronger Health System. In *OECD Health Policy Studies*. OECD Publishing.

Palmer, K., Marengoni, A., Forjaz, M. J., Jureviciene, E., Laatikainen, T., Mammarella, F., Muth, C., Navickas, R., Prados-Torres, A., Rijken, M., Rothe, U., Souchet, L., Valderas, J., Vontetsianos, T., Zaletel, J., & Onder, G. (2017). Multimorbidity care model: Recommendations from the consensus meeting of the Joint Action on Chronic Diseases and Promoting Healthy Ageing across the Life Cycle (JA-CHRODIS). *Health Policy (Amsterdam)*, 122(1), 4–11. DOI: 10.1016/j.healthpol.2017.09.006 PMID: 28967492

Palmer, K., Marengoni, A., Forjaz, M. J., Jureviciene, E., Laatikainen, T., Mammarella, F., Muth, C., Navickas, R., Prados-Torres, A., Rijken, M., Rothe, U., Souchet, L., Valderas, J., Vontetsianos, T., Zaletel, J., & Onder, G. (2017b). Multimorbidity care model: Recommendations from the consensus meeting of the Joint Action on Chronic Diseases and Promoting Healthy Ageing across the Life Cycle (JA-CHRODIS). *Health Policy (Amsterdam)*, 122(1), 4–11. DOI: 10.1016/j.healthpol.2017.09.006 PMID: 28967492

Palmer, K., Marengoni, A., Forjaz, M. J., Jureviciene, E., Laatikainen, T., Mammarella, F., Muth, C., Navickas, R., Prados-Torres, A., Rijken, M., Rothe, U., Souchet, L., Valderas, J., Vontetsianos, T., Zaletel, J., & Onder, G. (2017c). Multimorbidity care model: Recommendations from the consensus meeting of the Joint Action on Chronic Diseases and Promoting Healthy Ageing across the Life Cycle (JA-CHRODIS). *Health Policy (Amsterdam)*, 122(1), 4–11. DOI: 10.1016/j.healthpol.2017.09.006 PMID: 28967492

Peng, Y., Wang, H., Fang, Q., Xie, L., Shu, L., Sun, W., & Liu, Q. (2020). Effectiveness of Mobile Applications on Medication Adherence in Adults with Chronic Diseases: A Systematic Review and Meta-Analysis. *Journal of Managed Care & Specialty Pharmacy*, 26(4), 550–561. DOI: 10.18553/jmcp.2020.26.4.550 PMID: 32223596

Prayag, R. B., Agrawal, R., Nguyen, B., Jeong, E. W., Noble, H. K., Paster, A., & Prayaga, R. S. (2019). Impact of Social Determinants of Health and Demographics on Refill Requests by Medicare Patients Using a Conversational Artificial Intelligence Text Messaging Solution: Cross-Sectional Study. *JMIR mHealth and uHealth*, 7(11), e15771. DOI: 10.2196/15771 PMID: 31738170

Prayaga, R. B., Agrawal, R., Nguyen, B., Jeong, E. W., Noble, H. K., Paster, A., & Prayaga, R. S. (2019b). Impact of Social Determinants of Health and Demographics on Refill Requests by Medicare Patients Using a Conversational Artificial Intelligence Text Messaging Solution: Cross-Sectional Study. *JMIR mHealth and uHealth*, 7(11), e15771. DOI: 10.2196/15771 PMID: 31738170

Prayaga, R. B., Jeong, E. W., Feger, E., Noble, H. K., Kmiec, M., & Prayaga, R. S. (2018b). Improving Refill Adherence in Medicare Patients with Tailored and Interactive Mobile Text Messaging: Pilot Study. *JMIR mHealth and uHealth*, 6(1), e30. DOI: 10.2196/mhealth.8930 PMID: 29382623

Rasmussen, J. N., Chong, A., & Alter, D. A. (2007). Relationship Between Adherence to Evidence-Based Pharmacotherapy and Long-term Mortality After Acute Myocardial Infarction. *Journal of the American Medical Association*, 297(2), 177. DOI: 10.1001/jama.297.2.177 PMID: 17213401

Rolnick, S. J., Pawloski, P. A., Hedblom, B. D., Asche, S. E., & Bruzek, R. J. (2013). Patient Characteristics Associated with Medication Adherence. *Clinical Medicine & Research*, 11(2), 54–65. DOI: 10.3121/cmr.2013.1113 PMID: 23580788

Rubeis, G. (2020). The disruptive power of Artificial Intelligence. Ethical aspects of gerontechnology in elderly care. *Archives of Gerontology and Geriatrics*, 91, 104186. DOI: 10.1016/j.archger.2020.104186 PMID: 32688106

Rubeis, G. (2020b). The Disruptive Power of Artificial Intelligence. Ethical aspects of gerontechnology in elderly care. *Archives of Gerontology and Geriatrics*, 91, 104186. DOI: 10.1016/j.archger.2020.104186 PMID: 32688106

Sabaté, E. (2003). Adherence to long-term therapies: Evidence for action. *World Health Organization*. Retrieved from https://apps.who.int/iris/handle/10665/42682

Shortreed, S. M., Cook, A. J., Coley, R. Y., Bobb, J. F., & Nelson, J. C. (2019). Challenges and opportunities for using big healthcare data to advance medical science and public health. *American Journal of Epidemiology*, 188(5), 851–861. DOI: 10.1093/aje/kwy292 PMID: 30877288

Simpson, S. H., Eurich, D. T., Majumdar, S. R., Padwal, R. S., Tsuyuki, R. T., Varney, J., & Johnson, J. A. (2006). A meta-analysis of the association between adherence to drug therapy and mortality. *BMJ (Clinical Research Ed.)*, 333(7557), 15. DOI: 10.1136/bmj.38875.675486.55 PMID: 16790458

Solomon, D. H., Avorn, J., Katz, J. N., Weinblatt, M. E., Setoguchi, S., Levin, R., & Schneeweiss, S. (2008). Compliance with osteoporosis medications. *Archives of Internal Medicine*, 165(20), 2414–2419. DOI: 10.1001/archinte.165.20.2414 PMID: 16287772

Svensson, E., Nielsen, R. B., Hasvold, P., Lund, J. L., & Thomsen, R. W. (2015). Statin use and discontinuation in Denmark: A nationwide drug utilization study. *British Journal of Clinical Pharmacology*, 80(6), 1444–1452. DOI: 10.1111/bcp.12704

Vrijens, B., De Geest, S., Hughes, D. A., Przemyslaw, K., Demonceau, J., Ruppar, T., Dobbels, F., Fargher, E., Morrison, V., Lewek, P., Matyjaszczyk, M., Mshelia, C., Clyne, W., Aronson, J. K., & Urquhart, J. (2012). A new taxonomy for describing and defining adherence to medications. *British Journal of Clinical Pharmacology*, 73(5), 691–705. DOI: 10.1111/j.1365-2125.2012.04167.x PMID: 22486599

Walsh, C. A., Cahir, C., Mecklenburg, S., Byrne, C., Culbertson, M. A., & Bennett, K. E. (2019). The association between medication non-adherence and adverse health outcomes in aging populations: A systematic review and meta-analysis. *British Journal of Clinical Pharmacology*, 85(11), 2464–2478. DOI: 10.1111/bcp.14075 PMID: 31486099

Welcome to FHIR. HL7. URL: https://www.hl7.org/fhir/ [accessed 2020-04-13]

Wolff, J., Pauling, J., Keck, A., & Baumbach, J. (2019). Systematic Review of Economic Impact Studies of Artificial Intelligence in Health Care. *Journal of Medical Internet Research*, 22(2), e16866. DOI: 10.2196/16866 PMID: 32130134

Xie, Z., St Clair, P., Goldman, D. P., & Joyce, G. (2019). Racial and ethnic disparities in medication adherence among privately insured patients in the United States. *PLoS One*, 14(2), e0212117. DOI: 10.1371/journal.pone.0212117 PMID: 30763400

Yeaw, J., Benner, J. S., Walt, J. G., Sian, S., & Smith, D. B. (2009). Comparing adherence and persistence across six chronic medication classes. *Journal of Managed Care Pharmacy : JMCP*, 15(9), 728–740. DOI: 10.18553/jmcp.2009.15.9.728 PMID: 19954264

Zhu, Z., Heng, B. H., & Teow, K. L. (2018). Lifetime trajectory simulation of chronic disease progression and comorbidity development. *Journal of Biomedical Informatics*, 88, 29–36. DOI: 10.1016/j.jbi.2018.11.002 PMID: 30414473

Chapter 11
Cognizing Nature: The AI Frontier in Natural Product Drug Discovery

Rana Alonazi
https://orcid.org/0009-0008-2815-7823
Prince Sattam Bin Abdulaziz University, Saudi Arabia

ABSTRACT

Abstract: Natural products (NPs) are mostly understood to be unique structures that interact with therapeutic protein targets. Their unique characteristics and structural diversity continue to astound scientists with their capacity to produce medicines that are modeled after naturally occurring products, even if the pharmaceutical industry has mostly given up. Nowadays, a lot of sectors and research domains use artificial intelligence (AI) because of developments in computer technology, storage capacity, software accessibility, and affordable online education. Two subfields of artificial intelligence (AI), natural language processing and machine learning algorithms, have evolved in recent decades to address challenges in NP drug discovery and open up new options. This chapter looks at and discusses the practical applications of artificial intelligence (AI) methods developed to aid in the discovery of bioactive natural products (NPs) and to determine the molecular "patterns" of these favored structures for target selectivity or combinatorial design.

INTRODUCTION

The term artificial intelligence (AI) describes the capacity of computer systems (as well as human judgment) to take in, process, and identify patterns in vast amounts of intricate data. AI has advanced from theoretical research to practical applications because of the revolution in powerful computer hardware, large amounts of storage,

DOI: 10.4018/979-8-3693-6270-9.ch011

and easily accessible software. A branch of artificial intelligence called machine learning (ML) deals with the collection of sophisticated statistics and mathematical formulas that people use through algorithms to solve many kinds of problems. Machine learning algorithms can easily and affordably be implemented at very large scales in the cloud.

The Internet has been overwhelmed with what is sometimes referred to as "data deluge," which is the digitalization of various data kinds (such as images, text, soundwaves, and biometrics) from wearables or sensors into proprietary and public web databases. Building useful prediction applications, such recommendation systems, has been made possible by the abundance of information available in those databases and on the internet, (Berman, Fox, & Hey, 2003).

The usage of AI applications across a variety of industries, including banking, law, cybersecurity, transportation, manufacturing, entertainment, robotics, education, health, and services, has become more accessible thanks to open-source toolkits, massively multiplayer online courses, and instructional videos on social media platforms, (Jordan & Mitchell, 2015). The pharmaceutical sector has been increasingly interested in machine learning algorithms, and various supervised and unsupervised learning techniques are being implemented at various phases of the drug discovery process. Clustering techniques, for instance, have assisted de novo molecular design, projected protein target drug ability, and segmented cell type imaging. Regressions and classifications—supervised learning techniques—identified potential targets for the disease Huntington's. In order to construct drugs and for many other purposes, they conjectured about the biological activities and the features of absorption, distribution, metabolism, excretion, and toxicity (ADME/Tox). Finally, in medicinal chemistry, generative algorithms are currently helping with the molecular design of novel chemical entities. In just 46 days, the AI system known as GENTRL (for Generative Tensorial Reinforcement Learning) developed by the American company Insilco Medicine in 2019 was able to successfully discover six kinase inhibitors of discoid in domain receptor 1, which is connected to lung fibrosis. The main understanding of natural products (NPs) is that they are special structures that can interact with therapeutically important protein targets, (Vamathevan *et al.,* 2019) (Schneider *et al.,* 2020) (Walters & Murcko, 2020) (Brown *et al.,* 2020) (Zhavoronkov *et al.,* 2019).

The development of small compounds and macrocyclic medicines is still motivated by their structural variety and biological activity, (Rodrigues *et al.,* 2016). Since the middle of the 1970s, NPs have dominated the sources of new human therapies in the pharmaceutical drug pipeline. Between the 1980s and the 2010s, two-thirds of the medications came from either unaltered NPs (5%), NP analogues (28%), or comprised NP pharmacophores (35%), (Driggers *et al.,* 2008) (Newman & Cragg, 2020). The majority of large pharmaceutical firms have reduced their natural product research, despite it being a reliable source for contemporary small-molecule drug development. The lengthy dereplication procedure, intricate synthesis, and extracts that are not suitable for high-throughput screening are the primary points of contention, (Strohl, 2000) (Atanasov *et al.,* 2021). Additionally, a lot of NPs have physicochemical and ADME characteristics that go beyond the existing drug-like chemical space, such as fused ring systems, rotatable bonds, and high degrees of stereochemistry, (Saldívar-González *et al.,* 2022). The peculiarities of NPs never cease to astound computer scientists and lab personnel alike. Unsurprisingly, scientists have created and implemented a number of computational techniques across the pharmaceutical pipeline: (1) to help with the identification and structural clarification of bioactive nanoparticles.

Johnston *et al.* (2015) and Nugroho and Morita (2019) and (2) to obtain these favored structures' molecular patterns for target selectivity or combinatorial design, (Giordanetto & Kihlberg, 2014) (Rodrigues, 2017) (Merk *et al.*, 2018). Chemo informatics, bioinformatics, and other informatics-related fields have made significant contributions to NP-based drug development throughout the years. Their limits and effective uses have been examined recently, (Pereira & Aires-de-Sousa, 2018) (Romano & Tatonetti, 2019) (Medina-Franco & Saldívar-González, 2020). Machine learning algorithms and Artificial intelligence have gradually permeated natural product research, a reliable avenue for contemporary small molecule drug discovery. For instance, the majority of AI applications in the early 2000s included the digitalization of organic molecules and the mapping of the NP chemical space using dimensionality reduction techniques (principal component analysis, self-organizing maps, etc.). In order to forecast their biological roles, machine learning binary classifiers were developed within the next ten years. Neural network designs have recently been used by scientists in molecular design and genome mining. The recent contributions of ML and AI algorithms to aid in the identification of bioactive NPs, the creation of NP-inspired medications, and their potential future development are covered in this viewpoint essay.

ARTIFICIAL INTELLIGENCE AI

Stellar method development in machine learning, a subdomain of "artificial intelligence," and biotechnology has contributed to advancements in computer-assisted drug discovery. These developments hold promises for overcoming some of these limitations through the use of certain algorithms and Ai techniques that will be covered in this chapter. is a system-based technology that, through the use of several state-of-the-art tools and networks, is capable of mimicking human intellect, (Adeniyi & Soliman, 2017) (Boadu & Asase, 2017). Artificial Intelligence uses software and hardware that can learn from and interpret input data to make decisions on its own for the purpose of accomplishing predefined objectives, (Borquaye *et al.,* 2020). Because AI technology has real-world applications across a wide range of technological and scientific fields, it has become an increasingly significant part of business in recent years. There has already been a shift from hype to optimism in the growing movement to apply AI in pharmacy for drug discovery, formulation design for medication delivery, and other healthcare applications, (Busia, 2007). Innovative knowledge development, enhanced precision, automated predictions and simulations, continuous performance, and early sickness detection or monitoring are among the main advantages of artificial intelligence. Neural network modeling may be used to predict the physicochemical characteristics of organic molecules and explain their molecular structure. The prediction of in vivo responses, therapeutic medication pharmacokinetic characteristics, proper dose, etc. is also made possible by the use of AI models, (Gamieldien, Fielding, & Berry, 2015). Due to the importance of drug pharmacokinetic prediction, the use of silico models in drug research facilitates their efficacy and lowers their cost, (Berry, Fielding, & Gamieldien, 2015). The advances in AI technology may be divided into two primary areas. The first one is composed of conventional computing techniques, including expert systems, which may mimic human experiences and provide deductions made from basic concepts. The second one is made up of neural network (ANN) based brain function modeling systems, (Bisht & Singh, 2018). AI-based drug development has been widely employed in the pharmaceutical industry and is regarded as a potent replacement for the conventional method, (Chávez-Fumagalli *et al.,* 2018). Artificial intelligence is created via the use of mathematics, data analytics, and computer science, (Chen, 2011). To complete the AI modeling process, algorithms are written in Python, Lisp, C++, JavaScript, and Haskell, among other computer languages.

To perform different machine learning tasks, a range of commercially accessible tools and platforms may be used, such as Tensor Flow, Cortana, Azure Machine Learning Studio, Google Cloud Machine Learning Engine, and IBM Watson, (Chen, 2015). Biological data analysis, drug target identification, and drug discovery using AI platforms may result in more effective drug development in the biopharmaceutical sector. Early in the drug discovery process, it is critical to remove any potentially dangerous or inactive compounds. ML techniques have been applied to screen and classify drug or nondrug collections, anticipate toxicity, and supplement fast filtering or virtual screening, (Daina, Michielin, & Zoete, 2017; Danker & Möller, 2014; David, Wolfender, & Dias, 2015). Building chemical libraries, predicting the biological activities of proteins, and identifying novel drug candidates with the finest qualities are all made possible by deep learning (DL), (Dhiman, Malik, & Khatkar, 2018). Outcomes from the most effective ANN-based models have regularly matched well with real data using a variety of experimental techniques, indicating that they may be used in place of intricate equations. ANNs may be used for a variety of tasks, including the categorization of cancers, the prediction of protein secondary structures, the modeling of complex biological data and nonlinear systems, and the resolution of multivariate and multi-response system problems, (Gamieldien, Fielding, & Berry, 2015).

Figure 1. The normal way for natural products drug discovery

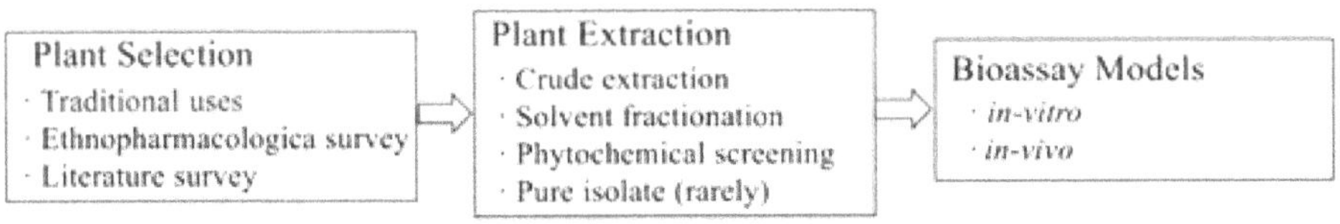

Figure 1 shows the workflow used by scientists who specialize in natural products, primarily in poor nations, to identify new drugs. Selection of plants, extractions, and bioassays of crude extracts or solvent fractions are the first steps in the process; pure component isolation, characterization, and bioassays are restricted.

Drug Discovery in the AI Era

Over the past two decades, artificial intelligence has played a significant role in the field of drug discovery. Machine learning models, including the widely used random forest (RF), have been effectively utilized for virtual screening (VS) and quantitative structure-activity relationship (QSAR) analyses since the early 2000s, (Madhavi et al., 2013) (Lavecchia, 2015). In 2012, Alex Net heralded the beginning of the age of deep learning, (Krizhevsky, Sutskever, & Hinton, 2012). Soon after, deep neural networks (DNNs) beat the conventional RF model in the competition in 2012 Merck Kaggle when it came to predicting chemical activity, (Ma *et al.,* 2015). The effectiveness of AI methods in computer vision and natural language processing has lately provided more insight into the drug development process, (Chen *et al.,* 2018; Vamathevan *et al.,* 2019; Öztürk *et al.,* 2020; Jiménez-Luna *et al.,* 2021).

It paved the way for the development of deep learning in chemistry, (Mater & Coote, 2019). Insilco Medicine researchers found powerful inhibitors of discoid in domain receptor 1 (DDR1) in 21 days in 2019, (Zhavoronkov *et al.,* 2019). In 2020, MIT researchers discovered halicin, a new antibiotic contender that fights bacteria resistant to antibiotics, (Stokes *et al.,* 2020). Keep in mind that AI may be used at several phases of the drug development process, from target selection and validation to determining the medication's response, (Vamathevan *et al.,* 2019). This survey focuses on lead identification, which entails two core tasks: molecule creation and chemical property prediction. Predicting a molecule's property value based on its structure or learnt representation is the fundamental function of molecular property prediction (VS), (Chuang, Gunsalus, & Keiser, 2020). It has several uses, including the prediction of drug-target interactions (DTIs), (Sydow *et al.,* 2019). Prediction the toxicity (Mayr *et al.,* 2016) in the prediction of drug-induced liver damage (DILI), (Andrade *et al.,* 2019). In addition to others. Creating molecules within the limitations set by chemical principles is known as realistic molecule generation, and creating chemically valid molecules with desired qualities is known as goal-directed molecule generation. These tasks are the foundation of drug design, (Elton *et al.,* 2019); Mercado *et al.,* 2020.)

Molecular Docking Use

The many active ingredients that make up a particular medicinal plant are what give it its biological action. When a plant's crude extract has strong biological activity, in-silico research can be used to investigate many possible therapeutic targets through compound separation and structural characterization of the active component. Docking studies often employ established database structures to investigate novel targets. It is possible to identify new applications for "old" medications by using docking for natural product repurposing, as is already done. When phytochemicals from a particular plant are docked against medication targets for new illnesses, for instance, it may become clear whether the plant has any kind of action against the ailment. As a result, the plant can be chosen for biological testing using suitable disease models and extraction. To put it simply, molecular docking is a modeling approach used to examine the interactions between a macromolecule (DNA, protein/enzyme, etc.) and a small molecule (ligand/drug). Essentially, posture prediction, binding affinity calculation, and virtual screening are the three main objectives of molecular docking, (Sastry *et al.,* 2013).

The preparation of the ligand and protein has a significant impact on the docking outcomes. Prior to docking, proteins and ligands are individually prepared using automated processes (such as the addition of hydrogens and charges). Even though some of the structures are produced by NMR, x-ray crystallography provides the majority of the macromolecules and ligands, (Sorokina *et al.,* 2021). Atomic collisions, hydrogen bond distortion, and hydrogen atom removal are among the outcomes of the procedures that produce an x-ray crystallographic structure. In order to carry out a docking exercise, it's necessary to correct a few abnormalities associated with the crystal structure. Adding hydrogen helps to enhance bonding contact saturation and stability, as well as ligand binding affinity versus target, (Kim *et al.,* 2011). It has been found that the binding energy and binding structures are dominated by the columbic interaction between partial atomic charges, (Adeniyi &

Soliman, 2017; Sorokina *et al.,* 2021). Any macromolecule's ability to recognize the ligand is dependent upon its three-dimensional orientation as well as its molecular connections. The protein and ligand are able to interact to produce a variety of postures with different binding affinities. Medicinal chemists can determine if a certain chemical is worth synthesizing because of its potential biological uses based on the outcomes of these in-silico experiments. All of the known phytochemicals of one or more herbal plants can be docked against one or more proteins and their interactions can be seen in studies on natural products. In drug discovery, there are essentially two forms of docking: 1) blind or global docking and 2) precision or focus docking. Building confidence in the docking outcomes requires validation of the docking techniques. Here, concentrated or precise docking is recommended. After making certain movements and acquiring distinct conformational forms, the ligand (native/experimental inhibitor) co-crystallized to the protein retrieved from the PDB databank is detached and re-docked into the active site. A good docking strategy has to be able to anticipate the native (experimental) position and its molecular interactions accurately, within a certain tolerance level. The docked outcomes are contrasted with this native interaction. A higher number of experimental interactions, particularly those involving catalytic residues—must be preserved for the docking approach to produce reliable results.

After the right drug target or targets have been chosen and a phytochemical library has been created, docking is carried out using either free or licensed molecular docking tools, such as PyRx Autodock vina, CCDC GOLD, GLIDE, MOE and Schrodinger, among others. Other server-based docking solutions are Swiss Dock and Patch Dock. Comparing several platforms and choosing the structures that the majority of the software predicts can be helpful at times. The probability of discovering active molecules is increased by using numerous docking techniques and their respective score systems. It is stated that this "consensus-based approach" yields a richer hit list than docking and scoring using a single algorithm, (Gamieldien, Fielding, & Berry, 2015; Kim *et al.,* 2011). Protein-ligand interaction types may often be usefully compared through the docking of standard reference molecules. The binding postures or binding energies of the docked phytochemicals are often selected using experimenter-set selection criteria before moving on to the next phase. (Figure 2)

Figure 2. Workflow of natural product-based drug discovery approach

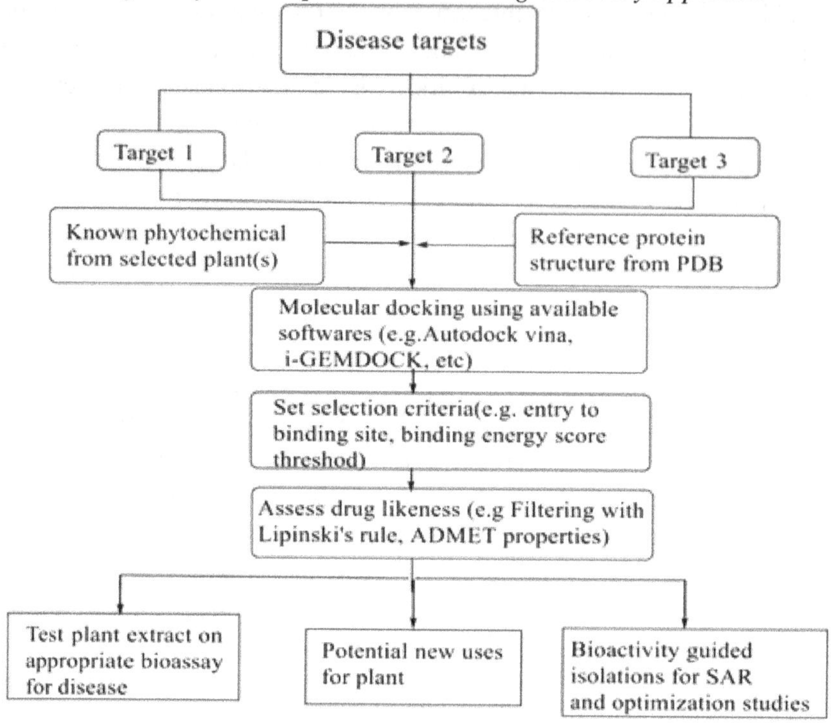

Figure 2 shows the workflow of a natural product-based drug discovery approach that includes the molecular docking of reference compounds and known phytochemicals on suitable disease targets. Target plants are chosen for biological screening, compound isolations, and compound characterizations using suitable selection criteria and compound filtering.

OVERVIEW OF ML/AI ALGORITHMS THAT ARE IMPLEMENTED ACROSS THE DIFFERENT STAGES OF THE NATURAL PRODUCT DRUG DISCOVERY PIPELINE

1. Computer-Assisted Discovery of Natural Products: Data Mining Into Traditional Medicines and Peer-Reviewed Articles

For a considerable amount of time, scientific compilations have been recorded in codices, dissertations, journals, patents, reports, or lab notebooks. An estimated 10,000 publications on chemistry are produced year; yet, the amount of knowledge that can be retrieved beyond human comprehension, and many discoveries are still unknown. It is imperative that the information be machine-readable. Data-mining technologies have gained momentum due to the recent shift from hard copy documents to digital versions and from constrained geographical locales to the World Wide Web. Many text-mining techniques are used in the discipline of chemistry alone to keep track of the 20,000 novel compounds that are published in journals of medicinal and biological chemistry each year, (Krallinger *et al.*, 2017). The best software system for optical chemical entity recognition was created in 2020 by Rajan and colleagues utilizing deep learning (DL) to identify chemical structures in scientific articles, (Tshitoyan *et al.*, 2019). A branch of machine learning known as "deep learning" makes use of three or more-layer neural network structures. Tshitoyan and colleagues revealed the finding of "forgotten" thermoelectric materials in peer-reviewed publications from 1922 to 2018 the previous year. The authors employed Word2vec, a natural language processing (NLP) tool, to create semantic associations from a corpus of 1.5 million abstracts that they had originally selected. Using word embeddings, or vector representations of words, they constructed a machine learning model to forecast the thermoelectric property of 7663 candidate materials and 1820 known materials, (Tshitoyan *et al.*, 2019).

NLP is an area of artificial intelligence that focuses on comprehending how computers and human languages interact. NLP techniques extract, classify, and analyze words or sentences to get information from unstructured documents (e.g., knowledge graphs, (Ernst, Siu, & Weikum, 2015). BioNLP is the domain in which natural language processing (NLP) techniques are required to handle molecular representations linked to biomedical research, in addition to textual data in English. (Rebholz-Schuhmann, Oellrich, & Hoehndorf, 2012; Öztürk *et al.*, 2020). As of right now, drug discovery subfields such protein docking (Badal, Kundrotas, & Vakser, 2015; Badal, Kundrotas, & Vakser, 2021) and protein–protein interactions, (Papanikolaou *et al.*, 2015) or disease-protein associations have benefited from the use of biomedical text mining as well. NLP, on the other hand, has only demonstrated a few uses in the search for bioactive NPs.

Thus far, BioNLP techniques have mostly been used to locate bioactive plants by decoding old texts from traditional remedies that are becoming extinct. Throughout history, traditional medicine has fueled the hunt for innovative medications and bioactive nanoparticles from a variety of sources. Early records, recorded in cuneiform on clay tablets, mentioned the medical usage of plants, (Sharma *et al.*, 2018). Due to its contribution to the discovery of therapies for rheumatoid arthritis and malaria, traditional Chinese medicine (TCM) has attracted interest from all around the world. An algorithm that could screen, extract, choose, categorize, and score data from ancient texts was created in 2014 by May and colleagues. With such technology at their disposal, the writers tracked throughout time how the names given to particular illnesses changed. They found common treatments and made it easier to find NPs in Zhong Yi Fang Ji Da Ci Dian (Great Compendium of Chinese Medical Formulae), the largest compilation of herbal formulas, and Zhong Hua Yi Dian (ZHYD; Encyclopedia of Traditional Chinese Medicine), the most comprehensive encyclopedia of TCM books, (Wells, 2011; Xia *et al.,* 2020; May *et al.,* 2014). Shergis and colleagues (2015) searched for natural remedies for persistent cough, a side effect of cancer, obstructive pulmonary illness, TB, and asthma in 2015 using text mining inside TCM codices. These semantic techniques are novel, yet they are still quite basic and have numerous shortcomings. The fact that medical paradigms and concepts have evolved throughout time is one of the primary disadvantages of researching old literature. For instance, Qi theory (also known as the yin-yang theory) and the five elements theory are two ancient philosophies from which TCM derived its diagnosis and treatment methods. TCM practitioners refer to a group of patient symptoms as a syndrome when they might be caused by several diseases and causes, making it difficult to determine the best course of action, (Zhou, Peng, & Liu, 2010). Forty Similar to conventional medicine, ethnobotanical research has led to the discovery of several NPs, (Porras *et al.,* 2020). In an effort to identify medicinal plants and their therapeutic applications, Sharma and colleagues examined the Palau and Pohnpei Primary Health Care Manuals in 2014, which are traditional botanical descriptions from Micronesian islands, (Sharma *et al.,* 2018).

To construct individual plants and medicinal notes, the writers first digitized the manuals using the Biodiversity Heritage Library. Using Meta Map, the retrieved data was cross-referenced with current biomedical terms, (Aronson & Lang, 2010). A website called Metamap.nlm.nih.gov. This BioNLP program looks up synonyms in the Unified Medical Language System using computational linguistic approaches. From the Primary Health Care Manuals, the team identified over 700 therapy indications and 129 distinct plant species. Of the (Wells, 2011) plant species that the Biodiversity Heritage Library regularly reported, 10 had similar symptoms (such as diarrhea, discomfort, or redness) that may be caused by pathogen infections or venomous stings.

2. Utilizing Molecular Descriptors to Vectorize Natural Products

In addition to fingerprints, which chemo informaticians often utilize, computational chemists would compute hundreds of characteristics, or variables, called molecular descriptors using molecular representations, (Wetzel *et al.,* 2009). The means of precise algorithms. These descriptors capture particular molecular characteristics that are simple for researchers to understand, such as atomic qualities, size, shape, flexibility, polarity, lipophilicity, and pharmacophore. A key component in the development of predictive QSA/PR modeling has been the use of molecular descriptors. They have proven crucial in characterizing the dispersions of artificial chemicals and NPs in low-dimensional chemical space representations (s). To quickly identify orally accessible small compounds from screening campaigns and combinatorial libraries, Lipinski and colleagues developed a set of empirical principles or recommendations known as the rule-of-five (Ro5) at the beginning of the twenty-first century. These rules or guidelines were based on important chemical characteristics, (Lipinski *et al.,* 1997). Several computational investigations compared and described the chemical spaces filled by NPs, combinatorial chemical libraries, synthesized compounds, and commercial pharmaceuticals using molecular descriptors in conjunction with their structural similarity analysis, (Schneider, 2018; Reutlinger & Schneider, 2012; Osolodkin *et al.*, 2015; Davison & Brimble, 2019). Despite being disregarded while establishing the Ro5 standards, natural compounds and macrocycles have been shown to breach one or more of these guidelines while still demonstrating oral bioavailability. Quinn and colleagues tried to create a set of guidelines exclusive to NPs in 2008.

In order to explain cell permeability and oral bioavailability of macrocycles, a number of research groups have followed suit and developed a new set of empirical guidelines known as "beyond the Ro5" (bRo5), which are based on molecular descriptors. Grisoni, Consonni, and Todeschini (2018) examined the influence of molecular descriptors on chemoinformatic applications in a recent chapter, (Grisoni, Consonni, & Todeschini, 2018). Primarily, the writers presented molecular representations that go beyond three dimensions, resulting in novel characteristics like flexibility in conformation and states or orientations of protons. The remaining descriptors are scaled and used for similarity search or QSA/PR modeling once the irrelevant features (missing values, low variance threshold, multicollinearity) are eliminated. When selecting the appropriate distance metrics and molecular descriptors to measure the (dis-)similarity of chemical entities in the previous application, the authors issued a warning. They suggested using the enrichment factor to quantify the best molecular descriptors and distance metrics before choosing them,, (Truchon & Bayly, 2007). In the latter application, the metrics (e.g., accuracy, root mean squared error) for model evaluation as well as the stability, performance, and interpretability of the employed algorithm are primarily responsible for determining which molecular descriptors will yield the best predictions of the biological activity or property of interest.

Deep learning (DL) techniques have gained widespread traction in fields like computer vision throughout the last ten years., (Rawat & Wang, 2017). As well as natural language processing. DL models have gained popularity recently because of their use in molecular informatics and drug development, (Paolini *et al.,* 2006). Neural networks are fundamentally capable of processing massive datasets and capturing the intricate connections between input information (like chemical descriptors or 2D/3D fingerprints) and output judgments (like biological activity or ADME/

Tox). In spite of its notable advancements over conventional machine learning algorithms, deep learning models are mostly constructed using a selected collection of features, or molecular representations, as opposed to acquiring knowledge from "raw" chemical data. Convolutional neural networks (CNNs) that are now in use for picture categorization are not well adapted to interpret 3D structures or 2D graph visualizations. Molecular graphs with erratic sizes and forms can be used to represent chemical substances such as pharmaceuticals, synthetic tiny molecules, or nanoparticles. Additionally, as CNNs often scan pictures in a certain sequence, the DL structures need to accurately read the atoms, or nodes and vertices, and chemical bonds, or edges, that make up molecular graphs.

The state-of-the-art methods for reading irregular and raw data from molecular graphs have been set by recent efforts toward the construction of graph convolutional networks (GCNs). Sun and colleagues have so far examined their applicability to the drug discovery pipeline's four domains: synthesis planning, de novo molecular design, drug-target/drug-drug interaction, and QSA/PR modeling, (Sun *et al.*, 2020). There have been several reports of studies using large and general chemical datasets to develop GCNs with domain-specific applications, such as the NCI dataset from the National Cancer Institute (https://cactus.nci.nih.gov/download/nci/), three datasets from the European Molecular Biology Laboratory (https://www.ebi.ac.uk – SIDER, STITCH, ChEMBL), or Binding DB from the University of California San Diego (https://www.bindingdb.org/bind/index.jsp). In 2019, Sanchez-Lengeling et al. revealed the odor profiles (138 labels) for about 5030 molecules from the Leffingwell 2001 PMP databases and the Good Scents perfume materials, which are close to NPs, (Sanchez-Lengeling *et al.*, 2019). Each molecule displayed one to fifteen odor markers on average. The significant correlations between odor labels and structures that the authors discovered allowed them to predict all 138 characteristics for all molecules at once using GCNs. It is still necessary to apply GCNs explicitly to NP databases such as COCONUT or LOTUS (see above).

3. Automating the Process of Dereplicating Natural Products

The process of dereplication, which produces single metabolites (or combinations of them) by repeated extractions, chromatography/spectrometry-guided fractionations, and purifications, is what defines the early stages of NP discovery from species across all kingdoms. The process of screening and ranking the extracts, fractions, and isolates containing the bioactive compounds is frequently guided by one or more biological tests. Dereplication is time-consuming, laborious, and may encounter issues that reduce the anticipated return on investments (time, equipment, and human resources), such as finding previously identified NPs, purifying purportedly novel structures insufficiently, or using high-throughput robotics to screen natural crude extracts (NCEs), (Strohl, 2000; Atanasov *et al.,* 2021; Koehn & Carter, 2005). Scientists have used early chemical characterization of (un-)targeted NPs to develop several strategies to decrease duplicate NCEs, (Hubert, Nuzillard, & Renault, 2017; Wolfender et al., 2019). Using cutting-edge analytical chemistry methods, such as mass spectrometry (MS), gas/liquid chromatography (GC/LC), nuclear magnetic resonance (NMR) spectroscopy, and combinations of these, they have particularly prioritized NCEs.

The use of statistical and mathematical techniques has been made possible by the growing digitalization of data. For the quick identification of known and unknown bioactive NPs from NCEs, the area of chemometrics has made use of multivariate statistical analysis of data from the studies and from the optical radiation (i.e., infrared, visible, and ultraviolet). Cornejo-Baez and colleagues (2020) published a list of the most used statistical methods for NP research in 2019. The list comprised supervised and unsupervised machine learning methods, such as partial least squares and orthogonal projection to latent structures, as well as principal component analysis, discriminant analysis, and hierarchical cluster analysis. Beyond NCEs, researchers have used machine learning (ML) techniques to glean biologically novel insights and information from metabolomic data. Because they can produce quantitative predictions, supervised machine learning (ML) techniques like random forest, support vector machine (SVM), artificial neural network, and genetic algorithms have demonstrated considerable promise in metabolomics research, (Liebal *et al.,* 2020). The utilization of these algorithms has promoted biological applications, integrated omics data, and eased analytical data processing. ML algorithms are utilized, for instance, to amputate missing data, forecast retention duration, and combine chromatogram peaks, (Risum & Bro, 2019; Witting & Böcker, 2020; Wolfer *et al.,* 2016; Bouwmeester, Martens, & Degroeve, 2019; Kokla *et al.,* 2019).

4. Natural Product Machine Learning: Converting Natural Goods Into Molecular Representations

Modeling and forecasting NPs' (or any chemical structure's) characteristics and bioactivities mostly involve translating them into computer-readable format(s), or so-called molecular representations. The majority of representations encode chemical data for a particular purpose. Chemical compounds with similar nomenclatures can be retrieved using original generic and IUPAC names. It was computationally hard to match chemical structures based on their representations in bidimensional molecular graphs. The original purpose of molecular representations was to store chemical information in a lightweight manner or to facilitate structural research. The international chemical identification (InChI), Daylight CIS, Open Eye Scientific Software, SMILES arbitrary target specification, and simplified input line entry system (SMILES), (Weininger, 1988; Heller *et al.*, 2015) were developed to discover common molecular traits or substructures from databases, as well as to store and retrieve molecular information. Fresh molecular depictions like SELFIES106 and DeepSMILES105 emerged lately due to their application in ML algorithms. Chemical and biomolecular databases are ubiquitous in informatics-related fields and are essential to many AI applications, (López-López, Bajorath, & Medina-Franco, 2020). Chemical databases (Cornejo- Báez *et al.,* 2020) contributed significantly to the improvement of the NP dereplication process through the use of chemical fingerprinting (calculated physical parameters, spectroscopic/chromatographic data, and preassembled NP libraries). The American Chemical Society's generalist Chemical Abstracts Service and the University of Canterbury, New Zealand's highly specialized Marin Lit, which are currently under the British Royal Society of Chemistry, are two examples of the commercial databases from curated literature reviews that public and private research entities launched in the mid-1990s. Nonetheless, many academic researchers are now considering free and open-access alternatives like ChemSpider due to the high fees and restricted access to commercial databases. There weren't many NP databases available to the general public a few years ago. But given the resurgence of interest in NP research, the quick progress in informatics, and

The creation and release of NP collections into the public domain were facilitated by data sharing, (Koch *et al.,* 2005). Commercial and open-access databases, industrial catalogs, publications, and collections that were still being mentioned in the scientific literature after 2000 were examined by Soronika *et al.* (2021) in search of NP information. The developers of several NP databases, both open-access and commercial, occasionally maintain them. Fewer than half of these databases had stereochemical information, and less than half allowed substructure searching using at least one of the previously described molecular representations. As a consequence, the authors created COCONUT (https://coconut.naturalproducts.net/), the biggest library of open-access natural products, which assembled the structures and associated data of more than 400 000 non-redundant NPs. The same research team has carried on creating and maintaining COCONUT and has made available an upgraded version known as LOTUS, (Rutz *et al.,* 2021).

Molecular fingerprints are also a result of the requirement for effective substructure research in expanding chemical databases and a demand for less storage space. The initial bitstring fingerprints were binary vectors that indicated whether substructures were present (1) or absent (0), (Ahrens, 1988; Christie, Leland, & Nourse, 1993). Bidimensional fingerprints were implemented to compare the molecular similarity of NPs against synthetic chemical libraries. The similarity of any two molecules is measured using one of many distance metrics, such as the Tanimoto coefficient. Subsequent topological fingerprints based on atom pairs, local circular neighborhoods, Extended Connectivity fingerprints (ECFP), Molecular ACCess System (MACCS) keys, to name a few, were specifically designed for bioactivity prediction and similarity analysis, (Carhart, Smith, & Venkataraghavan, 1985; Rogers & Hahn, 2010; Durant *et al.*, 2002; Chen & Reynolds, 2002; Todeschini *et al.*, 2012; Bajusz, Rácz, & Héberger, 2015).

In a groundbreaking 1999 study, Henzel and associates. 118 transformed, chemical compounds from the Available Chemicals Directory, 29 432 entries from the Bioactive Natural Product Database, 78 318 entries from the Database of Natural Products, 14 596 medications, and a few synthetic chemicals from Bayer AG into MACCS- and UNITY-format. Greater molecular weights and unique heteroatom distributions were shown by NPs, and more than 40% of NP-derived pharmacophores were absent from the synthesized libraries. Over the next twenty years, as numerous reviews have summarized, pharmaceutical companies and academic institutions have incorporated bioactive NP scaffolds into their combinatorial drug design strategies, resulting in the creation of NP-like libraries through diversity-oriented synthesis (DOS), diverted total synthesis (DTS), biology-oriented synthesis (BIOS), and function-oriented synthesis (FOS). Simultaneously, computer scientists have conducted repeated structural similarity studies, resulting in unique visual representations of the chemical space (see Mapping NPs in chemical space), using the previously stated fingerprints indifferently between NPs and synthetic molecules, (Boldi, 2004).

5. Charting Natural Products in the Realm of Chemistry

The geometric region is bounded by all potential chemical compounds and their structural and functional characteristics are known as the chemical space. The space inhabited by a group of recognized NPs is referred to as an NP chemical space. Decision-making and advancements in the drug-discovery process have greatly benefited by the visualization of this high-dimensional space using human-readable graphical representations (of one to three dimensions). Coordinate-based representations are often used to create visual representations of the chemical space, but they frequently need a reduction in the number of dimensions. Dimensionality reduction is a common strategy in artificial intelligence projects, which involves reducing the number of dimensions in high-dimensional data to improve comprehension and interpretation of the findings, (Maniyar *et al.*, 2006; Schneider, 2018; Arús-Pous *et al.*, 2019). In the past twenty years, a multitude of research teams have employed various dimensionality-reduction methods to investigate NP chemical space, which have been well discussed elsewhere, (Reutlinger & Schneider, 2012; Saldívar-González, Pilón-Jiménez, & Medina-Franco, 2019; Osolodkin *et al.,* 2015).

Dimensionality-reduction strategies reveal structure-activity/property connections (SA/PRs) between compounds and compound databases in addition to mapping chemical spaces. The depiction of SA/PRs is a tough endeavor due to the growing quantity of data collected in chemical databases.126 Lastly, the application domain of QSA/PR modeling—a certain area of the underlying chemical space where the model predictions are deemed credible—is defined with the use of dimensionality-reduction techniques. Dimensionality-reduction methods find outliers and produce strong models in that application. Principal component analysis (PCA), t-distributed stochastic neighbor embedding (t-SNE), and self-organizing map (SOM) are the three methods most frequently used to either map the chemical space, specify its bounds, or display SARs/SPRs.

6. Estimating the Functions of Biological Systems

Natural crude extracts (NCEs) include trace levels of bioactive NPs (mg to few mg); nevertheless, these concentrations are occasionally inadequate to perform biological assessments in several, consecutive phenotypic or target-based experiments. Conventional bioassay-guided fractionation examines just a few biological reactions; fractions that fail to react to the assay(s) are discarded, their NPs are not included, and their biological profile(s) is/are not determined. Recently, Atanasov and colleagues (2021) talked about how culture systems, metabolite engineering, and genome mining may be used to address that persistent problem. To make the most of their upcoming screening campaigns, research labs keep their purified NPs and NCEs in freezers (diluted at various quantities or lyophilized). To promote collaboration between chemical and biological laboratories, several nations have established national chemical repositories, such as Compound Australia (https://www.griffith.edu.au/griffith-sciences/compounds-australia) and France's Chimiothèque Nationale (https://chembiofrance.cn.cnrs.fr). Structure-based (e.g., docking and virtual screening) and ligand-based (e.g., QSA/PR modeling) in silico methods are utilized to forecast the biological or ADME/Tox profiles of unexplored chemical compounds. ML techniques, namely regressors and classifiers, are used in Quantitative Structure–Activity/Property Relationship (QSA/PR) models to establish a connection between changes in chemical moieties and the biological activity or physicochemical property of interest. QSA/PR modeling has evolved over the last fifty years from a specialized field in computational and theoretical chemistry to one of the main approaches for keeping an eye on sizable chemical libraries with uses in drug development, quantum mechanics, materials and nanomaterials science, regenerative medicine, and environmental toxicity, (Muratov *et al.,* 2020).

7. Creating a Chemical Inspired by a De Novo Natural Product

Natural products can be used as beginning, intermediate, or end products in the construction of synthetic chemical libraries because of their unique properties that allow them to interact with (protein) pharmacological targets. Despite these benefits, the majority of NPs require medicinal chemistry interventions since they do not fully meet the criteria of the drug development paradigm in terms of toxicity, selectivity, lipophilicity, and bioavailability (for example, 92% of NP-inspired medications were changed between 1980 and 2014), (Newman & Cragg, 2020). The intricate architectures of these compounds, such as their fused rings, heteroatom-containing functional groups, and stereo genic centers, have frequently impeded the development of analogues and the analysis of their structure-activity/property connection (SA/PR). Furthermore, in certain countries where the compounds were found, patenting bioactive NPs in their native form may not be permitted, (Harrison, 2014). As a result, several artificial techniques have resulted in the creation of lead structures that maintain the NP privileges, (Karageorgis *et al.*, 2020; Barnes, Kumar, & Davis, 2016; Davison & Brimble, 2019). The first method is called biology-oriented synthesis (BIOS), in which NPs are used as models to create derivatives and mimics that can be synthesized, (Breinbauder, Vetter, & Waldmann, 2002) (Karageorgis & Waldmann, 2018). Diverted total synthesis, also known as diversity-oriented or diverted total synthesis (DOS/DTS), aims to create novel chemical structures with NP, such as pharmacophores, to fill the underexplored chemical space, (Schreiber, 2000; Tan, 2005; Yi *et al.*, 2018). The complexity-to-diversity technique (CtD) is a synthetic approach that uses chemical functionalization and structurally diverse compound collections to simulate enzyme operations, (Huigens *et al.*, 2013; Rafferty *et al.*, 2014). Ultimately, the notion of BIOS is refined by function-oriented synthesis (FOS), which involves fine-tuning or recapitulating the function of a physiologically active lead structure. This process results in simpler scaffolds, makes them easier to synthesize, and fosters synthetic creativity, (Wender *et al.*, 2008; Wender, Quiroz, & Stevens, 2015). Recently, Waldmann and colleagues presented a set of guidelines to direct the creation of small molecular compound libraries known as "pseudo-NPs," which combine two or more NP-derived fragments (NPDFs) to create hitherto unheard-of scaffolds. According to their chemo-informatic assessments, compared to other libraries like BIOS and ChEMBL NPs, pseudo-NPs shared more properties (sizes, shapes, and lipophilicity) with medicines, (Karageorgis *et al.*, 2020; Karageorgis *et al.*, 2018; Grigalunas *et al.*, 2020).

CONCLUSION

Many drug discovery success stories have been sparked by natural products; however, the numerous obstacles that accompanied their discovery or design—tiny quantities, unfavorable extracts, unclear biological functions, absent biological targets, challenging chemical syntheses, intricate SA/PR studies, undruggable ADME/Tox properties—caused NP drug discovery programs to decline. But even with this limitation, computer scientists and lab scientists alike are still in awe of NPs' special ability to attach biological drug targets for possible therapeutic benefits. The various phases of NP drug development have gradually been merged by artificial intelligence and machine learning algorithms: (1) to help find and clarify bioactive structures; and (2) to record the molecular patterns of these favored structures for molecular design and target selectivity.

With regard to the early discovery of bioactive nanoparticles (NPs), natural language processing and text-mining tools have not been able to fully decipher the multitude of bioactive compounds that are concealed or overlooked in codices of traditional medicines and peer-reviewed articles. However, ML-fueled applications in genome mining and dereplication processes have decreased the screening of redundant producers or natural crude extracts and accelerated the discovery of novel natural chemical entities, such as the subclass V lanthipeptides. With reported NPs, new AI technologies began to be included at the turn of the twenty-first century with the task of encoding their structures into computer-readable formats (i.e., 1–3D molecular representations, molecular descriptors) and creating chemical space visualization techniques to manage and interpret the numerous nat

PCA, t-SNE, SOM, and most recently, TMAP are dimensionality reduction algorithms that have made it possible to compare NP privileged characteristics (i.e., physicochemical qualities, fragments, similarity scores) with those of synthetic libraries and medications. The creation of machine learning (ML) algorithms in the 2010s—regressions and classifications—to forecast the biological activity or property of natural products (NPs) has propelled candidates into further phases of medication development. It is important to note that because of their notable structural and physicochemical variance with the model training sets (i.e., medicines), many forecasts may unintentionally eliminate numerous bioactive NPs. The application areas, which are the limits of these prediction models, are not systematically determined.

An awareness of the extent and constraints of the available data should be a component of any future advances to predictive machine learning models. Beyond biological activities, de-orphanized NPs have been identified as therapeutically relevant protein partners through the use of prediction algorithms and derivative web servers, broadening the range of uses beyond their native functions. Finally, with the autonomous synthesis of novel drug candidates with reduced structures and biological activity inherited from NPs, deep generative models are rerouting NP-inspired de novo design. Similarly, combining de-orphanizing models with de novo design yields new isofunctional chemotypes (NP mimetics) that occupy previously unexplored and NP-exclusive parts of the chemical space. These tactics are increasing the potency, synthetic accessibility, and drug-likeness resemblance of compounds inspired by NPs.

REFERENCES

Adeniyi, A. A., & Soliman, M. E. (2017). Implementing QM in docking calculations: Is it a waste of computational time? *Drug Discovery Today*, *22*(8), 1216–1223. DOI: 10.1016/j.drudis.2017.06.012 PMID: 28689054

Ahrens, E. K. F. (1988). *Chemical Structures*. Springer Berlin Heidelberg. [Google Scholar]

Aronson, A. R., & Lang, F. M. (2010). An overview of MetaMap: Historical perspective and recent advances. *Journal of the American Medical Informatics Association : JAMIA*, *17*(3), 229–236. DOI: 10.1136/jamia.2009.002733 PMID: 20442139

Arús-Pous, J., Awale, M., Probst, D., & Reymond, J. L. (2019). Exploring chemical space with machine learning. *Chimia*, *73*(12), 1018–1018. DOI: 10.2533/chimia.2019.1018 PMID: 31883554

Atanasov, A. G., Zotchev, S. B., Dirsch, V. M., & Supuran, C. T. (2021). International natural product sciences taskforce. *Nature Reviews. Drug Discovery*, *20*(3), 200–216. DOI: 10.1038/s41573-020-00114-z PMID: 33510482

Atanasov, A. G., Zotchev, S. B., Dirsch, V. M., & Supuran, C. T. (2021). Natural products in drug discovery: Advances and opportunities. *Nature Reviews. Drug Discovery*, *20*(3), 200–216. DOI: 10.1038/s41573-020-00114-z PMID: 33510482

Badal, V. D., Kundrotas, P. J., & Vakser, I. A. (2015). Text mining for protein docking. *PLoS Computational Biology*, *11*(12), e1004630. DOI: 10.1371/journal.pcbi.1004630 PMID: 26650466

Badal, V. D., Kundrotas, P. J., & Vakser, I. A. (2021). Text mining for modeling of protein complexes enhanced by machine learning. *Bioinformatics, 37*(4), 497-505. 69Tsai F. S. *International Journal of Computational Biology and Drug Design*, *2011*(4), 239–244. DOI: 10.1504/IJCBDD.2011.041412

Bajusz, D., Rácz, A., & Héberger, K. (2015). Why is Tanimoto index an appropriate choice for fingerprint-based similarity calculations? *Journal of Cheminformatics*, *7*(1), 1–13. DOI: 10.1186/s13321-015-0069-3 PMID: 26052348

Barnes, E. C., Kumar, R., & Davis, R. A. (2016). The use of isolated natural products as scaffolds for the generation of chemically diverse screening libraries for drug discovery. *Natural Product Reports*, *33*(3), 372–381. DOI: 10.1039/C5NP00121H PMID: 26739749

Berman, F., Fox, G., & Hey, T. (2003). Overview of the book: grid computing–making the global infrastructure a reality. *Grid computing: Making the global infrastructure a reality*, 1-8.

Berry, M., Fielding, B. C., & Gamieldien, J. (2015). Potential broad spectrum inhibitors of the coronavirus 3CLpro: A virtual screening and structure-based drug design study. *Viruses*, *7*(12), 6642–6660. DOI: 10.3390/v7122963 PMID: 26694449

Bisht, N., & Singh, B. K. (2018). Role of computer aided drug design in drug development and drug discovery. *International Journal of Pharmaceutical Sciences and Research*, *9*(4), 1405–1415.

Boadu, A. A., & Asase, A. (2017). Documentation of herbal medicines used for the treatment and management of human diseases by some communities in southern Ghana. *Evidence-Based Complementary and Alternative Medicine : eCAM*, *2017*(1), 3043061. DOI: 10.1155/2017/3043061 PMID: 28684965

Boldi, A. M. (2004). Libraries from natural product-like scaffolds. *Current Opinion in Chemical Biology*, *8*(3), 281–286. DOI: 10.1016/j.cbpa.2004.04.010 PMID: 15183326

Borquaye, L. S., Gasu, E. N., Ampomah, G. B., Kyei, L. K., Amarh, M. A., Mensah, C. N., Nartey, D., Commodore, M., Adomako, A. K., Acheampong, P., Mensah, J. O., Mormor, D. B., & Aboagye, C. I. (2020). Alkaloids from Cryptolepis sanguinolenta as potential inhibitors of SARS-CoV-2 viral proteins: An in silico study. *BioMed Research International*, *2020*(1), 5324560. DOI: 10.1155/2020/5324560 PMID: 33029513

Bouwmeester, R., Martens, L., & Degroeve, S. (2019). Comprehensive and empirical evaluation of machine learning algorithms for small molecule LC retention time prediction. *Analytical Chemistry*, *91*(5), 3694–3703. DOI: 10.1021/acs.analchem.8b05820 PMID: 30702864

Breinbauer, R., Vetter, I. R., & Waldmann, H. (2002). From protein domains to drug candidates—Natural products as guiding principles in the design and synthesis of compound libraries. *Angewandte Chemie International Edition*, *41*(16), 2878–2890. DOI: 10.1002/1521-3773(20020816)41:16<2878::AID-ANIE2878>3.0.CO;2-B PMID: 12203413

Brown, N., Ertl, P., Lewis, R., Luksch, T., Reker, D., & Schneider, N. (2020). Artificial intelligence in chemistry and drug design. *Journal of Computer-Aided Molecular Design*, *34*(7), 709–715. DOI: 10.1007/s10822-020-00317-x PMID: 32468207

Busia, K. (Ed.). (2007). *Ghana herbal pharmacopoeia.* Science and Technology Policy Research Institute, Council for Scientific and Industrial Research.

Carhart, R. E., Smith, D. H., & Venkataraghavan, R. E. N. G. A. C. H. A. R. I. (1985). Atom pairs as molecular features in structure-activity studies: Definition and applications. *Journal of Chemical Information and Computer Sciences, 25*(2), 64–73. DOI: 10.1021/ci00046a002

Chávez-Fumagalli, M. A., Schneider, M. S., Lage, D. P., Tavares, G. D. S. V., Mendonça, D. V. C., Santos, T. T. D. O., Pádua, R. M., Machado-de-Ávila, R. A., Leite, J. P. V., & Coelho, E. A. F. (2018). A computational approach using bioinformatics to screening drug targets for Leishmania infantum species. *Evidence-Based Complementary and Alternative Medicine : eCAM, 2018*(1), 6813467. DOI: 10.1155/2018/6813467 PMID: 29785196

Chen, C. Y. C. (2011). TCM Database@ Taiwan: The world's largest traditional Chinese medicine database for drug screening in silico. *PLoS One, 6*(1), e15939. DOI: 10.1371/journal.pone.0015939 PMID: 21253603

Chen, H., Engkvist, O., Wang, Y., Olivecrona, M., & Blaschke, T. (2018). The rise of deep learning in drug discovery. *Drug Discovery Today, 23*(6), 1241–1250. DOI: 10.1016/j.drudis.2018.01.039 PMID: 29366762

Chen, X., & Reynolds, C. H. (2002). Performance of similarity measures in 2D fragment-based similarity searching: Comparison of structural descriptors and similarity coefficients. *Journal of Chemical Information and Computer Sciences, 42*(6), 1407–1414. DOI: 10.1021/ci025531g PMID: 12444738

Chen, Y., & Kirchmair, J. (2020). Cheminformatics in Natural Product-based Drug Discovery. *Molecular Informatics, 39*(12), e2000171. DOI: 10.1002/minf.202000171 PMID: 32725781

Chen, Y. C. (2015). Beware of docking! *Trends in Pharmacological Sciences, 36*(2), 78–95. DOI: 10.1016/j.tips.2014.12.001 PMID: 25543280

Christie, B. D., Leland, B. A., & Nourse, J. G. (1993). Structure searching in chemical databases by direct lookup methods. *Journal of Chemical Information and Computer Sciences, 33*(4), 545–547. DOI: 10.1021/ci00014a004

Chuang, K. V., Gunsalus, L. M., & Keiser, M. J. (2020). Learning molecular representations for medicinal chemistry: Miniperspective. *Journal of Medicinal Chemistry, 63*(16), 8705–8722. DOI: 10.1021/acs.jmedchem.0c00385 PMID: 32366098

Corley, D. G., & Durley, R. C. (1994). Strategies for database dereplication of natural products. *Journal of Natural Products*, *57*(11), 1484–1490. DOI: 10.1021/np50113a002

Cornejo-Báez, A. A., Peña-Rodríguez, L. M., Álvarez-Zapata, R., Vázquez-Hernández, M., & Sánchez-Medina, A. (2020). Chemometrics: A complementary tool to guide the isolation of pharmacologically active natural products. *Drug Discovery Today*, *25*(1), 27–37. DOI: 10.1016/j.drudis.2019.09.016 PMID: 31600581

Daina, A., Michielin, O., & Zoete, V. (2017). SwissADME: A free web tool to evaluate pharmacokinetics, drug-likeness and medicinal chemistry friendliness of small molecules. *Scientific Reports*, *7*(1), 42717. DOI: 10.1038/srep42717 PMID: 28256516

Danker, T., & Möller, C. (2014). Early identification of hERG liability in drug discovery programs by automated patch clamp. *Frontiers in Pharmacology*, *5*, 203. DOI: 10.3389/fphar.2014.00203 PMID: 25228880

David, B., Wolfender, J. L., & Dias, D. A. (2015). The pharmaceutical industry and natural products: Historical status and new trends. *Phytochemistry Reviews*, *14*(2), 299–315. DOI: 10.1007/s11101-014-9367-z

Davison, E. K., & Brimble, M. A. (2019). Natural product derived privileged scaffolds in drug discovery. *Current Opinion in Chemical Biology*, *52*, 1–8. DOI: 10.1016/j.cbpa.2018.12.007 PMID: 30682725

Dhiman, P., Malik, N., & Khatkar, A. (2018). 3D-QSAR and in-silico studies of natural products and related derivatives as monoamine oxidase inhibitors. *Current Neuropharmacology*, *16*(6), 881–900. DOI: 10.2174/1570159X15666171128143650 PMID: 29189167

Driggers, E. M., Hale, S. P., Lee, J., & Terrett, N. K. (2008). The exploration of macrocycles for drug discovery—An underexploited structural class. *Nature Reviews. Drug Discovery*, *7*(7), 608–624. DOI: 10.1038/nrd2590 PMID: 18591981

Durant, J. L., Leland, B. A., Henry, D. R., & Nourse, J. G. (2002). Reoptimization of MDL keys for use in drug discovery. *Journal of Chemical Information and Computer Sciences*, *42*(6), 1273–1280. DOI: 10.1021/ci010132r PMID: 12444722

Elton, D. C., Boukouvalas, Z., Fuge, M. D., & Chung, P. W. (2019). Deep learning for molecular design—A review of the state of the art. *Molecular Systems Design & Engineering, 4*(4), 828-849.

Mercado, , RRastemo, , TLindelöf, , EKlambauer, , GEngkvist, , OChen, , HBjerrum, , E. J. (2020). Practical notes on building molecular graph generative models. *Applied AI Letters*, *1*(2).

Ernst, P., Siu, A., & Weikum, G. (2015). Knowlife: A versatile approach for constructing a large knowledge graph for biomedical sciences. *BMC Bioinformatics*, *16*(1), 1–13. DOI: 10.1186/s12859-015-0549-5 PMID: 25971816

Gamieldien, J., Fielding, B. C., & Berry, M. (2015). Potential broad spectrum inhibitors of the coronavirus 3clpro: a virtual screening and structure-based drug design study.

Giordanetto, F., & Kihlberg, J. (2014). Macrocyclic drugs and clinical candidates: What can medicinal chemists learn from their properties? *Journal of Medicinal Chemistry*, *57*(2), 278–295. DOI: 10.1021/jm400887j PMID: 24044773

Grigalunas, M., Burhop, A., Christoforow, A., & Waldmann, H. (2020). Pseudo-natural products and natural product-inspired methods in chemical biology and drug discovery. *Current Opinion in Chemical Biology*, *56*, 111–118. DOI: 10.1016/j.cbpa.2019.10.005 PMID: 32362382

Grisoni, F., Consonni, V., & Todeschini, R. (2018). Impact of molecular descriptors on computational models. *Computational chemogenomics*, 171-209.

Harrison, C. (2014). Patenting natural products just got harder. *Nature Biotechnology*, *32*(5), 403–405. DOI: 10.1038/nbt0514-403a PMID: 24811496

Heller, S. R., McNaught, A., Pletnev, I., Stein, S., & Tchekhovskoi, D. (2015). InChI, the IUPAC international chemical identifier. *Journal of Cheminformatics*, *7*(1), 1–34. DOI: 10.1186/s13321-015-0068-4 PMID: 26136848

Hubert, J., Nuzillard, J. M., & Renault, J. H. (2017). Dereplication strategies in natural product research: How many tools and methodologies behind the same concept? *Phytochemistry Reviews*, *16*(1), 55–95. DOI: 10.1007/s11101-015-9448-7

Huigens, R. W.III, Morrison, K. C., Hicklin, R. W., Flood, T. A.Jr, Richter, M. F., & Hergenrother, P. J. (2013). A ring-distortion strategy to construct stereochemically complex and structurally diverse compounds from natural products. *Nature Chemistry*, *5*(3), 195–202. DOI: 10.1038/nchem.1549 PMID: 23422561

Jain, A. N., & Nicholls, A. (2008). Recommendations for evaluation of computational methods. *Journal of Computer-Aided Molecular Design*, *22*(3-4), 133–139. DOI: 10.1007/s10822-008-9196-5 PMID: 18338228

Jiménez-Luna, J., Grisoni, F., Weskamp, N., & Schneider, G. (2021). Artificial intelligence in drug discovery: Recent advances and future perspectives. *Expert Opinion on Drug Discovery*, *16*(9), 949–959. DOI: 10.1080/17460441.2021.1909567 PMID: 33779453

Johnston, C. W., Skinnider, M. A., Wyatt, M. A., Li, X., Ranieri, M. R., Yang, L., Zechel, D. L., Ma, B., & Magarvey, N. A. (2015). An automated Genomes-to-Natural Products platform (GNP) for the discovery of modular natural products. *Nature Communications*, *6*(1), 8421. DOI: 10.1038/ncomms9421 PMID: 26412281

Jordan, M. I., & Mitchell, T. M. (2015). Machine learning: Trends, perspectives, and prospects. *Science*, *349*(6245), 255–260. DOI: 10.1126/science.aaa8415 PMID: 26185243

Karageorgis, G., Foley, D. J., Laraia, L., & Waldmann, H. (2020). Principle and design of pseudo-natural products. *Nature Chemistry*, *12*(3), 227–235. DOI: 10.1038/s41557-019-0411-x PMID: 32015480

Karageorgis, G., Reckzeh, E. S., Ceballos, J., Schwalfenberg, M., Sievers, S., Ostermann, C., Pahl, A., Ziegler, S., & Waldmann, H. (2018). Chromopynones are pseudo natural product glucose uptake inhibitors targeting glucose transporters GLUT-1 and-3. *Nature Chemistry*, *10*(11), 1103–1111. DOI: 10.1038/s41557-018-0132-6 PMID: 30202104

Kim, J. H., Lim, J. W., Lee, S. W., Kim, K., & No, K. T. (2011). Ligand supported homology modeling and docking evaluation of CCR2: Docked pose selection by consensus scoring. *Journal of Molecular Modeling*, *17*(10), 2707–2716. DOI: 10.1007/s00894-010-0943-x PMID: 21213000

Koch, M. A., Schuffenhauer, A., Scheck, M., Wetzel, S., Casaulta, M., Odermatt, A., Ertl, P., & Waldmann, H. (2005). Charting biologically relevant chemical space: A structural classification of natural products (SCONP). *Proceedings of the National Academy of Sciences of the United States of America*, *102*(48), 17272–17277. DOI: 10.1073/pnas.0503647102 PMID: 16301544

Koehn, F. E., & Carter, G. T. (2005). The evolving role of natural products in drug discovery. *Nature Reviews. Drug Discovery*, *4*(3), 206–220. DOI: 10.1038/nrd1657 PMID: 15729362

Kokla, M., Virtanen, J., Kolehmainen, M., Paananen, J., & Hanhineva, K. (2019). Random forest-based imputation outperforms other methods for imputing LC-MS metabolomics data: A comparative study. *BMC Bioinformatics*, *20*(1), 1–11. DOI: 10.1186/s12859-019-3110-0 PMID: 31601178

Krallinger, M., Rabal, O., Lourenco, A., Oyarzabal, J., & Valencia, A. (2017). Information retrieval and text mining technologies for chemistry. *Chemical reviews, 117*(12), 7673-7761. 62

Rajan, K., Zielesny, A., & Steinbeck, C. J. (2020). *Cheminf* 12:65. [PMC free article] [PubMed] [Google Scholar]

Krenn, M., Häse, F., Nigam, A., Friederich, P., & Aspuru-Guzik, A. (2020). Self-referencing embedded strings (SELFIES): A 100% robust molecular string representation. *Machine Learning: Science and Technology, 1*(4), 045024. DOI: 10.1088/2632-2153/aba947

Krizhevsky, A., Sutskever, I., & Hinton, G. E. (2012). Imagenet classification with deep convolutional neural networks. *Advances in neural information processing systems, 25.*

Alom, M. Z., Taha, T. M., Yakopcic, C., Westberg, S., Sidike, P., Nasrin, M. S., ... & Asari, V. K. (2018). *The history began from alexnet: A comprehensive survey on deep learning approaches.* arXiv preprint arXiv:1803.01164.

Lavecchia, A. (2015). Machine-learning approaches in drug discovery: Methods and applications. *Drug Discovery Today, 20*(3), 318–331. DOI: 10.1016/j.drudis.2014.10.012 PMID: 25448759

Liebal, U. W., Phan, A. N., Sudhakar, M., Raman, K., & Blank, L. M. (2020). Machine learning applications for mass spectrometry-based metabolomics. *Metabolites, 10*(6), 243. DOI: 10.3390/metabo10060243 PMID: 32545768

Lipinski, C. A., Lombardo, F., Dominy, B. W., & Feeney, P. J. (1997). Experimental and computational approaches to estimate solubility and permeability in drug discovery and development settings. *Advanced Drug Delivery Reviews, 23*(1-3), 3–25. DOI: 10.1016/S0169-409X(96)00423-1 PMID: 11259830

López-López, E., Bajorath, J., & Medina-Franco, J. L. (2020). Informatics for chemistry, biology, and biomedical sciences. *Journal of Chemical Information and Modeling, 61*(1), 26–35. DOI: 10.1021/acs.jcim.0c01301 PMID: 33382611

Ma, J., Sheridan, R. P., Liaw, A., Dahl, G. E., & Svetnik, V. (2015). Deep neural nets as a method for quantitative structure–activity relationships. *Journal of Chemical Information and Modeling, 55*(2), 263–274. DOI: 10.1021/ci500747n PMID: 25635324

Madhavi Sastry, G., Adzhigirey, M., Day, T., Annabhimoju, R., & Sherman, W. (2013). Protein and ligand preparation: Parameters, protocols, and influence on virtual screening enrichments. *Journal of Computer-Aided Molecular Design*, *27*(3), 221–234. DOI: 10.1007/s10822-013-9644-8 PMID: 23579614

Maniyar, D. M., Nabney, I. T., Williams, B. S., & Sewing, A. (2006). Data visualization during the early stages of drug discovery. *Journal of Chemical Information and Modeling*, *46*(4), 1806–1818. DOI: 10.1021/ci050471a PMID: 16859312

Mater, A. C., & Coote, M. L. (2019). Deep learning in chemistry. *Journal of Chemical Information and Modeling*, *59*(6), 2545–2559. DOI: 10.1021/acs.jcim.9b00266 PMID: 31194543

May, B. H., Zhang, A., Lu, Y., Lu, C., & Xue, C. C. (2014). The systematic assessment of traditional evidence from the premodern Chinese medical literature: A text-mining approach. *Journal of Alternative and Complementary Medicine (New York, N.Y.)*, *20*(12), 937–942. DOI: 10.1089/acm.2013.0372 PMID: 25389563

Mayr, A., Klambauer, G., Unterthiner, T., & Hochreiter, S. (2016). DeepTox: Toxicity prediction using deep learning. *Frontiers in Environmental Science, 3*, 80.57

Andrade, , R. JChalasani, , NBjörnsson, , E. SSuzuki, , AKullak-Ublick, , G. AWatkins, , P. BAithal, , G. P. (2019). Drug-induced liver injury. *Nature Reviews. Disease Primers*, *5*(1), 58.

Medina-Franco, J. L., Naveja, J. J., & López-López, E. (2019). Reaching for the bright StARs in chemical space. *Drug Discovery Today*, *24*(11), 2162–2169. DOI: 10.1016/j.drudis.2019.09.013 PMID: 31557448

Medina-Franco, J. L., & Saldívar-González, F. I. (2020). Cheminformatics to characterize pharmacologically active natural products. *Biomolecules*, *10*(11), 1566. DOI: 10.3390/biom10111566 PMID: 33213003

Merk, D., Grisoni, F., Friedrich, L., & Schneider, G. (2018). Tuning artificial intelligence on the de novo design of natural-product-inspired retinoid X receptor modulators. *Communications Chemistry*, *1*(1), 68. DOI: 10.1038/s42004-018-0068-1

Morris, G. M., Huey, R., & Olson, A. J. (2008). Using autodock for ligand-receptor docking. *Current Protocols in Bioinformatics*, *24*(1), 8–14. DOI: 10.1002/0471250953.bi0814s24 PMID: 19085980

Muratov, E. N., Bajorath, J., Sheridan, R. P., Tetko, I. V., Filimonov, D., Poroikov, V., Oprea, T. I., Baskin, I. I., Varnek, A., Roitberg, A., Isayev, O., Curtalolo, S., Fourches, D., Cohen, Y., Aspuru-Guzik, A., Winkler, D. A., Agrafiotis, D., Cherkasov, A., & Tropsha, A. (2020). QSAR without borders. *Chemical Society Reviews*, *49*(11), 3525–3564. DOI: 10.1039/D0CS00098A PMID: 32356548

Newman, D. J., & Cragg, G. M. (2020). Natural products as sources of new drugs over the nearly four decades from 01/1981 to 09/2019. *Journal of Natural Products*, *83*(3), 770–803. DOI: 10.1021/acs.jnatprod.9b01285 PMID: 32162523

Nugroho, A. E., & Morita, H. (2019). Computationally-assisted discovery and structure elucidation of natural products. *Journal of Natural Medicines*, *73*(4), 687–695. DOI: 10.1007/s11418-019-01321-8 PMID: 31093833

O'Boyle, N., & Dalke, A. (2018). DeepSMILES: an adaptation of SMILES for use in machine-learning of chemical structures.

Osolodkin, D. I., Radchenko, E. V., Orlov, A. A., Voronkov, A. E., Palyulin, V. A., & Zefirov, N. S. (2015). Progress in visual representations of chemical space. *Expert Opinion on Drug Discovery*, *10*(9), 959–973. DOI: 10.1517/17460441.2015.1060216 PMID: 26094796

Öztürk, H., Özgür, A., Schwaller, P., Laino, T., & Ozkirimli, E. (2020). Exploring chemical space using natural language processing methodologies for drug discovery. *Drug Discovery Today*, *25*(4), 689–705. DOI: 10.1016/j.drudis.2020.01.020 PMID: 32027969

Paolini, G. V., Shapland, R. H., van Hoorn, W. P., Mason, J. S., & Hopkins, A. L. (2006). Global mapping of pharmacological space. *Nature Biotechnology*, *24*(7), 805–815. DOI: 10.1038/nbt1228 PMID: 16841068

Papanikolaou, N., Pavlopoulos, G. A., Theodosiou, T., & Iliopoulos, I. (2015). Protein–protein interaction predictions using text mining methods. *Methods (San Diego, Calif.)*, *74*, 47–53. DOI: 10.1016/j.ymeth.2014.10.026 PMID: 25448298

Pereira, F., & Aires-de-Sousa, J. (2018). Computational methodologies in the exploration of marine natural product leads. *Marine Drugs*, *16*(7), 236. DOI: 10.3390/md16070236 PMID: 30011882

Porras, G., Chassagne, F., Lyles, J. T., Marquez, L., Dettweiler, M., Salam, A. M., Samarakoon, T., Shabih, S., Farrokhi, D. R., & Quave, C. L. (2020). Ethnobotany and the role of plant natural products in antibiotic drug discovery. *Chemical Reviews*, *121*(6), 3495–3560. DOI: 10.1021/acs.chemrev.0c00922 PMID: 33164487

Rafferty, R. J., Hicklin, R. W., Maloof, K. A., & Hergenrother, P. J. (2014). Synthesis of complex and diverse compounds through ring distortion of abietic acid. *Angewandte Chemie*, *126*(1), 224–228. DOI: 10.1002/ange.201308743 PMID: 24273016

Rawat, W., & Wang, Z. (2017). Deep convolutional neural networks for image classification: A comprehensive review. *Neural Computation*, *29*(9), 2352–2449. DOI: 10.1162/neco_a_00990 PMID: 28599112

Rebholz-Schuhmann, D., Oellrich, A., & Hoehndorf, R. (2012). Text-mining solutions for biomedical research: Enabling integrative biology. *Nature Reviews. Genetics*, *13*(12), 829–839. DOI: 10.1038/nrg3337 PMID: 23150036

Renner, S., Van Otterlo, W. A., Dominguez Seoane, M., Möcklinghoff, S., Hofmann, B., Wetzel, S., Schuffenhauer, A., Ertl, P., Oprea, T. I., Steinhilber, D., Brunsveld, L., Rauh, D., & Waldmann, H. (2009). Bioactivity-guided mapping and navigation of chemical space. *Nature Chemical Biology*, *5*(8), 585–592. DOI: 10.1038/nchembio.188 PMID: 19561619

Reutlinger, M., & Schneider, G. (2012). Nonlinear dimensionality reduction and mapping of compound libraries for drug discovery. *Journal of Molecular Graphics & Modelling*, *34*, 108–117. DOI: 10.1016/j.jmgm.2011.12.006 PMID: 22326864

Risum, A. B., & Bro, R. (2019). Using deep learning to evaluate peaks in chromatographic data. *Talanta*, *204*, 255–260. DOI: 10.1016/j.talanta.2019.05.053 PMID: 31357290

Rodrigues, T. (2017). Harnessing the potential of natural products in drug discovery from a cheminformatics vantage point. *Organic & Biomolecular Chemistry*, *15*(44), 9275–9282. DOI: 10.1039/C7OB02193C PMID: 29085945

Rodrigues, T., Reker, D., Schneider, P., & Schneider, G. (2016). Counting on natural products for drug design. *Nature Chemistry*, *8*(6), 531–541. DOI: 10.1038/nchem.2479 PMID: 27219696

Rogers, D., & Hahn, M. (2010). Extended-connectivity fingerprints. *Journal of Chemical Information and Modeling*, *50*(5), 742–754. DOI: 10.1021/ci100050t PMID: 20426451

Romano, J. D., & Tatonetti, N. P. (2019). Informatics and computational methods in natural product drug discovery: A review and perspectives. *Frontiers in Genetics*, *10*, 368. DOI: 10.3389/fgene.2019.00368 PMID: 31114606

Rosén, J., Gottfries, J., Muresan, S., Backlund, A., & Oprea, T. I. (2009). Novel chemical space exploration via natural products. *Journal of Medicinal Chemistry*, *52*(7), 1953–1962. DOI: 10.1021/jm801514w PMID: 19265440

Rutz, A., Sorokina, M., Galgonek, J., Mietchen, D., Willighagen, E., Gaudry, A., . . . Allard, P. M. (2021). The LOTUS initiative for open natural products research: knowledge management through Wikidata. BioRxiv, 2021-02.

Saldívar-González, F. I., Aldas-Bulos, V. D., Medina-Franco, J. L., & Plisson, F. (2022). Natural product drug discovery in the artificial intelligence era. *Chemical Science (Cambridge)*, *13*(6), 1526–1546. DOI: 10.1039/D1SC04471K PMID: 35282622

Saldívar-González, F. I., Pilón-Jiménez, B. A., & Medina-Franco, J. L. (2019). Chemical space of naturally occurring compounds. *Physical Sciences Reviews*, *4*(5), 20180103.

Sanchez-Lengeling, B., Wei, J. N., Lee, B. K., Gerkin, R. C., Aspuru-Guzik, A., & Wiltschko, A. B. (2019). Machine learning for scent: Learning generalizable perceptual representations of small molecules. *arXiv preprint arXiv:1910.10685.*

Schäfer, T., Kriege, N., Humbeck, L., Klein, K., Koch, O., & Mutzel, P. (2017). Scaffold Hunter: A comprehensive visual analytics framework for drug discovery. *Journal of Cheminformatics*, *9*(1), 28. DOI: 10.1186/s13321-017-0213-3 PMID: 29086162

Schneider, G. (2018). Automating drug discovery. *Nature Reviews. Drug Discovery*, *17*(2), 97–113. DOI: 10.1038/nrd.2017.232 PMID: 29242609

Schneider, P., Walters, W. P., Plowright, A. T., Sieroka, N., Listgarten, J., Goodnow, R. A.Jr, Fisher, J., Jansen, J. M., Duca, J. S., Rush, T. S., Zentgraf, M., Hill, J. E., Krutoholow, E., Kohler, M., Blaney, J., Funatsu, K., Luebkemann, C., & Schneider, G. (2020). Rethinking drug design in the artificial intelligence era. *Nature Reviews. Drug Discovery*, *19*(5), 353–364. DOI: 10.1038/s41573-019-0050-3 PMID: 31801986

Schreiber, S. L. (2000). Target-oriented and diversity-oriented organic synthesis in drug discovery. *Science*, *287*(5460), 1964–1969. DOI: 10.1126/science.287.5460.1964 PMID: 10720315

Sharma, V., Law, W., Balick, M. J., & Sarkar, I. N. (2018, April). Harnessing biomedical natural language processing tools to identify medicinal plant knowledge from historical texts. *AMIA ... Annual Symposium Proceedings - AMIA Symposium. AMIA Symposium*, *2017*, 1537. PMID: 29854223

Shergis, J. L., Wu, L., May, B. H., Zhang, A. L., Guo, X., Lu, C., & Xue, C. C. (2015). Natural products for chronic cough: Text mining the East Asian historical literature for future therapeutics. *Chronic Respiratory Disease*, *12*(3), 204–211. DOI: 10.1177/1479972315583043 PMID: 25901012

Sorokina, M., Merseburger, P., Rajan, K., Yirik, M. A., & Steinbeck, C. (2021). COCONUT online: Collection of open natural products database. *Journal of Cheminformatics*, *13*(1), 2. DOI: 10.1186/s13321-020-00478-9 PMID: 33423696

Stokes, J. M., Yang, K., Swanson, K., Jin, W., Cubillos-Ruiz, A., Donghia, N. M., MacNair, C. R., French, S., Carfrae, L. A., Bloom-Ackermann, Z., Tran, V. M., Chiappino-Pepe, A., Badran, A. H., Andrews, I. W., Chory, E. J., Church, G. M., Brown, E. D., Jaakkola, T. S., Barzilay, R., & Collins, J. J. (2020). A deep learning approach to antibiotic discovery. *Cell*, *180*(4), 688–702. DOI: 10.1016/j.cell.2020.01.021 PMID: 32084340

Strohl, W. R. (2000). The role of natural products in a modern drug discovery program. *Drug Discovery Today*, *5*(2), 39–41. DOI: 10.1016/S1359-6446(99)01443-9 PMID: 10652450

Sun, M., Zhao, S., Gilvary, C., Elemento, O., Zhou, J., & Wang, F. (2020). Graph convolutional networks for computational drug development and discovery. *Briefings in Bioinformatics*, *21*(3), 919–935. DOI: 10.1093/bib/bbz042 PMID: 31155636

Sydow, D., Burggraaff, L., Szengel, A., van Vlijmen, H. W., IJzerman, A. P., van Westen, G. J., & Volkamer, A. (2019). Advances and challenges in computational target prediction. *Journal of Chemical Information and Modeling*, *59*(5), 1728–1742. DOI: 10.1021/acs.jcim.8b00832 PMID: 30817146

Tan, D. S. (2005). Diversity-oriented synthesis: Exploring the intersections between chemistry and biology. *Nature Chemical Biology*, *1*(2), 74–84. DOI: 10.1038/nchembio0705-74 PMID: 16408003

Todeschini, R., Consonni, V., Xiang, H., Holliday, J., Buscema, M., & Willett, P. (2012). Similarity coefficients for binary chemoinformatics data: Overview and extended comparison using simulated and real data sets. *Journal of Chemical Information and Modeling*, *52*(11), 2884–2901. DOI: 10.1021/ci300261r PMID: 23078167

Truchon, J. F., & Bayly, C. I. (2007). Evaluating virtual screening methods: Good and bad metrics for the "early recognition" problem. *Journal of Chemical Information and Modeling*, *47*(2), 488–508. DOI: 10.1021/ci600426e PMID: 17288412

Tshitoyan, V., Dagdelen, J., Weston, L., Dunn, A., Rong, Z., Kononova, O., Persson, K. A., Ceder, G., & Jain, A. (2019). Unsupervised word embeddings capture latent knowledge from materials science literature. *Nature*, *571*(7763), 95–98. DOI: 10.1038/s41586-019-1335-8 PMID: 31270483

Vamathevan, J., Clark, D., Czodrowski, P., Dunham, I., Ferran, E., Lee, G., Li, B., Madabhushi, A., Shah, P., Spitzer, M., & Zhao, S. (2019). Applications of machine learning in drug discovery and development. *Nature Reviews. Drug Discovery*, *18*(6), 463–477. DOI: 10.1038/s41573-019-0024-5 PMID: 30976107

Walters, W. P., & Murcko, M. (2020). Assessing the impact of generative AI on medicinal chemistry. *Nature Biotechnology*, *38*(2), 143–145. DOI: 10.1038/s41587-020-0418-2 PMID: 32001834

Weininger, D. (1988). SMILES, a chemical language and information system. 1. Introduction to methodology and encoding rules. *Journal of Chemical Information and Computer Sciences*, *28*(1), 31–36. DOI: 10.1021/ci00057a005

Wells, T. N. (2011). Natural products as starting points for future anti-malarial therapies: Going back to our roots? *Malaria Journal*, *10*(S1), 1–12. DOI: 10.1186/1475-2875-10-S1-S3 PMID: 21411014

Wender, P. A., Quiroz, R. V., & Stevens, M. C. (2015). Function through synthesis-informed design. *Accounts of Chemical Research*, *48*(3), 752–760. DOI: 10.1021/acs.accounts.5b00004 PMID: 25742599

Wender, P. A., Verma, V. A., Paxton, T. J., & Pillow, T. H. (2008). Function-oriented synthesis, step economy, and drug design. *Accounts of Chemical Research*, *41*(1), 40–49. DOI: 10.1021/ar700155p PMID: 18159936

Wetzel, S., Klein, K., Renner, S., Rauh, D., Oprea, T. I., Mutzel, P., & Waldmann, H. (2009). Interactive exploration of chemical space with Scaffold Hunter. *Nature Chemical Biology*, *5*(8), 581–583. DOI: 10.1038/nchembio.187 PMID: 19561620

Witting, M., & Böcker, S. (2020). Current status of retention time prediction in metabolite identification. *Journal of Separation Science*, *43*(9-10), 1746–1754. DOI: 10.1002/jssc.202000060 PMID: 32144942

Wolfender, J. L., Litaudon, M., Touboul, D., & Queiroz, E. F. (2019). Innovative omics-based approaches for prioritisation and targeted isolation of natural products–new strategies for drug discovery. *Natural Product Reports*, *36*(6), 855–868. DOI: 10.1039/C9NP00004F PMID: 31073562

Wolfer, A. M., Lozano, S., Umbdenstock, T., Croixmarie, V., Arrault, A., & Vayer, P. (2016). UPLC–MS retention time prediction: A machine learning approach to metabolite identification in untargeted profiling. *Metabolomics*, *12*(1), 8. DOI: 10.1007/s11306-015-0888-2

Xia, X., May, B. H., Zhang, A. L., Guo, X., Lu, C., Xue, C. C., & Huang, Q. (2020). Chinese Herbal Medicines for Rheumatoid Arthritis: Text-Mining the Classical Literature for Potentially Effective Natural Products. *Evidence-Based Complementary and Alternative Medicine : eCAM, 2020*(1), 7531967. DOI: 10.1155/2020/7531967 PMID: 32419824

Yi, S., Varun, B. V., Choi, Y., & Park, S. B. (2018). A brief overview of two major strategies in diversity-oriented synthesis: Build/couple/pair and ring-distortion. *Frontiers in Chemistry*, *6*, 507. DOI: 10.3389/fchem.2018.00507 PMID: 30406085

Zhavoronkov, A., Ivanenkov, Y. A., Aliper, A., Veselov, M. S., Aladinskiy, V. A., Aladinskaya, A. V., Terentiev, V. A., Polykovskiy, D. A., Kuznetsov, M. D., Asadulaev, A., Volkov, Y., Zholus, A., Shayakhmetov, R. R., Zhebrak, A., Minaeva, L. I., Zagribelnyy, B. A., Lee, L. H., Soll, R., Madge, D., & Aspuru-Guzik, A. (2019). Deep learning enables rapid identification of potent DDR1 kinase inhibitors. *Nature Biotechnology*, *37*(9), 1038–1040. DOI: 10.1038/s41587-019-0224-x PMID: 31477924

Zhou, X., Peng, Y., & Liu, B. (2010). Text mining for traditional Chinese medical knowledge discovery: A survey. *Journal of Biomedical Informatics*, *43*(4), 650–660. DOI: 10.1016/j.jbi.2010.01.002 PMID: 20074663

Chapter 12
From Concept to Reality: Implementing Blockchain Solutions in Pharmaceutical Supply Chains

G. Sowmya
https://orcid.org/0000-0002-9275-7726
MLR Institute of Technology, India

R. Sridevi
Jawaharlal Nehru Technological University, India

K. S. Sadasiva Rao
Sri Indu Institute of Technology, India

ABSTRACT

The pharmaceutical supply chain is fraught with challenges, including counterfeit drugs, lack of transparency, and stringent regulatory compliance. Blockchain technology offers a transformative solution to these issues through its decentralized, immutable, and transparent nature. This chapter explores the implementation of blockchain in pharmaceutical supply chains, detailing the technology's fundamentals, types, and the specific challenges it addresses within the industry. Case studies illustrate successful blockchain applications, highlighting enhanced traceability, reduced counterfeiting, and improved regulatory compliance. Furthermore, the chapter discusses the practical aspects of blockchain implementation, including feasibility studies, stakeholder involvement, technical integration, and data privacy concerns. Finally, it delves into future prospects, emphasizing the integration of emerging technologies like IoT and AI, and predicting trends that will shape the future of blockchain in the pharmaceutical industry.

DOI: 10.4018/979-8-3693-6270-9.ch012

1. INTRODUCTION

Pharmaceutical supply chains are intricate networks involving multiple stakeholders, including raw material suppliers, manufacturers, wholesalers, distributors, pharmacies, and healthcare providers. The journey of a pharmaceutical product from the manufacturing facility to the patient encompasses several critical stages, such as production, quality control, packaging, transportation, and storage. Ensuring safety, efficacy, and timely delivery of medications is paramount in this highly regulated industry, (Gruchmann, Elgazzar, & Ali, 2023).

The complexity of pharmaceutical supply chains arises from various factors:

a. Diverse Raw Materials: Pharmaceuticals often require a wide range of raw materials sourced from different parts of the world.
b. Stringent Regulatory Requirements: Compliance with regulatory standards, such as Good Manufacturing Practices (GMP) and Good Distribution Practices (GDP), is mandatory to ensure product safety and quality.
c. Temperature Sensitivity: Many pharmaceuticals, particularly biologics and vaccines, require specific temperature conditions throughout the supply chain.
d. Global Distribution: Pharmaceuticals are distributed globally, making the supply chain susceptible to geopolitical and logistical challenges.
e. Counterfeit Risk: The prevalence of counterfeit drugs poses significant risks to patient safety and brand integrity, (Abdullah & Nizamuddin, 2023).

1.1 Introduction to Blockchain Technology

Blockchain technology, initially conceptualized as the underlying framework for cryptocurrencies like Bitcoin, is a decentralized digital ledger system that securely records transactions across multiple computers. Key features of blockchain include:

a. Decentralization: Unlike traditional centralized databases, blockchain operates on a peer-to-peer network where each participant maintains a copy of the entire ledger.
b. Immutability: Once recorded, transactions on a blockchain cannot be altered or deleted, ensuring data integrity, (Estrada *et al.,* 2024).
c. Transparency: All transactions are visible to participants with access rights, promoting accountability and traceability.
d. Consensus Mechanisms: Blockchain employs various consensus algorithms (e.g., Proof of Work, Proof of Stake) to validate transactions and maintain the integrity of the ledger.

Blockchain's unique attributes offer promising solutions to many of the challenges faced by modern supply chains, particularly in industries like pharmaceuticals where security, transparency, and traceability are crucial, (Moosivand, Ghatari, & Rasekh, 2019).

1.2 Importance of the Topic

1.2.1 Challenges in Current Pharmaceutical Supply Chains

Pharmaceutical supply chains face several critical challenges that can compromise the delivery of safe and effective medications to patients:

a. Counterfeit Drugs: The infiltration of counterfeit drugs into the supply chain is a major concern. These fake products can be ineffective or harmful, posing severe risks to patient health and undermining public trust, (Moosivand, Ghatari, & Rasekh, 2019).
b. Lack of Transparency and Traceability: Traditional supply chain systems often suffer from fragmented and siloed data, making it difficult to trace the origin and journey of pharmaceutical products. This opacity can lead to inefficiencies, errors, and delays.
c. Regulatory Compliance: Meeting regulatory requirements across different regions is complex and costly. Non-compliance can result in legal penalties and market withdrawal.
d. Supply Chain Inefficiencies: Inefficiencies such as delayed shipments, inventory mismanagement, and logistical bottlenecks can disrupt the timely delivery of medications, impacting patient care, (Nguyen *et al.,* 2021).

1.2.2 Potential Benefits of Blockchain Technology

Implementing blockchain technology in pharmaceutical supply chains can address many of these challenges and offer several significant benefits:

a. Enhanced Security and Counterfeit Prevention: Blockchain's immutable ledger can help verify the authenticity of drugs at each stage of the supply chain, reducing the risk of counterfeit products reaching patients.
b. Improved Transparency and Traceability: Blockchain enables end-to-end visibility of the supply chain, allowing stakeholders to trace the movement and handling of products in real-time. This transparency ensures accountability and can quickly identify and resolve issues, (Habib *et al.,* 2022).

c. Streamlined Regulatory Compliance: Automated, tamper-proof records on the blockchain can simplify compliance with regulatory standards, making audits more efficient and reducing the risk of non-compliance.
d. Operational Efficiency: By providing a single source of truth, blockchain can eliminate data silos, reduce paperwork, and streamline processes such as recalls and inventory management, leading to more efficient and responsive supply chain operations.

As the pharmaceutical industry continues to evolve, embracing innovative technologies like blockchain can transform supply chain management, enhance patient safety, and drive overall industry growth. This chapter will explore the journey from conceptualizing blockchain applications to their practical implementation in pharmaceutical supply chains, providing insights and real-world examples of this transformative technology in action.

2. UNDERSTANDING BLOCKCHAIN TECHNOLOGY

2.1 Fundamentals of Blockchain

2.1.1 Definition and Key Characteristics

Blockchain is a decentralized digital ledger technology that records transactions across multiple computers in such a way that the registered transactions cannot be altered retroactively. This technology was initially designed for digital currencies like Bitcoin but has since evolved to serve a variety of applications across different industries.

a. **Decentralization**: Unlike traditional centralized systems where a single entity controls the database, blockchain operates on a peer-to-peer network. Every participant (node) in the network has access to the entire ledger, ensuring that no single point of failure or control exists. This decentralization enhances security and reduces the risk of data manipulation.
b. **Immutability:** Once data is recorded on the blockchain, it is nearly impossible to alter or delete. Each block contains a cryptographic hash of the previous block, a timestamp, and transaction data. This chaining of blocks ensures that any attempt to alter a block would require changes to all subsequent blocks, which is computationally infeasible, (Vadapalli, 2020).

c. **Transparency**: Blockchain transactions are transparent to all participants in the network. While the details of the transactions are encrypted, the metadata (such as transaction timestamps and involved parties) is visible, promoting accountability and trust among users.

2.1.2 How Blockchain Works: Blocks, Chains, and Consensus Mechanisms

a. **Blocks:** A block in the blockchain contains a list of transactions. Each block has a unique identifier known as a hash and contains the hash of the previous block, linking them together in a chain. This structure ensures the chronological order of transactions and the integrity of the entire chain.
b. **Chains:** The chain is formed by linking blocks through their hashes. The blockchain grows as new blocks are added to it. The linkage through hashes makes the chain secure and tamper-evident, (Zhou *et al.,* 2023).
c. **Consensus Mechanisms**: To ensure that all participants agree on the validity of transactions, blockchain uses consensus mechanisms. The most common consensus algorithms include:
d. **Proof of Work (PoW):** Nodes (miners) compete to solve complex mathematical problems. The first to solve the problem gets to add the next block to the chain and is rewarded. This method is secure but energy-intensive.
e. **Proof of Stake (PoS):** Participants (validators) lock up a certain amount of cryptocurrency as a stake. Validators are chosen to add new blocks based on their stake and other factors, making this method more energy-efficient than PoW.
f. **Practical Byzantine Fault Tolerance (PBFT):** Designed for private blockchains, PBFT allows nodes to reach consensus through a majority vote, making it efficient and suitable for environments where participants are known and trusted.

2.2 Types of Blockchain

2.2.1 Public vs. Private Blockchains

a. **Public Blockchains**: These are open to anyone who wishes to participate. Examples include Bitcoin and Ethereum. Public blockchains are fully decentralized and rely on consensus mechanisms like PoW or PoS to validate transactions. They offer high transparency and security but can suffer from scalability issues and high energy consumption, (Sharma, Jindal, & Borah, 2022).

b. **Private Blockchains**: These are restricted networks where only authorized participants can join. They are often used by businesses and organizations that require privacy and control over their data. Private blockchains can operate more efficiently as they typically use consensus mechanisms like PBFT, which are faster and less resource-intensive.

2.2.2 Permissioned vs. Permissionless Blockchains

a. **Permissioned Blockchains**: These blockchains restrict who can participate in the network and what transactions they can perform. They are used in scenarios where trust among participants is established, such as in enterprise settings. Permissioned blockchains can achieve higher performance and compliance with regulatory requirements, (Solat & Naït-Abdesselam, 2020).
b. **Permissionless Blockchains**: Anyone can join and participate in a permissionless blockchain network without any restrictions. They are inherently decentralized and democratic, making them suitable for applications where openness and censorship resistance are critical.

Understanding these fundamental aspects of blockchain technology is crucial for appreciating its potential applications and benefits in various industries, including the pharmaceutical supply chain. By leveraging the unique characteristics of blockchain, businesses can enhance transparency, security, and efficiency in their operations.

3. CHALLENGES IN PHARMACEUTICAL SUPPLY CHAINS

3.1 Counterfeit Drugs

3.1.1 Statistics and Impact on Health and Economy

Counterfeit drugs are a significant and growing threat to global health and economies. According to the World Health Organization (WHO), approximately 10% of medicines in low- and middle-income countries are counterfeit or substandard. This figure can be higher in certain regions, particularly in areas with less stringent regulatory oversight.

The impact of counterfeit drugs is profound:

a. **Health Risks**: Counterfeit drugs often contain incorrect dosages, harmful substances, or no active ingredients at all. This can lead to treatment failure, adverse reactions, and in severe cases, death, (Ziavrou, Noguera, & Boumba, 2022).
b. **Economic Costs**: The global market for counterfeit drugs is estimated to be worth $200 billion annually. This not only represents lost revenue for legitimate pharmaceutical companies but also increased costs for healthcare systems dealing with the consequences of counterfeit medications.
c. **Public Trust:** The presence of counterfeit drugs undermines public trust in healthcare systems and pharmaceutical brands, potentially leading to hesitancy in medication adherence and vaccination uptake.

3.1.2 Current Methods of Addressing Counterfeits

To combat counterfeit drugs, various strategies are currently employed:

a. **Regulatory Measures**: Governments and regulatory bodies have implemented stringent laws and regulations to control the production and distribution of pharmaceuticals. Agencies like the U.S. Food and Drug Administration (FDA) and the European Medicines Agency (EMA) enforce strict guidelines.
b. **Serialization and Barcoding**: Pharmaceuticals are often serialized, with unique identifiers assigned to each product unit. Barcoding allows for scanning and tracking at different points in the supply chain, (Butticè *et al.,* 2020).
c. **Anti-Counterfeiting Technologies**: Advanced technologies such as holograms, RFID tags, and tamper-evident packaging are used to secure pharmaceutical products.
d. **Public Awareness Campaigns**: Educating consumers about the dangers of counterfeit drugs and how to identify legitimate medications is also a crucial preventive measure.

3.2 Lack of Transparency and Traceability

3.2.1 Issues With Current Tracking Systems

The pharmaceutical supply chain is notoriously complex, with products often passing through multiple hands before reaching the end consumer. Current tracking systems face several issues:

a. **Data Fragmentation**: Information is often siloed across different stakeholders, making it difficult to maintain a cohesive view of the supply chain.

b. **Manual Processes**: Reliance on manual entry and paper-based documentation can lead to errors, delays, and data manipulation, (Assiri *et al.,* 2020).
c. **Limited Visibility**: Many existing systems do not provide real-time visibility, making it challenging to trace the journey of a product promptly and accurately.

3.2.2 Examples of Traceability Challenges

Several scenarios illustrate the traceability challenges in pharmaceutical supply chains:

a. **Product Recalls**: When a defective or contaminated batch of drugs needs to be recalled, lack of traceability can delay the process, risking patient safety and increasing costs.
b. **Cold Chain Management**: For temperature-sensitive products like vaccines, maintaining the required conditions throughout the supply chain is critical. Inadequate tracking can lead to compromised product efficacy and safety.
c. **Cross-Border Shipments**: International shipments involve multiple regulatory environments and logistical handovers, complicating traceability efforts.

3.3 Regulatory Compliance

3.3.1 Overview of Regulatory Requirements

Regulatory bodies across the world enforce stringent guidelines to ensure the safety, efficacy, and quality of pharmaceuticals:

a. **FDA (U.S.):** The FDA mandates compliance with Good Manufacturing Practices (GMP) and Good Distribution Practices (GDP), along with serialization requirements under the Drug Supply Chain Security Act (DSCSA).
b. **EMA (European Union):** The EMA requires adherence to similar GMP and GDP standards and mandates the implementation of the Falsified Medicines Directive (FMD) for serialization and verification, (Klessascheck, Knoche, & Pufahl, 2024).
c. **WHO (Global):** The WHO provides international guidelines and supports initiatives to strengthen regulatory systems in low- and middle-income countries.

3.3.2 Compliance Challenges and Costs

Meeting these regulatory requirements presents several challenges:

a. **Complexity**: The regulatory landscape is continually evolving, requiring companies to stay updated and adapt quickly.
b. **Costs:** Implementing and maintaining compliance systems can be costly, involving investments in technology, training, and process reengineering.
c. **Global Variability**: Different regions have varying regulations, making it difficult for multinational companies to achieve uniform compliance, (Haelterman, 2022).
d. **Documentation and Reporting**: Comprehensive documentation and regular reporting are mandatory, necessitating robust data management systems.

By addressing these challenges with innovative solutions such as blockchain, the pharmaceutical industry can enhance the integrity, transparency, and efficiency of its supply chains, ultimately improving patient safety and trust.

4. BLOCKCHAIN SOLUTIONS FOR PHARMACEUTICAL SUPPLY CHAINS

4.1 Enhanced Traceability and Transparency

4.1.1 How Blockchain Improves Product Tracking

Blockchain technology significantly enhances the traceability and transparency of pharmaceutical supply chains through several mechanisms:

a. **Immutable Ledger**: Every transaction and movement of pharmaceutical products is recorded on a blockchain. This ledger is immutable, meaning it cannot be altered or deleted once recorded, ensuring data integrity.
b. **Real-Time Visibility**: Blockchain provides real-time access to product data for all authorized stakeholders. This transparency allows for immediate tracking of a product's journey from manufacturer to consumer, (Ghadge *et al.,* 2023).
c. **End-to-End Traceability**: Blockchain can trace the entire lifecycle of a product, including raw material sourcing, manufacturing, distribution, and retail. Each step is documented, providing a comprehensive history.
d. **Smart Contracts**: These are self-executing contracts with the terms of the agreement directly written into code. Smart contracts automate and enforce the execution of transactions, reducing delays and human error, (Abdullah & Nizamuddin, 2023).

Figure 1. Blockchain solutions for pharmaceutical supply chains

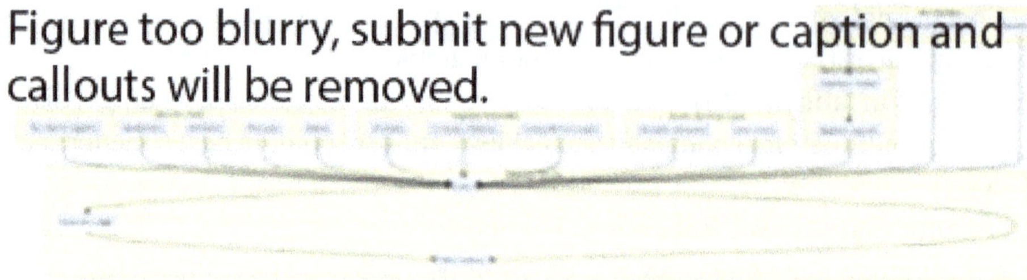

4.1.2 Case Studies and Examples

a. **MediLedger Project**: This blockchain-based network brings together major pharmaceutical companies to enhance drug traceability and compliance with the Drug Supply Chain Security Act (DSCSA). It enables secure and interoperable data sharing, ensuring that drugs can be tracked through their entire journey.
b. **IBM and Merck**: In collaboration with the FDA, IBM and Merck have piloted a blockchain project to track vaccines and medications. The project aims to improve the visibility and integrity of the pharmaceutical supply chain, demonstrating blockchain's potential to enhance traceability.

Chronicled: Chronicled uses blockchain to provide secure and verifiable product information. Their solutions help pharmaceutical companies and regulators to trace the provenance of drugs, ensuring authenticity and safety, (Zakari *et al.,* 2022).

4.2 Combating Counterfeit Drugs

4.2.1 Blockchain-Enabled Anti-Counterfeiting Measures

Blockchain can combat counterfeit drugs through several innovative measures:

a. **Unique Digital Identities**: Each pharmaceutical product can be assigned a unique digital identity on the blockchain. This ID is recorded and updated with every transaction, making it easy to verify authenticity.

b. **Tamper-Evident Features:** Products can be equipped with blockchain-enabled tags or QR codes that consumers and stakeholders can scan to verify the product's history and legitimacy, (Yiu, 2021a).
c. **Secure Data Sharing:** Blockchain facilitates secure data sharing between manufacturers, distributors, and regulators, ensuring that only verified products are circulated in the market.

4.2.2 Real-World Applications and Success Stories

a. **GSK and VeChain**: GlaxoSmithKline (GSK) partnered with VeChain to use blockchain for verifying the authenticity of its products. By scanning QR codes, customers can access detailed information about the product's origin and supply chain journey, ensuring it is genuine.
b. **Walgreens and IBM**: Walgreens has collaborated with IBM to implement a blockchain solution that tracks the movement of pharmaceuticals through the supply chain. This initiative helps in identifying and removing counterfeit drugs, protecting consumers and maintaining trust.

4.3 Improving Regulatory Compliance

4.3.1 Blockchain's Role in Meeting Regulatory Requirements

Blockchain technology can streamline compliance with regulatory requirements by:

a. **Automated Record-Keeping:** Blockchain automates the recording of transactions and processes, ensuring accurate and timely documentation for regulatory audits.
b. **Data Integrity and Security**: The immutable nature of blockchain records ensures data integrity, which is crucial for compliance with regulations like the DSCSA and the Falsified Medicines Directive (FMD), (Yiu, 2021b).
c. **Audit Trails**: Blockchain provides a clear and verifiable audit trail of all transactions and product movements, simplifying the process of demonstrating compliance to regulators.

4.3.2 Examples of Blockchain-Based Compliance Solutions

a. **Modum**: This company offers a blockchain-based solution that monitors and records the conditions (such as temperature and humidity) of pharmaceutical shipments. This ensures that products comply with Good Distribution Practices (GDP) and regulatory requirements throughout their journey.
b. **Provenance**: Provenance uses blockchain to create a transparent and tamper-proof record of a product's supply chain. Their platform helps pharmaceutical companies comply with regulatory standards by providing detailed and verifiable product histories, (Zhang *et al.*, 2019).
c. **Farmatrust**: This blockchain-based platform ensures compliance with global pharmaceutical regulations by tracking drugs from production to patient delivery. It provides real-time data to regulators and supply chain participants, ensuring transparency and accountability.

By leveraging blockchain technology, the pharmaceutical industry can overcome significant challenges in traceability, anti-counterfeiting, and regulatory compliance. These solutions not only enhance the efficiency and security of supply chains but also ensure that patients receive safe and authentic medications.

5. IMPLEMENTING BLOCKCHAIN: FROM CONCEPT TO REALITY

5.1 Feasibility Studies and Pilot Projects

5.1.1 Importance of Initial Studies and Pilots

Feasibility studies and pilot projects are critical steps in implementing blockchain solutions in pharmaceutical supply chains. These initial phases help in:

a. **Assessing Viability**: Determining whether blockchain can effectively address specific challenges within the supply chain.
b. **Identifying Challenges**: Highlighting potential technical, operational, and regulatory hurdles.
c. **Resource Allocation**: Understanding the financial and human resources required for full-scale implementation.
d. **Proof of Concept**: Demonstrating the potential benefits and practicalities of blockchain applications in real-world settings, (Zhang *et al.*, 2019).

5.1.2 Examples of Successful Pilot Projects in the Pharmaceutical Industry

a. **Pfizer and Chronicled**: Pfizer partnered with Chronicled to pilot a blockchain solution for drug traceability. The project demonstrated improved transparency and efficiency in tracking drug shipments.
b. **Merck and IBM**: In a pilot project with the FDA, Merck and IBM used blockchain to track vaccines and medication. The project highlighted blockchain's capability to enhance supply chain integrity and regulatory compliance.
c. **Boehringer Ingelheim and IBM**: Boehringer Ingelheim conducted a pilot with IBM to use blockchain for tracking clinical trials, ensuring data integrity and improving the transparency of trial results.

5.2 Stakeholder Involvement

5.2.1 Identifying and Engaging Key Stakeholders

Successful blockchain implementation requires the involvement of all key stakeholders in the pharmaceutical supply chain:

a. **Manufacturers**: To ensure the authenticity and quality of the products from the point of production.
b. **Distributors**: To maintain accurate and real-time records of product movement and storage conditions.
c. **Pharmacies**: To verify the authenticity of received products and provide transparency to consumers.
d. **Regulators**: To ensure compliance with legal and regulatory requirements and to facilitate a secure and transparent oversight mechanism.

5.2.2 Importance of Collaboration and Consensus

Collaboration among stakeholders is essential for several reasons:

a. **Standardization**: Developing and adopting industry-wide standards for data formats and communication protocols.
b. **Interoperability**: Ensuring different systems and platforms can work together seamlessly.
c. **Trust and Transparency**: Building trust among stakeholders through transparent and verifiable data sharing.

d. **Shared Responsibility**: Distributing the responsibility of maintaining the blockchain network and ensuring its integrity.

5.3 Technical Implementation

5.3.1 Choosing the Right Blockchain Platform

Selecting an appropriate blockchain platform involves considering several factors:

a. **Scalability**: The platform must handle the volume of transactions typical in pharmaceutical supply chains.
b. **Security**: Robust security features to protect sensitive data.
c. **Interoperability**: Compatibility with existing systems and potential for integration with other technologies.
d. **Cost**: Evaluating the cost of implementation and operation.

Popular blockchain platforms suitable for pharmaceutical supply chains include:

a. **Hyperledger Fabric:** Known for its modular architecture and permissioned network, making it suitable for enterprise applications.
b. **Ethereum:** Offers smart contract functionality and has a large developer community.
c. **Corda:** Designed specifically for businesses, focusing on privacy and interoperability, (Sáez, 2020).

5.3.2 Integration With Existing Systems and Infrastructure

Integrating blockchain with current systems involves

a. Data Migration: Transferring existing data to the blockchain without loss of integrity or functionality.
b. System Compatibility: Ensuring that blockchain solutions can interface with current IT infrastructure, such as ERP and supply chain management systems.
c. Training and Support: Providing training for staff to manage and operate the new system effectively.

5.4 Data Privacy and Security

5.4.1 Ensuring Patient and Product Data Privacy

Protecting sensitive data is paramount in pharmaceutical supply chains. Blockchain can enhance privacy through:

a. **Encryption:** Encrypting data on the blockchain to prevent unauthorized access.
b. **Access Controls**: Implementing permissioned access to ensure that only authorized parties can view or modify data, (Xiang & Cai, 2021).
c. **Anonymization**: Using techniques to anonymize patient data, ensuring privacy while maintaining data utility for analysis.

5.4.2 Security Measures and Best Practices

To secure blockchain applications, several best practices should be followed:

a. **Regular Audits**: Conducting regular security audits to identify and mitigate vulnerabilities.
b. **Multi-Signature Transactions**: Requiring multiple approvals for critical transactions to prevent fraud and unauthorized changes.
c. **Disaster Recovery Plans**: Establishing comprehensive disaster recovery plans to ensure data integrity and availability in case of system failures.
d. **Compliance with Standards**: Adhering to industry standards and regulations, such as GDPR for data protection and DSCSA for drug supply chain security.

By meticulously planning and executing feasibility studies, engaging stakeholders, selecting the right technology, and prioritizing data privacy and security, pharmaceutical companies can successfully implement blockchain solutions. These implementations can lead to more secure, transparent, and efficient supply chains, ultimately benefiting all stakeholders, including patients.

6. CASE STUDIES AND REAL-WORLD EXAMPLES

6.1 Case Study 1: Company A's Blockchain Implementation

6.1.1 Background

Company A, a leading pharmaceutical manufacturer, faced significant challenges in ensuring the authenticity and traceability of its products. The company was experiencing issues with counterfeit drugs entering the supply chain, which posed risks to patient safety and brand reputation. To address these challenges, Company A decided to implement a blockchain solution to enhance supply chain transparency and security, (Varma *et al.*, 2024).

6.1.2 Implementation Process

a. Feasibility Study: Company A began with a thorough feasibility study to assess the potential benefits and challenges of using blockchain technology. This involved evaluating different blockchain platforms and consulting with experts to understand the technical and regulatory implications.
b. Pilot Project: A pilot project was launched in collaboration with a select group of suppliers, distributors, and retailers. The pilot aimed to track a high-value medication from production to delivery using a blockchain-based system.
c. Platform Selection: Hyperledger Fabric was chosen for its scalability, security features, and suitability for enterprise use. The platform's permissioned nature ensured that only authorized participants could access sensitive data.
d. Integration: The blockchain solution was integrated with existing ERP and supply chain management systems. This integration allowed seamless data flow between blockchain and legacy systems, ensuring continuity and minimizing disruptions.
e. Training and Onboarding: Key stakeholders were trained on how to use the new system. Workshops and training sessions were conducted to familiarize staff with the blockchain platform and its benefits.

6.1.3 Outcomes

a. Enhanced Traceability: The blockchain system provided end-to-end traceability of the medication, allowing Company A to monitor each step in the supply chain in real-time.

b. Counterfeit Reduction: The unique digital identifiers and immutable records on the blockchain significantly reduced the risk of counterfeit drugs entering the supply chain.
c. Regulatory Compliance: Automated, tamper-proof records helped Company A comply more efficiently with regulatory requirements, streamlining audits and inspections.
d. Operational Efficiency: The pilot revealed improvements in supply chain efficiency, including faster recall processes and reduced paperwork.

6.1.4 Lessons Learned

a. Stakeholder Engagement: Successful implementation required active engagement and collaboration among all stakeholders, including suppliers, distributors, and regulators.
b. Scalability: While the pilot was successful, scaling the solution required addressing technical challenges related to data volume and transaction speed.
c. Continuous Improvement: Ongoing monitoring and feedback were essential for refining the system and addressing any issues that arose during the pilot.

6.2 Case Study 2: Industry-Wide Blockchain Initiative: Overview of a Collaborative Blockchain Project

An industry-wide initiative, known as the PharmaLedger Project, was launched to create a blockchain-based platform for the pharmaceutical supply chain. The project involved multiple stakeholders, including major pharmaceutical companies, logistics providers, regulatory agencies, and technology partners, (Chang & Chen, 2020).

6.2.1 Challenges

a. Interoperability: Ensuring interoperability between different stakeholders' systems and the blockchain platform was a major technical challenge. The project required developing standardized data formats and protocols.
b. Data Privacy: Protecting sensitive data while ensuring transparency and traceability was a critical concern. The project had to balance these requirements to gain the trust of all participants.

c. Regulatory Alignment: Aligning the blockchain solution with varying regulatory requirements across different regions posed significant hurdles. The project needed to ensure compliance with regulations like the DSCSA in the U.S. and the FMD in Europe.

6.2.2 Successes

a. Collaborative Framework: The initiative established a collaborative framework that brought together diverse stakeholders to work towards a common goal. This collaboration fostered innovation and shared learning.
b. Pilot Programs: Several pilot programs were conducted to test different aspects of the blockchain platform, including drug traceability, anti-counterfeiting measures, and patient safety applications. These pilots provided valuable insights and demonstrated the feasibility of blockchain solutions.
c. Regulatory Endorsement: The project gained endorsement from regulatory bodies, which recognized the potential of blockchain to enhance supply chain security and compliance.
d. Scalability and Adoption: The platform demonstrated scalability, with several companies expressing interest in adopting the solution for their supply chains. The initiative paved the way for broader industry adoption of blockchain technology.

6.2.3 Lessons Learned

a. Standardization is Key: Developing and adopting industry-wide standards for data sharing and blockchain protocols was essential for interoperability and success.
b. Collaboration and Trust: Building trust among stakeholders through transparent and secure data sharing was crucial for the project's success. Continuous engagement and communication were key.
c. Regulatory Involvement: Early and ongoing involvement of regulatory bodies helped ensure that the blockchain solution met compliance requirements and gained regulatory support.

These case studies highlight the potential of blockchain technology to transform pharmaceutical supply chains by enhancing traceability, combating counterfeit drugs, and improving regulatory compliance. The lessons learned from these implementations can guide future projects and foster wider adoption of blockchain in the industry.

7. CHALLENGES AND CONSIDERATIONS

7.1 Technical Challenges

7.1.1 Scalability

One of the primary technical challenges in implementing blockchain solutions in pharmaceutical supply chains is scalability:

a. Transaction Throughput: Blockchain networks, particularly public ones, can suffer from limited transaction throughput. This bottleneck can lead to delays in processing the large volumes of transactions typical in pharmaceutical supply chains.
b. Latency: High latency in blockchain networks can impact the real-time tracking and traceability of pharmaceutical products, (Rijal *et al.,* 2023).
c. Data Storage: Storing extensive supply chain data on a blockchain can be costly and inefficient. Efficient off-chain storage solutions need to be integrated with blockchain systems.

7.1.2 Interoperability

Interoperability between different blockchain platforms and existing systems is another critical challenge:

a. Standards and Protocols: The lack of standardized protocols for data exchange between various blockchain platforms and traditional supply chain systems can hinder seamless integration.
b. Legacy Systems: Many pharmaceutical companies rely on legacy IT systems that may not be easily compatible with blockchain technology, requiring extensive modifications and integration efforts.

7.1.3 Technological Limitations

Blockchain technology itself has certain inherent limitations:

a. Energy Consumption: Some blockchain consensus mechanisms, like Proof of Work (PoW), are energy-intensive and may not be sustainable for large-scale supply chain applications.

b. Privacy Concerns: While blockchain provides transparency, it must also ensure that sensitive data, especially patient and proprietary information, remains private and secure.
c. Complexity: Implementing and maintaining a blockchain system can be complex and requires specialized knowledge and skills, which might not be readily available within the organization.

7.2 Economic and Financial Considerations

7.2.1 Cost-Benefit Analysis of Blockchain Implementation

Implementing blockchain in pharmaceutical supply chains involves significant financial considerations:

a. Initial Investment: High initial costs for setting up the blockchain infrastructure, including software, hardware, and integration with existing systems.
b. Operational Costs: Ongoing costs for maintaining the blockchain network, including transaction fees, energy consumption, and system upgrades.
c. ROI and Benefits: Evaluating the return on investment (ROI) is crucial. The potential benefits include reduced costs from decreased counterfeiting, improved efficiency, and better regulatory compliance. However, these benefits must be weighed against the implementation and operational costs, (Xu, Chen, & Kou, 2019).

7.2.2 Financial Risks

a. Investment Risk: The financial risk associated with investing in a new and evolving technology that may not yield immediate returns.
b. Market Acceptance: The success of blockchain solutions also depends on widespread acceptance and adoption by all stakeholders in the supply chain, which can be uncertain.

7.3 Regulatory and Legal Issues

7.3.1 Navigating the Regulatory Landscape

The pharmaceutical industry is highly regulated, and implementing blockchain solutions must align with various regulatory requirements:

a. Compliance Requirements: Ensuring that blockchain solutions comply with regulations like the FDA's DSCSA in the U.S. and the EMA's FMD in Europe. This includes maintaining accurate and tamper-proof records that meet regulatory standards.
b. Cross-Border Regulations: Navigating different regulatory environments in different countries can be challenging. Blockchain solutions must be flexible enough to adapt to various regional regulations.

7.3.2 Legal Considerations and Intellectual Property

i. Data Ownership and Privacy:
   a. Ownership: Determining who owns the data recorded on the blockchain can be complex, especially in a decentralized network involving multiple stakeholders.
   b. Privacy: Ensuring compliance with data privacy regulations like GDPR in Europe, which mandates strict guidelines on the handling and sharing of personal data. Blockchain solutions must incorporate privacy-preserving technologies to comply with these regulations.
ii. Intellectual Property:
   a. Patents and IP Rights: Protecting intellectual property rights associated with blockchain innovations. Companies must consider patenting their blockchain solutions to safeguard their technological advancements.
   b. Legal Framework: The legal framework for blockchain technology is still evolving, and there are uncertainties regarding its use and enforceability in different jurisdictions. Companies must stay updated on legal developments and be prepared to navigate these uncertainties.
iii. Contractual Obligations:
   a. Smart Contracts: While smart contracts automate and enforce transactions, they also introduce legal complexities. Ensuring that smart contracts are legally binding and enforceable requires careful legal scrutiny.

Addressing these challenges and considerations is crucial for the successful implementation of blockchain in pharmaceutical supply chains. A comprehensive approach that includes technical solutions, financial planning, and legal compliance will help in overcoming these hurdles and realizing the full potential of blockchain technology.

8. FUTURE PROSPECTS AND TRENDS

8.1 Emerging Technologies and Innovations

8.1.1 Integration with IoT, AI, and Other Emerging Technologies

The future of pharmaceutical supply chains will likely see increased integration with emerging technologies such as:

a. Internet of Things (IoT): IoT devices can provide real-time data on temperature, humidity, and location, ensuring the integrity of pharmaceutical products throughout the supply chain. Integrating blockchain with IoT can enhance transparency and traceability.
b. Artificial Intelligence (AI): AI-powered analytics can analyze vast amounts of supply chain data to identify patterns, optimize processes, and predict potential disruptions. Combining AI with blockchain can improve decision-making and risk management, (Gouiza, Jebari, & Reklaoui, 2024).
c. Big Data Analytics: Leveraging big data analytics can provide valuable insights into supply chain performance, demand forecasting, and customer behavior. Blockchain can ensure the integrity and security of this data, enabling more informed decision-making.

8.2 Future of Blockchain in Pharma Supply Chains

8.2.1 Predictions and Potential Developments

The future of blockchain in pharmaceutical supply chains holds several promising developments:

a. Widespread Adoption: As blockchain technology matures and becomes more accessible, its adoption in pharmaceutical supply chains is expected to increase. More companies will recognize the benefits of blockchain for enhancing transparency, traceability, and security.
b. Interoperability Standards: Industry-wide standards for blockchain interoperability will likely emerge, enabling seamless data exchange between different blockchain platforms and supply chain systems. This will facilitate collaboration and data sharing among diverse stakeholders.

c. Regulatory Integration: Regulatory agencies may increasingly embrace blockchain technology to improve drug traceability, combat counterfeit drugs, and ensure compliance with regulatory requirements. Blockchain-based solutions may become a regulatory requirement for pharmaceutical companies.
d. Supply Chain Digitization: The adoption of blockchain will accelerate the digitization of pharmaceutical supply chains, leading to greater efficiency, reduced costs, and improved patient safety. Smart contracts and automated processes will streamline supply chain operations.
e. Enhanced Patient Care: Blockchain-enabled supply chains will empower patients with access to transparent information about the origin, quality, and authenticity of medications. Patients will have greater confidence in the drugs they consume, leading to improved medication adherence and health outcomes.

As these trends unfold, blockchain technology will play an increasingly significant role in revolutionizing pharmaceutical supply chains, driving innovation, and improving the overall efficiency and safety of the industry. Companies that embrace blockchain early and invest in innovative solutions will be well-positioned to thrive in this rapidly evolving landscape.

CONCLUSION

Blockchain technology holds immense promise for revolutionizing pharmaceutical supply chains by enhancing traceability, combating counterfeit drugs, and improving regulatory compliance. Despite the challenges of scalability, interoperability, and regulatory complexities, successful implementations like Company A's showcase the tangible benefits of blockchain adoption. As the industry embraces emerging technologies like IoT and AI, we can anticipate widespread blockchain adoption, interoperability standards, and regulatory integration, ultimately leading to greater transparency, efficiency, and patient safety within the pharmaceutical ecosystem.

REFERENCES

Abdallah, S., & Nizamuddin, N. Blockchain-based solution for Pharma Supply Chain Industry, Computers & Industrial Engineering, Volume 177,2023,108997,ISSN 0360-8352,DOI: 10.1016/j.cie.2023.108997

Assiri, S., Alyamani, M., Mansour, A., Fakieh, B., Badri, S., & Babour, A. 2020. Current Shipment Tracking Technologies and Trends in Research. In *Proceedings of the 2020 the 4th International Conference on Information System and Data Mining (ICISDM '20)*. Association for Computing Machinery, New York, NY, USA, 113–117. https://doi.org/DOI: 10.1145/3404663.3404683

Butticè, V., Caviggioli, F., Franzoni, C., Scellato, G., Stryszowski, P., & Thumm, N. (2020). Counterfeiting in digital technologies: An empirical analysis of the economic performance and innovative activities of affected companies, Research Policy, Volume 49, Issue 5, 103959,ISSN 0048-7333,DOI: 10.1016/j.respol.2020.103959

Chang, S. E., & Chen, Y. (2020, August 31). Blockchain in Health Care Innovation: Literature Review and Case Study From a Business Ecosystem Perspective. *Journal of Medical Internet Research*, 22(8), e19480. DOI: 10.2196/19480 PMID: 32865501

Estrada, C. A., Naranjo, S. S., Toasa, V. J., & Yoo, S. G. 2024. A Systematic Literature Review of Blockchain Technology: Applications Fields, Platforms, and Consensus Protocols. In *Proceedings of the 2023 7th International Conference on Computer Science and Artificial Intelligence (CSAI '23)*. Association for Computing Machinery, New York, NY, USA, 123–131. https://doi.org/DOI: 10.1145/3638584.3638632

Ghadge, A., Bourlakis, M., Kamble, S., & Seuring, S. (2023). Blockchain implementation in pharmaceutical supply chains: A review and conceptual framework. *International Journal of Production Research*, 61(19), 6633–6651. DOI: 10.1080/00207543.2022.2125595

Godyn, M., Kedziora, M., Ren, Y., Liu, Y., & Song, H. H. (2022). Analysis of solutions for a blockchain compliance with GDPR. *Scientific Reports*, 12(1), 15021. DOI: 10.1038/s41598-022-19341-y PMID: 36056166

Gouiza, N., Jebari, H., & Reklaoui, K. (2024). INTEGRATION OF IOT-ENABLED TECHNOLOGIES AND ARTIFICIAL INTELLIGENCE IN DIVERSE DOMAINS: RECENT ADVANCEMENTS AND FUTURE TRENDS. *Journal of Theoretical and Applied Information Technology*, 102, 1975–2029.

Gruchmann, T., Elgazzar, S., & Ali, A. H. (2023). Blockchain technology in pharmaceutical supply chains: A transaction cost perspective. *Modern Supply Chain Research and Applications*, 5(2), 115–133. DOI: 10.1108/MSCRA-10-2022-0023

Habib, G., Sharma, S., Ibrahim, S., Ahmad, I., Qureshi, S., & Ishfaq, M. (2022). Blockchain Technology: Benefits, Challenges, Applications, and Integration of Blockchain Technology with Cloud Computing. *Future Internet*, 14(11), 341. DOI: 10.3390/fi14110341

Haelterman, H. (2022). Breaking Silos of Legal and Regulatory Risks to Outperform Traditional Compliance Approaches. *European Journal on Criminal Policy and Research*, 28(1), 19–36. DOI: 10.1007/s10610-020-09468-x

Klessascheck, Finn, Knoche, Tom, & Pufahl, Luise. (2024). Reviewing Conformance Checking Uses for Run-Time Regulatory Compliance. . DOI: 10.1007/s10610-020-09468-x

Kumar, K. P. V., Lakshmi, B., & Sai Kumar, S. M. V, N. R. Sai and V. Nagamalleswara, "Blockchain Technology: A Comprehensive Review and Future Directions," *2023 Second International Conference on Augmented Intelligence and Sustainable Systems (ICAISS)*, Trichy, India, 2023, pp. 1362-1368, DOI: 10.1109/ICAISS58487.2023.10250707

Moosivand, A., Rajabzadeh Ghatari, A., & Rasekh, H. R. (2019, Spring). Supply Chain Challenges in Pharmaceutical Manufacturing Companies: Using Qualitative System Dynamics Methodology. *Iranian Journal of Pharmaceutical Research : IJPR*, 18(2), 1103–1116. DOI: 10.22037/ijpr.2019.2389 PMID: 31531092

Nguyen, A., Lamouri, S., Pellerin, R., & Giraldo, T. (2021). Data analytics in pharmaceutical supply chains: State of the art, opportunities, and challenges. *International Journal of Production Research*, 60(22), 6888–6907. Advance online publication. DOI: 10.1080/00207543.2021.1950937

Rijal, Syamsu, Saranani, Fajar, & Joseph, Amal & C, Midhun & Ajibade, Samuel & Salvia, Vijay & Nazir, Mamona. (2023). Block chain Technology: Challenges, Opportunities and Future Direction. *European Chemical Bulletin*, 12, 3494–3515.

Sáez, M. (2020). Blockchain-Enabled Platforms: Challenges and Recommendations. *International Journal of Interactive Multimedia and Artificial Intelligence*, 6(3), 73. DOI: 10.9781/ijimai.2020.08.005

Sharma, P., Jindal, R., & Borah, M. D. (2022). A Review of Blockchain-Based Applications and Challenges. *Wireless Personal Communications*, 123(2), 1201–1243. DOI: 10.1007/s11277-021-09176-7

Solat, S., Calvez, P., & Naït-Abdesselam, F. (2020). Permissioned vs. Permissionless Blockchain: How and Why There Is Only One Right Choice. *Journal of Software*, 16, 95–106. DOI: 10.17706/jsw.16.3.95-106

Vadapalli, Ravindhar. (2020). BLOCKCHAIN FUNDAMENTALS TEXT BOOK Fundamentals of Blockchain. DOI: 10.17706/jsw.16.3.95-106

Varma, A., Dixit, N., Ray, S., & Kaur, J. (2024). Blockchain technology for sustainable supply chains: A comprehensive review and future prospects. *World Journal of Advanced Research and Reviews.*, 21(3), 980–994. DOI: 10.30574/wjarr.2024.21.3.0804

Xiang, D., & Cai, W. (2021, October 7). Privacy Protection and Secondary Use of Health Data: Strategies and Methods. *BioMed Research International*, 6967166(1), 6967166. Advance online publication. DOI: 10.1155/2021/6967166 PMID: 34660798

Xu, M., Chen, X., & Kou, G. (2019). A systematic review of blockchain. *Financial Innovation*, 5(1), 27. DOI: 10.1186/s40854-019-0147-z

Yiu, N. C. K. (2021). Toward Blockchain-Enabled Supply Chain Anti-Counterfeiting and Traceability. *Future Internet*, 13(4), 86. DOI: 10.3390/fi13040086

Zakari, N., Al-Razgan, M., Alsaadi, A., Alshareef, H., Al Saigh, H., Alashaikh, L., Alharbi, M., Alomar, R., & Alotaibi, S. (2022, March 11). Blockchain technology in the pharmaceutical industry: A systematic review. *PeerJ. Computer Science*, 8, e840. DOI: 10.7717/peerj-cs.840 PMID: 35634106

Zhang, W., (2019). Blockchain-Based Distributed Compliance in Multinational Corporations' Cross-Border Intercompany Transactions. In Arai, K., Kapoor, S., & Bhatia, R. (Eds.), *Advances in Information and Communication Networks. FICC 2018. Advances in Intelligent Systems and Computing* (Vol. 887). Springer., DOI: 10.1007/978-3-030-03405-4_20

Zhou, S., Li, K., Xiao, L., Cai, J., Liang, W., & Castiglione, A. (2023). A Systematic Review of Consensus Mechanisms in Blockchain. *Mathematics*, 11(10), 2248. DOI: 10.3390/math11102248

Ziavrou, K. S., Noguera, S., & Boumba, V. A. (2022, September). Trends in counterfeit drugs and pharmaceuticals before and during COVID-19 pandemic. *Forensic Science International*, 338, 111382. DOI: 10.1016/j.forsciint.2022.111382 PMID: 35882074

Chapter 13 The Economic Implications of AI in Pharmaceuticals and Research

Sarah A. Alajlan
https://orcid.org/0000-0003-0050-4164
Almaarefa University, Saudi Arabia

Miltiadis D. Lytras
Effat Unversity, Saudi Arabia

ABSTRACT

This chapter provides an overview of the history and impact of artificial intelligence on businesses, with a specific focus on the pharmaceutical industry and research. It discusses the basic principles of pharmacoeconomics, explores ways AI can enhance business processes, and examines various applications of AI in pharmaceutical research, such as drug development, digital therapy, personalized treatment, clinical trials, epidemic forecasting, and supply chain management. The chapter also addresses challenges and considerations related to ethics, safety, data privacy, and liability in AI implementation. Finally, the discussion provides insights into AI's economic opportunities and implications in pharmaceutical research.

DOI: 10.4018/979-8-3693-6270-9.ch013

1.0 INTRODUCTION

The economic consequences of artificial intelligence (AI) for the pharmaceutical and research sectors have surfaced as both an extraordinary opportunity and a challenging disruption. The economic implications of artificial intelligence (AI) in the pharmaceutical and research sectors present both exceptional opportunities and significant challenges. AI can transform drug discovery, clinical trials, and market entry within an industry characterized by substantial research investments, complex regulatory environments, and lengthy development timelines.

This exploration focuses on the financial implications of AI in the pharmaceutical industry, particularly regarding how AI-driven advancements are reshaping cost structures, enhancing productivity, and creating new growth opportunities. It also addresses the potential benefits of AI adoption, such as improved efficiency and reduced costs, alongside the financial risks and challenges, particularly regarding investment, policy, and workforce considerations. Lastly, it examines the potential economic trajectory of AI in pharmaceutical research, providing insights into how these technological innovations could affect the industry's competitive landscape and long-term sustainability.

AI can significantly alter the economic dynamics surrounding drug discovery, clinical trials, and market entry. Nevertheless, the precise nature and extent of these changes remain unclear. This analysis will delve into the financial effects of AI on the pharmaceutical industry, focusing on how AI advancements are modifying cost structures, enhancing productivity, and fostering new growth opportunities. Additionally, it will explore the financial risks and challenges tied to AI adoption, particularly regarding investment, policy, and workforce implications. Finally, it will investigate the potential economic path of AI in pharmaceutical research, offering insights into how these technological innovations may influence the industry's competitive environment and long-term sustainability. The financial consequences of artificial intelligence (AI) in the pharmaceutical and research sectors present extraordinary opportunities and significant challenges. AI can transform drug discovery, clinical trials, and market entry within an industry characterized by substantial research investments, complex regulatory environments, and lengthy development timelines.

This exploration focuses on the financial implications of AI in the pharmaceutical industry, particularly regarding how specific AI-driven advancements, such as machine learning algorithms and data analytics tools, are reshaping cost structures, enhancing productivity, and creating new growth opportunities. It also addresses the financial risks and challenges associated with AI adoption, particularly regarding investment, policy, and workforce considerations. Lastly, it examines the potential economic trajectory of AI in pharmaceutical research, providing insights into how these technological innovations could affect the industry's competitive landscape and long-term sustainability.

AI can significantly alter the economic dynamics surrounding drug discovery, clinical trials, and market entry. Nevertheless, the precise nature and extent of these changes remain unclear. This analysis will delve into the financial effects of AI on the pharmaceutical industry, focusing on how AI advancements are modifying cost structures, enhancing productivity, and fostering new growth opportunities. Additionally, it will explore the financial risks and challenges tied to AI adoption, particularly regarding investment, policy, and workforce implications. Finally, it will investigate the potential economic path of AI in pharmaceutical research, offering insights into how these technological innovations may influence the industry's competitive environment and long-term sustainability. The financial impact of artificial intelligence (AI) on the pharmaceutical and research sectors presents both remarkable opportunities and significant challenges. AI can transform drug discovery, clinical trials, and market entry in an industry known for its heavy research investments, complex regulatory environments, and lengthy development timelines.

This exploration focuses on the financial implications of AI in the pharmaceutical industry, particularly how AI-driven advancements are reshaping cost structures, improving productivity, and creating new growth opportunities. It also addresses the financial risks and challenges related to AI adoption, especially regarding investment, policy, and workforce considerations. Lastly, it examines the potential economic trajectory of AI in pharmaceutical research, providing insights into how this technological innovation.

2.0 HISTORY OF AI

Artificial Intelligence, in its contemporary definition, entails a system's capacity to accurately analyze external data, assimilate knowledge from said data, and apply these acquired insights to accomplish objectives and tasks using adaptable adjustment (Berlinski, 2000). The concept's origins can be traced back to mythology, with tales of brilliant beings or philosophers attempting to comprehend human cognition's intricacies through mechanical symbolism. Within the 1940s, the development of the computerized computer propelled the concept of building an electronic brain, as this development started the potential for mechanizing human thought. It peaked in the summer of 1956 when AI was formally recognized as an academic field. A group of scientists convened at a workshop held at Dartmouth College, financed by the Rockefeller Foundation, titled "Dartmouth Summer Research Project on Artificial Intelligence (DSRPAI)," to pursue the objective of developing an artificial brain. That is where Marvin Minsky and John McCarthy, distinguished American computer and cognitive scientists, coined "Artificial Intelligence" and directed their research toward developing machines endowed with human-like intelligence (Kaplan, 2022). Nearly two decades of successful AI development were followed. A multitude of new projects resulted in significant progress in the field. In 1970, Minsky forecasted that a device capable of human intelligence would be attainable within three to eight years. However, significant criticisms were raised regarding this positive perspective. In 1973, the governments of the Joined Together States and the Joined Together Kingdom ended their backing of manufactured insights inquire about. This started what is now recognized as the Primary AI Winter (Haenlein & Kaplan, 2019). During the early 1980s, another phase of significant development in artificial intelligence was documented. This surge was initiated by intense financial support from the Japanese government towards its fifth-generation computer project, thus motivating the United States to enhance its funding in artificial intelligence. Consequently, advancements were observed in expert systems and connectionism. Nonetheless, the recession of the early 1990s resulted in significant funding reductions for this sector, thereby leading to a second AI Winter. (Newquist, 1994). The contemporary surge in artificial intelligence commenced in 2016, with the establishment being focused on harnessing generative AI systems. In late 2022, various AI tools and software were introduced to the public. This development sparked enthusiasm for their advanced capabilities yet simultaneously instilled apprehension due to their disruptive potential. Nevertheless, the opportunities presented by these AI tools, particularly within the business realm, were deemed highly promising. Many companies perceived this disruptive potential as a valuable resource that should be leveraged. (Firth-Butterfield, 2023; Kaplan & Haenlein, 2019). The type of intelligence exhibited by AI can be categorized into three groups: analytical (cognitive intelligence), human-inspired (emotional intelligence), and humanized (social intelligence). Furthermore, it can also be categorized into three groups according to its evolutionary stage: Artificial Narrow, General, and Super Intelligence. After artificial intelligence is incorporated into common usage, all these categories blend because of the "AI Effect," which proposes that the public diminishes AI as not constituting "true" intelligence or cognition as it hinges on mathematical computation (Haenlein & Kaplan, 2019; Fanti et al., 2022).

3.0 OVERVIEW OF AI'S IMPACT ON BUSINESSES

Historically, artificial intelligence has predominantly captured the attention of academic researchers rather than business professionals (Nilsson, 2010). With the most recent advancements, enterprises have acknowledged the potential of AI in creating value, particularly in industries with high volumes of data (Greenstein, 2001;

Åström et al., 2022).AI, akin to other transformative technology-based tools of the past, presents a potential for heightened efficiency and productivity. Nevertheless, it also can fundamentally alter the structuring and execution of processes. Therefore, it is imperative to evaluate the disruptive potential of AI, as well as the benefits it pledges. The alignment of companies' economic objectives, such as enhancing efficiency and reducing costs, is crucial in clarifying the widespread adoption of AI technologies (Rakočević & Marković, 2024). In the manufacturing sectors, incorporating intelligent machines that can learn and recognize images and sounds further bolsters the path of lean production. Several channels are currently operational, namely:(i) the reduction of labor input utilized in production;(ii) the maximization of efficiency for both humans and machines in task execution;(iii) the creation of new prospects for activities combining machines and human assistance;(iv) the resolution of bottlenecks and the implementation of information feedback mechanisms that enable sustained enhancements in quality (Rikap & Lundvall, 2021). As artificial intelligence advances, the potential for reducing labor costs through automation and robotization increases significantly. Companies can replicate routine tasks based on specific rules by stimulating AI tools' design, adoption, and use. However, due to its learning systems, AI's capacity to develop into reproducing non-routine complex tasks is unparalleled (Tyson & Zysman, 2022). For industries that heavily rely on technology, Artificial Intelligence (AI) plays a crucial role in their strategic planning. Depending on learning frameworks and data handling serve as a strategy for optimizing esteem by upgrading control over all its components (Dosi & Virgillito, 2019). Big Data companies can predict demand patterns, while machine learning enables the management of the supply network. This may significantly restructure organizational engagement patterns with customers, suppliers, and competitors (Rikap & Lundvall, 2021; Obschonka & Audretsch, 2020). A significant discrepancy exists between the demand and supply of artificial intelligence, resulting in a notable consolidation of enterprises equipped with the necessary resources for advancing and governance AI technology. What we observe is that artificial intelligence companies function within highly concentrated markets. Due to the importance of accessing digital markets and the capability to digitize processes to enhance productivity as essential factors for gaining a competitive edge, there has been a significant increase in the demand for AI products (UNCTAD, 2021). Considering the multifaceted and overarching impact of AI and business processes, it is not easy, nor would it be correct, to a priori label AI as having a bidirectional impact on a business, either as a tool for improvement or as a disruptive agent (Rakočević & Marković, 2024). While optimistic perspectives regarding the contributions of artificial intelligence to businesses are prevalent, a cautious examination of its negative impacts on the current business landscape necessitates thorough scrutiny. The literature elucidates the diverse effects that technology can have on a specific company. The foundation of a company's competitive advantage lies in its resources and capabilities (Grant, 2018). Henceforth, should a business's competitive advantage be influenced by the emergence of artificial intelligence, this influence will be manifested through the resources and capabilities possessed by the business. Technological radical and revolutionary change tends to disrupt the incumbent's leading position by rendering its resources and capabilities obsolete (Tushman & Anderson, 1986). The larger the technological shift, the more challenging it becomes for the incumbents to adapt or replace their resources and capabilities without jeopardizing their competitive standing. Companies that encounter a groundbreaking technological transformation typically demonstrate superior adaptability and sustain their competitive advantage, provided the technological shift entails a component innovation rather than an architectural one (Henderson & Clark, 1990). An architectural shift necessitates a significant restructuring and redesign of the company's processes and projects to leverage the advantages of the new technology. If the new technology can be integrated into the current product or process design, the incumbents will experience shorter adoption times. Moreover, implementing innovative technology will enhance a specific aspect of the issue or stage of the operation, thereby advancing the overall product or procedure.

REFERENCES

Abbas, K., Afaq, M., Ahmed Khan, T., & Song, W. C. (2020). A blockchain and machine learning-based drug supply chain management and recommendation system for the smart pharmaceutical industry. *Electronics (Basel)*, 9(5), 852. DOI: 10.3390/electronics9050852

Akhtar, M., Kraemer, M. U. G., & Gardner, L. M. (2019). A dynamic neural network model for predicting risk of Zika in real-time. *BMC Medicine*, 17(1), 171. DOI: 10.1186/s12916-019-1389-3 PMID: 31474220

Albu, A., & Ungureanu, L. (2005). Artificial Neural Network in Medicine. DOI: 10.1186/s12916-019-1389-3 PMID: 31474220

Amadin, F. I., & Bello, M. E. (2018). Prediction of yellow fever using multilayer perceptron neural network classifier. *Journal of Emerging Trends in Engineering and Applied Sciences*, 9, 282–286.

Åström, J., Reim, W., & Parida, V. (2022). Value creation and value capture for AI business model innovation: A three-phase process framework. *Review ofManagerial Science*, 16(7), 2111–2133. DOI: 10.1007/s11846-022-00521-z

Berlinski, D. (2000). *The advent of the algorithm*. Harcourt Books. Dosi, G., & Virgillito, M. E. (2019). What is the evolution of the contemporary social fabric? New technologies and old socio-economic trends. *International Labour Review*, 158(4), 593–625. DOI: 10.1111/ilr.12179

Burke, R. M., Shah, M. P., Wikswo, M. E., Barclay, L., Kambhampati, A., Marsh, Z., Cannon, J. L., Parashar, U. D., Vinjé, J., & Hall, A. J. (2018). The norovirus epidemiologic triad: Predictors of severe outcomes in US norovirus outbreaks, 2009–2016. *The Journal of Infectious Diseases*, 219(9), 1364–1372. DOI: 10.1093/infdis/jiy569 PMID: 30445538

Cheng, H.-Y., Wu, Y.-C., Lin, M.-H., Liu, Y.-L., Tsai, Y.-Y., Wu, J.-H., Pan, K.-H., Ke, C.-J., Chen, C.-M., Liu, D.-P., Lin, I.-F., & Chuang, J.-H. (2020). Applying Machine Learning Models with An Ensemble Approach for Accurate Real-Time Influenza Forecasting in Taiwan: Development and Validation Study. [CrossRef]. *Journal of Medical Internet Research*, 22(8), e15394. DOI: 10.2196/15394 PMID: 32755888

Dill, K. A., & MacCallum, J. L. (2012). The protein-folding problem, 50 years on. [DOI:10.1126/sciencc.1219021] [PMID]. *Science*, 338(6110), 1042–1046. DOI: 10.1126/science.1219021 PMID: 23180855

Drummond, M. F., Sculpher, M. J., Claxton, K., Stoddart, G. L., & Torrance, G. W. (2015). *Methods for the economic evaluation of health care programs* (4th ed.). Oxford University Press.

Fanti, L., Guarascio, D., & Moggi, M. (2022). From Heron of Alexandria to Amazon's Alexa: A stylized history of AI and its impact on business models, organization and work. *Economia e Politica Industriale*, 49(3), 495–518. DOI: 10.1007/s40812-022-00222-4

Firth-Butterfield, K. (2023, January 18). 2022 was a big year for AI development. In 2023, we must decide how best to use it. *Asia News Network*. https://asianews.network/2022-was-a-big-year-for-ai-developmentin-2023-we-must-decide-how-best-to-use-it

Fogel, D. B. (2000). What is evolutionary computation? *IEEE Spectrum*, 37(5), 26–32. DOI: 10.1109/6.819926

Fong, S. J., Li, G., Dey, N., Gonzalez-Crespo, R., & Herrera-Viedma, E. (2020). Finding an Accurate Early Forecasting Model from Small Dataset: A Case of 2019-nCoV Novel Coronavirus Outbreak. [CrossRef]. *International Journal of Interactive Multimedia and Artificial Intelligence*, 6(1), 132. DOI: 10.9781/ijimai.2020.02.002

Goldsack, J. (2019). Synthetic control arms can save time and money in clinical trials. *STAT News*.https://www.statnews.com/2019/02/05/synthetic-control-arms-clinical-trials/ (accessed November 5, 2021)

Gopinath, N. (2021). Artificial intelligence: Potential tool to subside SARS-CoV-2 pandemic. [CrossRef]. *Process Biochemistry (Barking, London, England)*, 110, 94–99. DOI: 10.1016/j.procbio.2021.08.001 PMID: 34366689

Grant, R. M. (2018). *Contemporary Strategy Analysis* (10th ed.). Wiley.

Greenstein, S. (2001). The commercialization of the Internet: The interaction. *Innovation Policy and the Economy*, 1, 151–186. DOI: 10.1086/ipe.1.25056144

Guo, P., Liu, T., Zhang, Q., Wang, L., Xiao, J., Zhang, Q., Luo, G., Li, Z., He, J., Zhang, Y., & Ma, W. (2017). Developing a dengue forecast model using machine learning: A case study in China. [CrossRef] [PubMed]. *PLoS Neglected Tropical Diseases*, 11(10), e0005973. DOI: 10.1371/journal.pntd.0005973 PMID: 29036169

Haenlein, M., & Kaplan, A. M. (2019). A brief history of artificial intelligence: On artificial intelligence's past, present, and future. *California Management Review*, 61(4), 5–14. DOI: 10.1177/0008125619864925

Hanson, C. W.III, & Marshall, B. E. (2001). Artificial intelligence applications in the intensive care unit. *Critical Care Medicine*, 29(4), 427–435. DOI: 10.1097/00003246-200102000-00038 PMID: 11269246

Harrer, S., Menard, J., Rivers, M., Green, D. V., Karpiak, J., & Jeliazkov, J. R.. (2024). Artificial intelligence drives the digital transformation of pharma. In Krittanawong, I. (Ed.), *Artificial intelligence in clinical practice*. Elsevier. [DOI:10.1016/B978-0-443-15688-5.00049-8] DOI: 10.1016/B978-0-443-15688-5.00049-8

Harrer, S., Shah, P., Antony, B., & Hu, J. (2019). Artificial intelligence for clinical trial design. *Trends in Pharmacological Sciences*, 40(8), 577–591. DOI: 10.1016/j.tips.2019.05.005 PMID: 31326235

Hemedan, A. A., Abd Elaziz, M., Jiao, P., Alavi, A. H., Bahgat, M., Ostaszewski, M., Schneider, R., Ghazy, H. A., Ewees, A. A., & Lu, S. (2020). Prediction of the Vaccine-derived Poliovirus Outbreak Incidence: A Hybrid Machine Learning Approach. [CrossRef] [PubMed]. *Scientific Reports*, 10(1), 5058. DOI: 10.1038/s41598-020-61853-y PMID: 32193487

Henderson, R. M., & Clark, K. B. (1990). Architectural innovation: The reconfiguration of existing. *Administrative Science Quarterly*, 35(1), 9. DOI: 10.2307/2393549

Hu, Z., Ge, Q., Li, S., Jin, S., & Xiong, M. (2020). Artificial intelligence forecasting of COVID-19 in China. *arXiv*. https://arxiv.org/abs/2002.07112

Huang, C. J., Chen, Y. H., Ma, Y., & Kuo, P. H. (2020). Multiple-input deep convolutional neural network model for COVID-19 forecasting in China. *medRxiv*. DOI: 10.1101/2020.03.23.20041608

Huss, R. (2016, October 3). The high price of failed clinical trials: Time to rethink the model. *Clinical Leader*.https://www.clinicalleader.com/doc/the-high-price-of-failed-clinical-trials-time-to-rethink-the-model-0001 (accessed November 10, 2022)

Jain, A., Mao, J., & Mohiuddin, K. (1996). Artificial neural networks: A tutorial. *Computer*, 29(3), 31–44. DOI: 10.1109/2.485891

Kaplan, A. M. (2022). *Artificial intelligence, business, and civilization: Our fate made in machines*. Routledge. DOI: 10.4324/9781003244554

Kaplan, A. M., & Haenlein, M. (2019). Siri, Siri, in my hand: Who is the fairest in the land? On the interpretations, illustrations, and implications of artificial intelligence. *Business Horizons*, 62(1), 15–25. DOI: 10.1016/j.bushor.2018.08.004

Kasaraneni, R. K. (2021). AI-enhanced pharmacoeconomics: Evaluating cost-effectiveness and budget impact of new pharmaceuticals. *Australian Journal of Machine Learning Research & Applications*, 1(1), 291–327. https://sydneyacademics.com/index.php/ajmlra/article/view/136

Khan, M. T., Kaushik, A. C., Ji, L., Malik, S. I., Ali, S., & Wei, D.-Q. (2019). Artificial Neural Networks for Prediction of Tuberculosis Disease. [CrossRef]. *Frontiers in Microbiology*, 10, 395. DOI: 10.3389/fmicb.2019.00395 PMID: 30886608

Kit-Kay, M., & Mallikarjuna, R. P. (2019). Artificial intelligence in drug development: Present status and prospects. *Drug Discovery Today*, 24(3), 773–780. https://doi.org/. drudis.2018.11.014. DOI: 10.3389/fmicb.2019.00395 PMID: 30886608

Kleiven, E.F., Henden, J.-A., Ims, R.A., & Yoccoz, N.G. Seasonal difference in temporal transferability of an ecological model: Near-term predictions of lemming outbreak abundances. Sci. Rep. 2018, 8, 15252. [CrossRef] 133. DOI: 10.3389/fmicb.2019.00395 PMID: 30886608

Kolluri, S., Lin, J., Liu, R., Zhang, Y., & Zhang, W. (2022). Machine learning and artificial intelligence in pharmaceutical research and development: A review. *The AAPS Journal*, 24(1), 19. DOI: 10.1208/s12248-021-00644-3 PMID: 34984579

Kostkova, P., Pinheiro dos Santos, W., & Massoni, T. (2019). ZIKA: Improved surveillance and forecast of Zika virus in Brazil. [CrossRef]. *European Journal of Public Health*, 29(Suppl. 4), ckz186–ckz085. DOI: 10.1093/eurpub/ckz186.085

Li, M., Liu, R., Lin, J., Bunn, V., & Zhao, H. (2020). Bayesian semi-parametric design (BSD) for adaptive dose-finding with multiple strata. *Journal of Biopharmaceutical Statistics*, 30(5), 806–820. DOI: 10.1080/10543406.2020.1730870 PMID: 32129133

Liu, R., Lin, J., & Li, P. (2020). Design considerations for phase I/II dose-finding clinical trials in immuno-oncology and cell therapy. *Contemporary Clinical Trials*, 96, 106083. DOI: 10.1016/j.cct.2020.106083 PMID: 32659438

Madhav, N., Oppenheim, B., Gallivan, M., Mulembakani, P., Rubin, E., & Wolfe, N. (2017). Pandemics: Risks, impacts, and mitigation. In *Disease control priorities: Improving health and reducing poverty* (3rd ed., Vol. 9, pp. 315–345). The International Bank for Reconstruction and Development/The World Bank.

Mandal, L., & Jana, N. D. (2019). Prediction of active drug molecule using back-propagation neural network. In *Proceedings of the 8th International Conference System Modeling and Advancement in Research Trends (SMART)* (pp. 22–26). Moradabad, India DOI: 10.1109/SMART46866.2019.9117378

Marcus, J. L., Sewell, W. C., Balzer, L. B., & Krakower, D. S. (2020). Artificial Intelligence and Machine Learning for HIV Prevention: Emerging Approaches to Ending the Epidemic. [CrossRef]. *Current HIV/AIDS Reports*, 17(3), 171–179. DOI: 10.1007/s11904-020-00490-6 PMID: 32347446

Marini, M., Chokani, N., & Abhari, R. S. COVID-19 Epidemic in Switzerland: Growth Prediction and Containment Strategy Using Artificial Intelligence and Big Data. *medRxiv* 2020. *medRxiv*:2020.03.30.20047472. DOI: 10.1101/2020.03.30.20047472

Muehlematter, U. J., Daniore, P., & Vokinger, K. N. (2021). Approval of artificial intelligence and machine learning-based medical devices in the USA and Europe (2015-20): A comparative analysis. [DOI:10.1016/ S2589-7500(20)30292-2] [PMID]. *The Lancet. Digital Health*, 3(3), e195–e203. DOI: 10.1016/S2589-7500(20)30292-2 PMID: 33478929

Newquist, H. P. (1994). *The brain makers: Genius, ego, and greed in the quest for machines that think*. Macmillan/SAMS. DOI: 10.1016/S2589-7500(20)30292-2 PMID: 33478929

Nilsson, N. J. (2010). *The quest for artificial intelligence: A history of ideas and achievements*. Cambridge University Press.

O'Sullivan, S., Nevejans, N., Allen, C., Blyth, A., Leonard, S., Pagallo, U., Holzinger, K., Holzinger, A., Sajid, M. I., & Ashrafian, H. (2019). Legal, regulatory, and ethical frameworks for developing standards in artificial intelligence (AI)and autonomous robotic surgery. [DOI:10.1002/rcs.1968] [PMID]. *International Journal of Medical Robotics and Computer Assisted Surgery*, 15(1), e1968. DOI: 10.1002/rcs.1968 PMID: 30397993

Obschonka, M., & Audretsch, D. B. (2020). Artificial intelligence and big data in entrepreneurship: A new era has begun. *Small Business Economics*, 55(3), 529–539. DOI: 10.1007/s11187-019-00202-4

OECD. (2019). *Artificial Intelligence in Society*. OECD.

Raja, D. B., Mallol, R., Ting, C. Y., Kamaludin, F., Ahmad, R., Ismail, S., Jayaraj, V. J., & Sundaram, B. M. (2019). Artificial intelligence model as a predictor for dengue outbreaks. *Malaysian Journal of Public Health Medicine*, 19(2), 103–108. DOI: 10.37268/mjphm/vol.19/no.2/art.176

Rakočević, T., & Markovic, M. (2024). Assessing the impact of AI: The case of the pharmaceutical industry. *European Journal of Business and Management Research*, 9(5), 70–75. DOI: 10.24018/ejbmr.2024.9.5.1124

Rakočević, T., & Markovic, M. (2024). Assessing the Impact of AI: The Case of the Pharmaceutical Industry. *European Journal of Business and Management Research, 9*5), 70-75.)

Ramesh, A. N., Kambhampati, C., Monson, J. R., & Drew, P. J. (2004). Artificial intelligence in medicine. *Annals of the Royal College of Surgeons of England*, 86(5), 334–338. DOI: 10.1308/147870804290 PMID: 15333167

Ravali, R. S., Auguskani, J. P. L., Reddy, L. K. V., Narapureddy, B. R., Chellathurai, A., & Mavaluru, D. (2023). Pioneering ethical boundaries: Empowering AI governance for the future of pharmaceutical and nursing sectors. *Latin American Journal of Pharmacy*, 42(3), 695–701.

Rikap, C., & Lundvall, B. (2021). *The Digital Innovation Race*. Springer Books. DOI: 10.1007/978-3-030-89443-6

Rikap, C., & Lundvall, B. Å. (2021). *The digital innovation race*. Springer. DOI: 10.1007/978-3-030-89443-6

Salim, N. A. M., Wah, Y. B., Reeves, C., Smith, M., Yaacob, W. F. W., Mudin, R. N., Dapari, R., Sapri, N. N. F. F., & Haque, U. (2021). Sapri, NNFF; Haque, U. Prediction of dengue outbreak in Selangor Malaysia using machine learning techniques. [CrossRef]. *Scientific Reports*, 11(1), 939. DOI: 10.1038/s41598-020-79193-2 PMID: 33441678

Schwendicke, F., Samek, W., & Krois, J. (2020). Artificial intelligence in dentistry: Chances and challenges. [DOI:10.1177/0022034520915714] [PMID]. *Journal of Dental Research*, 99(7), 769–774. DOI: 10.1177/0022034520915714 PMID: 32315260

Sharma, R., Shishodia, A., Gunasekaran, A., Min, H., & Munim, Z. H. (2022). The role of artificial intelligence in supply chain management: Mapping the territory. [DOI:10.1080/00207543.2022.2029611]. *International Journal of Production Research*, 60(24), 7527–7550. DOI: 10.1080/00207543.2022.2029611

Sinha, A., & Rathi, M. (2021). COVID-19 prediction using AI analytics for South Korea. [CrossRef] [PubMed]. *Applied Intelligence*, 51(12), 8579–8597. DOI: 10.1007/s10489-021-02352-z PMID: 34764592

Soni, U., Gupta, N., & Sakshi, . (2021). Sakshi. An Artificial Intelligence Approach for Forecasting Ebola Disease. [CrossRef]. *Journal of Physics: Conference Series*, 1950(1), 012038. DOI: 10.1088/1742-6596/1950/1/012038

Steele, L., Orefuwa, E., Bino, S., Singer, S. R., Lutwama, J., & Dickmann, P. (2020). Earlier outbreak detection—A generic model and novel methodology to guide earlier detection supported by data from low- and mid-income countries. *Frontiers in Public Health*, 8, 452. DOI: 10.3389/fpubh.2020.00452 PMID: 33014967

Su, K., Xu, L., Li, G., Ruan, X., Li, X., Deng, P., Li, X., Li, Q., Chen, X., Xiong, Y., Lu, S., Qi, L., Shen, C., Tang, W., Rong, R., Hong, B., Ning, Y., Long, D., Xu, J., & Li, Y. (2019). Forecasting influenza activity using a self-adaptive AI model and multi-source data in Chongqing, China. [CrossRef]. *EBioMedicine*, 47, 284–292. DOI: 10.1016/j.ebiom.2019.08.024 PMID: 31477561

Thorlund, K., Haggstrom, J., Park, J. J., & Mills, E. J. (2018). Key design considerations for adaptive clinical trials: A primer for clinicians. [CrossRef]. *BMJ (Clinical Research Ed.)*, 360, k698. DOI: 10.1136/bmj.k698 PMID: 29519932

Tufts Center for the Study of Drug Development. (2014). *The cost of developing a new drug*. Tufts University. https://csdd.tufts.edu

Tushman, M. L., & Anderson, P. (1986). Technological discontinuities and organizational environments. *Administrative Science Quarterly*, 31(3), 439–465. DOI: 10.2307/2392832

Tyson, L. D., & Zysman, J. (2022). Automation, AI, and work. *Daedalus*, 151(2), 256–271. https://www.jstor.org/stable/48662040. DOI: 10.1162/daed_a_01914

UNCTAD. (2021). *Digital Economy Report. Cross-Border Data Flows and Development: For Whom the Data Flows*. United Nations Publication.

Unger, J. M. (2019). Vaidya, R.; Hershman, D.L.; Minasian, L.M.; E Fleury, M. Systematic Review and Meta-Analysis of the Magnitude of Structural, Clinical, and Physician and Patient Barriers to Cancer Clinical Trial Participation. [CrossRef]. *Gynecologic Oncology*, 111, 245–255. PMID: 30856272

Venkatramanan, S., Sadilek, A., Fadikar, A., Barrett, C. L., Biggerstaff, M., Chen, J., Dotiwalla, X., Eastham, P., Gipson, B., Higdon, D., Kucuktunc, O., Lieber, A., Lewis, B. L., Reynolds, Z., Vullikanti, A. K., Wang, L., & Marathe, M. (2021). Forecasting Influenza Activity Using Machine-Learned Mobility Map. [CrossRef] [PubMed]. *Nature Communications*, 12(1), 726. DOI: 10.1038/s41467-021-21018-5 PMID: 33563980

Whitley, D. (1994). A genetic algorithm tutorial. *Statistics and Computing*, 4(1), 65–85.

Xiong, Y., Ba, X., Hou, A., Zhang, K., Chen, L., & Li, T. (2018). Automatic detection of mycobacterium tuberculosis using artificial intelligence. [CrossRef]. *Journal of Thoracic Disease*, 10(3), 1936–1940. DOI: 10.21037/jtd.2018.01.91 PMID: 29707349

Yu, C. S., Chang, S. S., Chang, T. H., Wu, J. L., Lin, Y. J., Chien, H. F., & Chen, R. J. A. (2021). COVID-19 Pandemic Artificial Intelligence–Based System with Deep Learning Forecasting and Automatic Statistical Data Acquisition: Development and Implementation Study. [CrossRef]. *Journal of Medical Internet Research*, 23(5), e27806. DOI: 10.2196/27806 PMID: 33900932

Zhang, P., Chen, B., Ma, L., Li, Z., Song, Z., Duan, W., & Qiu, X. (2015). The Large Scale Machine Learning in an Artificial Society: Prediction of the Ebola Outbreak in Beijing. [CrossRef] [PubMed]. *Computational Intelligence and Neuroscience*, 2015, 1–12. DOI: 10.1155/2015/531650 PMID: 26457078

Compilation of References

Abbas, K., Afaq, M., Ahmed Khan, T., & Song, W. C. (2020). A blockchain and machine learning-based drug supply chain management and recommendation system for the smart pharmaceutical industry. *Electronics (Basel)*, *9*(5), 852. DOI: 10.3390/electronics9050852

Abdallah, S., & Nizamuddin, N. Blockchain-based solution for Pharma Supply Chain Industry, Computers & Industrial Engineering, Volume 177,2023,108997,ISSN 0360-8352,DOI: 10.1016/j.cie.2023.108997

Abdullahi, M., Adeniji, S. E., Arthur, D. E., & Musa, S. (2020). Quantitative structure-activity relationship (QSAR) modelling study of some novel carboxamide series as new anti-tubercular agents. *Bulletin of the National Research Center*, *44*(1), 136. DOI: 10.1186/s42269-020-00389-7

Abdullah, Z. (2023). Transforming Healthcare through AI: Unleashing the Power of Personalized Medicine. DOI: DOI: 10.47709/ijmdsa.v2i1.2424

Abulibdeh, A., Zaidan, E., & Abulibdeh, R. (2024). Navigating the confluence of artificial intelligence and education for sustainable development in the era of industry 4.0: Challenges, opportunities, and ethical dimensions. *Journal of Cleaner Production*. https://doi.org/10.1016/j.jclepro.2023.140527

Abusamaan, M. S., Ballreich, J., Dobs, A., Kane, B., Maruthur, N., McGready, J., Riekert, K., Wanigatunga, A. A., Alderfer, M., Alver, D., Lalani, B., Ringham, B., Vandi, F., Zade, D., & Mathioudakis, N. N. (2024). Effectiveness of artificial intelligence vs. human coaching in diabetes prevention: A study protocol for a randomized controlled trial. *Trials*, *25*(1), 325. DOI: 10.1186/s13063-024-08177-8 PMID: 38755706

Adeniyi, A. A., & Soliman, M. E. (2017). Implementing QM in docking calculations: Is it a waste of computational time? *Drug Discovery Today*, *22*(8), 1216–1223. DOI: 10.1016/j.drudis.2017.06.012 PMID: 28689054

Afzal, A. M., Mussa, H. Y., Turner, R. E., Bender, A., & Glen, R. C. (2015). A Multi-Label Approach to Target Prediction Taking Ligand Promiscuity into Account. *Journal of Cheminformatics*, *7*(1), 24. DOI: 10.1186/s13321-015-0071-9 PMID: 26064191

Ahmed, S. F., Bin, S., Hassan, M., Rozbu, M. R., Ishtiak, T., Rafa, N., Mofijur, M., Ali, A. B. M. S., & Gandomi, A. H. (2023). Deep learning modelling techniques: Current progress, applications, advantages, and challenges. *Artificial Intelligence Review*, *56*(11), 13521–13617. Advance online publication. DOI: 10.1007/s10462-023-10466-8

Ahmed, Z., & Barber, N., Yogini, Sara, J. ;, Bryony, G. ;, & Franklin, D. (n.d.). *Elsevier Editorial System(tm) for International Journal of Medical Informatics Manuscript Draft Title: Economic impact of electronic prescribing in the hospital setting: a systematic review*. DOI: 10.1186/s13195-021-00951-z PMID: 35012639

Ahrens, E. K. F. (1988). *Chemical Structures*. Springer Berlin Heidelberg. [Google Scholar]

Akhoon, N. (2021). Precision medicine: a new paradigm in therapeutics. International journal of preventive medicine. lww.comDOI: 10.3390/pr10061107

Akhtar, M., Kraemer, M. U. G., & Gardner, L. M. (2019). A dynamic neural network model for predicting risk of Zika in real-time. *BMC Medicine*, *17*(1), 171. DOI: 10.1186/s12916-019-1389-3 PMID: 31474220

Alexander, M., Solomon, B., Ball, D. L., Sheerin, M., Dankwa-Mullan, I., Preininger, A. M., Jackson, G. P., & Herath, D. M. (2020). Evaluation of an artificial intelligence clinical trial matching system in Australian lung cancer patients. *JAMIA Open*, *3*(2), 209–215. DOI: 10.1093/jamiaopen/ooaa002 PMID: 32734161

Aliper, A., Plis, S., Artemov, A., Ulloa, A., Mamoshina, P., & Zhavoronkov, A. (2016). Deep Learning Applications for Predicting Pharmacological Properties of Drugs and Drug Repurposing Using Transcriptomic Data. *Molecular Pharmaceutics*, *13*(7), 2524–2530. DOI: 10.1021/acs.molpharmaceut.6b00248 PMID: 27200455

Alom, M. Z., Taha, T. M., Yakopcic, C., Westberg, S., Sidike, P., Nasrin, M. S., ... & Asari, V. K. (2018). *The history began from alexnet: A comprehensive survey on deep learning approaches*. arXiv preprint arXiv:1803.01164.

Alonso, A. K. M., Hirt, J., Woelfle, T., Janiaud, P., & Hemkens, L. G. (2023). Definitions of digital biomarkers: a systematic mapping of the biomedical literature. *medRxiv. medrxiv*.org DOI: 10.1101/2023.09.01.23294897

Alowais, S. A., Alghamdi, S. S., Alsuhebany, N., Alqahtani, T., Alshaya, A. I., Almohareb, S. N., Aldairem, A., Alrashed, M., Bin Saleh, K., Badreldin, H. A., Al Yami, M. S., Al Harbi, S., & Albekairy, A. M. (2023). Revolutionizing healthcare: The role of artificial intelligence in clinical practice. *BMC Medical Education*, *23*(1), 689. DOI: 10.1186/s12909-023-04698-z PMID: 37740191

Alskaf, E., Frey, S. M., Scannell, C. M., Suinesiaputra, A., Vilic, D., Dinu, V., Masci, P. G., Perera, D., Young, A., & Chiribiri, A. (2024). Machine learning outcome prediction using stress perfusion cardiac magnetic resonance reports and natural language processing of electronic health records. *Informatics in Medicine Unlocked*, *44*, 101418. DOI: 10.1016/j.imu.2023.101418 PMID: 38173908

Al-Taee, M. A., Kapoor, R., Garrett, C., & Choudhary, P. (2016). Acceptability of Robot Assistant in Management of Type 1 Diabetes in Children. *Diabetes Technology & Therapeutics*, *18*(9), 551–554. DOI: 10.1089/dia.2015.0428 PMID: 27479198

Amadin, F. I., & Bello, M. E. (2018). Prediction of yellow fever using multilayer perceptron neural network classifier. *Journal of Emerging Trends in Engineering and Applied Sciences*, *9*, 282–286.

Andrade, , R. JChalasani, , NBjörnsson, , E. SSuzuki, , AKullak-Ublick, , G. AWatkins, , P. BAithal, , G. P. (2019). Drug-induced liver injury. *Nature Reviews. Disease Primers*, *5*(1), 58.

Arin, H. (2023). *AI and the Human Experience: Embracing the Age of Intelligent Machines*.

Aronson, A. R., & Lang, F. M. (2010). An overview of MetaMap: Historical perspective and recent advances. *Journal of the American Medical Informatics Association : JAMIA*, *17*(3), 229–236. DOI: 10.1136/jamia.2009.002733 PMID: 20442139

Arús-Pous, J., Awale, M., Probst, D., & Reymond, J. L. (2019). Exploring chemical space with machine learning. *Chimia*, *73*(12), 1018–1018. DOI: 10.2533/chimia.2019.1018 PMID: 31883554

Asad, M., Mahmood, A., & Usman, M. (2020). A machine learning-based framework for predicting treatment failure in tuberculosis: A case study of six countries. *Tuberculosis (Edinburgh, Scotland)*, *123*, 101944. DOI: 10.1016/j.tube.2020.101944 PMID: 32741529

Asare, P., Otchere, I. D., Bedeley, E., Brites, D., Loiseau, C., Baddoo, N. A., Asante-Poku, A., Osei-Wusu, S., Prah, D. A., Borrell, S., Reinhard, M., Forson, A., Koram, K. A., Gagneux, S., & Yeboah-Manu, D. (2020). Whole genome sequencing and spatial analysis identifies recent tuberculosis transmission hotspots in Ghana. *Frontiers of Medicine*, *7*, 161. DOI: 10.3389/fmed.2020.00161 PMID: 32509791

Askin, S., Burkhalter, D., Calado, G., & El Dakrouni, S. (2023). Artificial Intelligence Applied to clinical trials: Opportunities and challenges. *Health and Technology*, *13*(2), 203–213. DOI: 10.1007/s12553-023-00738-2 PMID: 36923325

Assiri, S., Alyamani, M., Mansour, A., Fakieh, B., Badri, S., & Babour, A. 2020. Current Shipment Tracking Technologies and Trends in Research. In *Proceedings of the 2020 the 4th International Conference on Information System and Data Mining (ICISDM '20)*. Association for Computing Machinery, New York, NY, USA, 113–117. https://doi.org/DOI: 10.1145/3404663.3404683

Åström, J., Reim, W., & Parida, V. (2022). Value creation and value capture for AI business model innovation: A three-phase process framework. *Review of Managerial Science*, *16*(7), 2111–2133. DOI: 10.1007/s11846-022-00521-z

Atanasov, A. G., Zotchev, S. B., Dirsch, V. M., & Supuran, C. T. (2021). International natural product sciences taskforce. *Nature Reviews. Drug Discovery*, *20*(3), 200–216. DOI: 10.1038/s41573-020-00114-z PMID: 33510482

Auffray, C., Balling, R., Barroso, I., Bencze, L., Benson, M., Bergeron, J., Bernal-Delgado, E., Blomberg, N., Bock, C., Conesa, A., Del Signore, S., Delogne, C., Devilee, P., Di Meglio, A., Eijkemans, M., Flicek, P., Graf, N., Grimm, V., Guchelaar, H., & Zanetti, G. (2016c). Making sense of big data in health research: Towards an EU action plan. *Genome Medicine*, *8*(1), 71. Advance online publication. DOI: 10.1186/s13073-016-0323-y PMID: 27338147

Avacharmal, R., Pamulaparthyvenkata, S., & Gudala, L. (2023). Unveiling the Pandora's Box: A Multifaceted Exploration of Ethical Considerations in Generative AI for Financial Services and Healthcare. *Hong Kong Journal of AI and Medicine*, *3*(1), 84–99.

Azad, A. K., Sadee, W., & Schlesinger, L. S. (2012). Innate immune gene polymorphisms in tuberculosis. *Infection and Immunity*, *80*(10), 3343–3359. DOI: 10.1128/IAI.00443-12 PMID: 22825450

Aznar-Lou, I., Fernández, A., Gil-Girbau, M., Fajó-Pascual, M., Moreno-Peral, P., Peñarrubia-María, M. T., Serrano-Blanco, A., Sánchez-Niubó, A., March-Pujol, M. A., Jové, A. M., & Rubio-Valera, M. (2017). Initial medication non-adherence: Prevalence and predictive factors in a 1.6 million primary care patients cohort. *British Journal of Clinical Pharmacology, 83*(6), 1328–1340. DOI: 10.1111/bcp.13215 PMID: 28229476

Badal, V. D., Kundrotas, P. J., & Vakser, I. A. (2015). Text mining for protein docking. *PLoS Computational Biology, 11*(12), e1004630. DOI: 10.1371/journal.pcbi.1004630 PMID: 26650466

Badal, V. D., Kundrotas, P. J., & Vakser, I. A. (2021). Text mining for modeling of protein complexes enhanced by machine learning. *Bioinformatics, 37*(4), 497-505. 69Tsai F. S. *International Journal of Computational Biology and Drug Design, 2011*(4), 239–244. DOI: 10.1504/IJCBDD.2011.041412

Bade, S. O., & Tomomewo, O. S. (2024). A review of governance strategies, policy measures, and regulatory framework for hydrogen energy in the United States. *International Journal of Hydrogen Energy, 78*, 1363–1381. DOI: 10.1016/j.ijhydene.2024.06.338

Bain, E. E., Shafner, L., Walling, D. P., Othman, A. A., Chuang-Stein, C., Hinkle, J., & Hanina, A. (2017). Use of a Novel Artificial Intelligence Platform on Mobile Devices to Assess Dosing Compliance in a Phase 2 Clinical Trial in Subjects with Schizophrenia. *JMIR mHealth and uHealth, 5*(2), e18. DOI: 10.2196/mhealth.7030 PMID: 28223265

Bajusz, D., Rácz, A., & Héberger, K. (2015). Why is Tanimoto index an appropriate choice for fingerprint-based similarity calculations? *Journal of Cheminformatics, 7*(1), 1–13. DOI: 10.1186/s13321-015-0069-3 PMID: 26052348

Bakuła, Z., Marczak, M., Bluszcz, A., Proboszcz, M., Kościuch, J., Krenke, R., Stakėnas, P., Mokrousov, I., & Jagielski, T. (2023). Phylogenetic relationships of *Mycobacterium tuberculosis*isolates in Poland: The emergence of Beijing genotype among multiRifampicin-resistant cases. *Frontiers in Cellular and Infection Microbiology, 13*, 1161905. DOI: 10.3389/fcimb.2023.1161905 PMID: 37009494

Barnes, E. C., Kumar, R., & Davis, R. A. (2016). The use of isolated natural products as scaffolds for the generation of chemically diverse screening libraries for drug discovery. *Natural Product Reports, 33*(3), 372–381. DOI: 10.1039/C5NP00121H PMID: 26739749

Baron, R., Dickenson, A. H., Calvo, M., Dib-Hajj, S. D., & Bennett, D. L. (2023). Maximizing treatment efficacy through patient stratification in neuropathic pain trials. *Nature Reviews. Neurology*, *19*(1), 53–64. DOI: 10.1038/s41582-022-00741-7 PMID: 36400867

Bateson, A., Ortiz Canseco, J., Mchugh, T. D., Witney, A. A., Feuerriegel, S., Merker, M., Kohl, T. A., Utpatel, C., Niemann, S., Andres, S., Kranzer, K., Maurer, F. P., Ghodousi, A., Borroni, E., Cirillo, D. M., Wijkander, M., Toro, J. C., Groenheit, R., Werngren, J., & Timm, J. (2022). Ancient and recent differences in the intrinsic susceptibility of *Mycobacterium tuberculosis* complex to pretomanid. *The Journal of Antimicrobial Chemotherapy*, *77*(6), 1685–1693. DOI: 10.1093/jac/dkac070 PMID: 35260883

Batko, K., & Ślęzak, A. (2022). The Use of Big Data Analytics in Healthcare. *Journal of Big Data*, *9*(1), 3. Advance online publication. DOI: 10.1186/s40537-021-00553-4 PMID: 35013701

Beck, B. R., Shin, B., Choi, Y., Park, S., & Kang, K. (2020). Predicting commercially available antiviral drugs that may act on the novel coronavirus (SARS-CoV-2) through a drug-target interaction deep learning model. *Computational and Structural Biotechnology Journal*, *18*, 784–790. DOI: 10.1016/j.csbj.2020.03.025 PMID: 32280433

Begam, B. F., & Kumar, J. S. (2012). A Study on Cheminformatics and Its Applications on Modern Rifampicin Discovery. *Procedia Engineering*, *38*, 1264–1275. DOI: 10.1016/j.proeng.2012.06.156

Begum, M. S., Haris, R., Vetrimaran, V., & Raj, P. A. "Prediction of Herbs with its Benefits using Deep Learning Techniques," *2022 International Conference on Sustainable Computing and Data Communication Systems (ICSCDS)*, Erode, India, 2022, pp. 307-310, doi: DOI: 10.1109/ICSCDS53736.2022.9760850

Belue, M. J., Harmon, S. A., Chappidi, S., Zhuge, Y., Tasci, E., Jagasia, S., Joyce, T., Camphausen, K., Turkbey, B., & Krauze, A. V. (2024). Diagnosing progression in glioblastoma—Tackling a neuro-oncology problem using artificial-intelligence-derived volumetric change over time on magnetic resonance imaging to examine progression-free survival in glioblastoma. *Diagnostics (Basel)*, *14*(13), 1374. DOI: 10.3390/diagnostics14131374 PMID: 39001264

Benchimol, E. I., Smeeth, L., Guttmann, A., Harron, K., Moher, D., Petersen, I., Sørensen, H. T., von Elm, E., & Langan, S. M. (2015). The REporting of studies Conducted using Observational Routinely-collected health Data (RECORD) Statement. *PLoS Medicine*, *12*(10), e1001885. DOI: 10.1371/journal.pmed.1001885 PMID: 26440803

Benjamens, S., Dhunnoo, P., & Meskó, B. (2020). The state of artificial intelligence-based FDA-approved medical devices and algorithms: an online database. *NPJ digital medicine*.

Berlinski, D. (2000). *The advent of the algorithm*. Harcourt Books. Dosi, G., & Virgillito, M. E. (2019). What is the evolution of the contemporary social fabric? New technologies and old socio-economic trends. *International Labour Review*, *158*(4), 593–625. DOI: 10.1111/ilr.12179

Berman, F., Fox, G., & Hey, T. (2003). Overview of the book: grid computing–making the global infrastructure a reality. *Grid computing: Making the global infrastructure a reality*, 1-8.

Berrocal-Almanza, L. C., Harris, R. J., Collin, S. M., Muzyamba, M. C., Conroy, O. D., Mirza, A., O'Connell, A.-M., Altass, L., Anderson, S. R., Thomas, H. L., Campbell, C., Zenner, D., Phin, N., Kon, O. M., Smith, E. G., & Lalvani, A. (2022). Effectiveness of nationwide programmatic testing and treatment for latent tuberculosis infection in migrants in England: A retrospective, population-based cohort study. *The Lancet. Public Health*, *7*(4), e305–e315. DOI: 10.1016/S2468-2667(22)00031-7 PMID: 35338849

Berry, M., Fielding, B. C., & Gamieldien, J. (2015). Potential broad spectrum inhibitors of the coronavirus 3CLpro: A virtual screening and structure-based drug design study. *Viruses*, *7*(12), 6642–6660. DOI: 10.3390/v7122963 PMID: 26694449

Bertsimas, D., Antonios Margonis, G., Sujichantararat, S., Koulouras, A., Ma, Y., Antonescu, C. R., & Singer, S. (2024). Interpretable artificial intelligence to optimize use of imatinib after resection in patients with localized gastrointestinal stromal tumors: An observational cohort study. *The Lancet. Oncology*. DOI: 10.1016/S1470-2045(24)00259-6 PMID: 38976997

Bhatt, A. (2019). Conducting real-world evidence studies in India. *Perspectives in Clinical Research*, *10*(2), 51. DOI: 10.4103/picr.PICR_8_19 PMID: 31008069

Bhattamisra, S. K., Banerjee, P., Gupta, P., Mayuren, J., Patra, S., & Candasamy, M. (2023). Artificial intelligence in pharmaceutical and healthcare research. *Big Data and Cognitive Computing*, *7*(1), 10. DOI: 10.3390/bdcc7010010

Bindra, S., & Jain, R. (2024). Artificial intelligence in medical science: A review. *Irish Journal of Medical Science*, *193*(3), 1419–1429. DOI: 10.1007/s11845-023-03570-9 PMID: 37952245

Bishop, C. M. (2013). Model-based machine learning. *Philosophical Transactions. Series A, Mathematical, Physical, and Engineering Sciences*, •••, 371. PMID: 23277612

Bisht, N., & Singh, B. K. (2018). Role of computer aided drug design in drug development and drug discovery. *International Journal of Pharmaceutical Sciences and Research*, *9*(4), 1405–1415.

Bizzarri, M., Fedeli, V., Monti, N., Cucina, A., Jalouli, M., Alwasel, S. H., & Harrath, A. H. (2021). Personalization of medical treatments in oncology: Time for rethinking the disease concept to improve individual outcomes. [springer.com]. *The EPMA Journal*, *12*(4), 1–14. DOI: 10.1007/s13167-021-00254-1 PMID: 34642594

Blalock, S. J. (2011). The theoretical basis for practice-relevant medication use research: Patient-centered/behavioral theories. *Research in Social & Administrative Pharmacy*, *7*(4), 317–329. DOI: 10.1016/j.sapharm.2010.11.001 PMID: 21272552

Blanco-Gonzalez, A., Cabezon, A., Seco-Gonzalez, A., Conde-Torres, D., Antelo-Riveiro, P., Pineiro, A., & Garcia-Fandino, R. (2023). The role of AI in drug discovery: Challenges, opportunities, and strategies. *Pharmaceuticals (Basel, Switzerland)*, *16*(6), 891. DOI: 10.3390/ph16060891 PMID: 37375838

Blei, D., Ng, A., & Jordan, M. (2003). Latent Dirichlet Allocation. *Journal of Machine Learning Research*, *3*, 993–1022. https://www.jmlr.org/papers/volume3/blei03a/blei03a.pdf

Boadu, A. A., & Asase, A. (2017). Documentation of herbal medicines used for the treatment and management of human diseases by some communities in southern Ghana. *Evidence-Based Complementary and Alternative Medicine : eCAM*, *2017*(1), 3043061. DOI: 10.1155/2017/3043061 PMID: 28684965

Boldi, A. M. (2004). Libraries from natural product-like scaffolds. *Current Opinion in Chemical Biology*, *8*(3), 281–286. DOI: 10.1016/j.cbpa.2004.04.010 PMID: 15183326

Bonnet, I., Enouf, V., Morel, F., Ok, V., Jaffré, J., & Jarlier, V.. (2021). A comprehensive evaluation of GeneLEAD VIII DNA platform combined to Deeplex Myc-TB® assay to detect in 8 days Rifampicin resistance to 13 antituberculous Rifampicins and transmission of *Mycobacterium tuberculosis* complex directly from clinical samples. *Frontiers in Cellular and Infection Microbiology, 11*, 707244. DOI: 10.3389/fcimb.2021.707244 PMID: 34778100

Borgelt, C. (2005). An implementation of the FP-growth algorithm. *Proceedings of the 1st International Workshop on Open Source Data Mining Frequent Pattern Mining Implementations - OSDM '05*. DOI: 10.1145/1133905.1133907

Borquaye, L. S., Gasu, E. N., Ampomah, G. B., Kyei, L. K., Amarh, M. A., Mensah, C. N., Nartey, D., Commodore, M., Adomako, A. K., Acheampong, P., Mensah, J. O., Mormor, D. B., & Aboagye, C. I. (2020). Alkaloids from Cryptolepis sanguinolenta as potential inhibitors of SARS-CoV-2 viral proteins: An in silico study. *BioMed Research International, 2020*(1), 5324560. DOI: 10.1155/2020/5324560 PMID: 33029513

Botha, G. H. R., Theron, G., Warren, R. M., Klopper, M., Dheda, K., Van Helden, P. D., & Niesler, T. R. (2018). Detection of tuberculosis by automatic cough sound analysis. *Physiological Measurement, 39*(4), 045005. DOI: 10.1088/1361-6579/aab6d0 PMID: 29543189

Bouwmeester, R., Martens, L., & Degroeve, S. (2019). Comprehensive and empirical evaluation of machine learning algorithms for small molecule LC retention time prediction. *Analytical Chemistry, 91*(5), 3694–3703. DOI: 10.1021/acs.analchem.8b05820 PMID: 30702864

Breiman, L. (2001). Random Forests. *Machine Learning, 45*(1), 5–32. DOI: 10.1023/A:1010933404324

Breinbauer, R., Vetter, I. R., & Waldmann, H. (2002). From protein domains to drug candidates—Natural products as guiding principles in the design and synthesis of compound libraries. *Angewandte Chemie International Edition, 41*(16), 2878–2890. DOI: 10.1002/1521-3773(20020816)41:16<2878::AID-ANIE2878>3.0.CO;2-B PMID: 12203413

Briesacher, B. A., Andrade, S. E., Fouayzi, H., & Chan, K. A. (2008). Comparison of drug adherence rates among patients with seven different medical conditions. *Pharmacotherapy, 28*(4), 437–443. DOI: 10.1592/phco.28.4.437 PMID: 18363527

Brom, H., Brooks Carthon, J. M., Ikeaba, U., & Chittams, J. (2020). Leveraging Electronic Health Records and Machine Learning to Tailor Nursing Care for Patients at High Risk for Readmissions. *Journal of Nursing Care Quality*, *35*(1), 27–33. DOI: 10.1097/NCQ.0000000000000412 PMID: 31136529

Brown, M. T., & Bussell, J. K. (2011). Medication adherence: WHO cares? *Mayo Clinic Proceedings*, *86*(4), 304–314. DOI: 10.4065/mcp.2010.0575 PMID: 21389250

Brown, N., Ertl, P., Lewis, R., Luksch, T., Reker, D., & Schneider, N. (2020). Artificial intelligence in chemistry and drug design. *Journal of Computer-Aided Molecular Design*, *34*(7), 709–715. DOI: 10.1007/s10822-020-00317-x PMID: 32468207

Burke, R. M., Shah, M. P., Wikswo, M. E., Barclay, L., Kambhampati, A., Marsh, Z., Cannon, J. L., Parashar, U. D., Vinjé, J., & Hall, A. J. (2018). The norovirus epidemiologic triad: Predictors of severe outcomes in US norovirus outbreaks, 2009–2016. *The Journal of Infectious Diseases*, *219*(9), 1364–1372. DOI: 10.1093/infdis/jiy569 PMID: 30445538

Busia, K. (Ed.). (2007). *Ghana herbal pharmacopoeia*. Science and Technology Policy Research Institute, Council for Scientific and Industrial Research.

Butticè, V., Caviggioli, F., Franzoni, C., Scellato, G., Stryszowski, P., & Thumm, N. (2020). Counterfeiting in digital technologies: An empirical analysis of the economic performance and innovative activities of affected companies, Research Policy, Volume 49, Issue 5, 103959,ISSN 0048-7333,DOI: 10.1016/j.respol.2020.103959

Cabibbe, A. M., Spitaleri, A., Battaglia, S., Colman, R. E., Suresh, A., Uplekar, S., Rodwell, T. C., & Cirillo, D. M. (2020). Application of targeted next-generation sequencing assay on a portable sequencing platform for culture-free detection of Rifampicin-resistant tuberculosis from clinical samples. *Journal of Clinical Microbiology*, *58*(10), e00632–e00620. DOI: 10.1128/JCM.00632-20 PMID: 32727827

Cabitza, F., Locoro, A., & Banfi, G. (2018). Machine Learning in Orthopedics: A Literature Review. *Frontiers in Bioengineering and Biotechnology*, *6*, 75. Advance online publication. DOI: 10.3389/fbioe.2018.00075 PMID: 29998104

Cai, C., Xu, L., Fang, J., Dai, Z., Wu, Q., Liu, X., Wang, Q., Fang, J., Liu, A.-L., & Du, G. H. (2021). In silico prediction and bioactivity evaluation of chemical ingredients against influenza a virus from Isatis tinctoria L. *Frontiers in Pharmacology*, *12*, 755396. DOI: 10.3389/fphar.2021.755396 PMID: 34950027

Cañamero, L., & Lewis, M. (2016). Making New "New AI" Friends: Designing a Social Robot for Diabetic Children from an Embodied AI Perspective. *International Journal of Social Robotics*, *8*(4), 523–537. DOI: 10.1007/s12369-016-0364-9

Carhart, R. E., Smith, D. H., & Venkataraghavan, R. E. N. G. A. C. H. A. R. I. (1985). Atom pairs as molecular features in structure-activity studies: Definition and applications. *Journal of Chemical Information and Computer Sciences*, *25*(2), 64–73. DOI: 10.1021/ci00046a002

Carmo-Fonseca, M. (2021). *Precision Medicine: Enabling Healthcare Progress in the Twenty-First Century*. Precision Medicine in Stroke. [HTML]

Caruana, R., Lou, Y., Gehrke, J., Koch, P., Sturm, M., & Elhadad, N. (2015). Intelligible Models for HealthCare. *Proceedings of the 21th ACM SIGKDD International Conference on Knowledge Discovery and Data Mining - KDD '15*. DOI: 10.1145/2783258.2788613

Cavaco, M. J., Alcobia, C., Oliveiros, B., Mesquita, L. A., Carvalho, A., Matos, F., Carvalho, J. M., Villar, M., Duarte, R., Mendes, J., Ribeiro, C., Cordeiro, C. R., Regateiro, F., & Silva, H. C. (2022). Clinical and genetic risk factors for Rifampicin-induced liver injury associated with anti-tuberculosis treatment—A study from patients of Portuguese health centers. *Journal of Personalized Medicine*, *12*(5), 790. DOI: 10.3390/jpm12050790 PMID: 35629211

Centers for Disease Control and Prevention. (2023). *Chronic diseases in America*. National Center for Chronic Disease Prevention and Health Promotion. https://www.cdc.gov/chronicdisease/pdf/infographics/chronic-disease-in-america-H.pdf

Chaix, B., Bibault, J., Pienkowski, A., Delamon, G., Guillemassé, A., Nectoux, P., & Brouard, B. (2019). When Chatbots Meet Patients: One-Year Prospective Study of Conversations Between Patients with Breast Cancer and a Chatbot. *JMIR Cancer*, *5*(1), e12856. DOI: 10.2196/12856 PMID: 31045505

Chandola, V., Banerjee, A., & Kumar, V. (2009). Anomaly Detection: A Survey. *ACM Computing Surveys*, *41*(3), 1–58. DOI: 10.1145/1541880.1541882

Chandra, S., Prakash, P. K. S., Samanta, S., & Chilukuri, S. (2024). ClinicalGAN: Powering patient monitoring in clinical trials with patient digital twins. *Scientific Reports*, *14*(1), 12236. DOI: 10.1038/s41598-024-62567-1 PMID: 38806536

Chang, S. E., & Chen, Y. (2020, August 31). Blockchain in Health Care Innovation: Literature Review and Case Study From a Business Ecosystem Perspective. *Journal of Medical Internet Research*, *22*(8), e19480. DOI: 10.2196/19480 PMID: 32865501

Chaoyong, W. (2022). Jianxin, Chen., Elaine, Lai-Han, Leung., Hang, Chang., Xu, Wang. Editorial: Artificial Intelligence in Traditional Medicine. *Frontiers in Pharmacology*, *13*, 933133. Advance online publication. DOI: 10.3389/fphar.2022.933133

Chávez-Fumagalli, M. A., Schneider, M. S., Lage, D. P., Tavares, G. D. S. V., Mendonça, D. V. C., Santos, T. T. D. O., Pádua, R. M., Machado-de-Ávila, R. A., Leite, J. P. V., & Coelho, E. A. F. (2018). A computational approach using bioinformatics to screening drug targets for Leishmania infantum species. *Evidence-Based Complementary and Alternative Medicine : eCAM*, *2018*(1), 6813467. DOI: 10.1155/2018/6813467 PMID: 29785196

Cheen, M. H., Tan, Y. Z., Ng, S. W., Chan, H. K., & Lim, L. M. (2019). A systematic review of medication adherence and health outcomes in patients with chronic disease. *Journal of Clinical Pharmacy and Therapeutics*, *44*(1), 1–10. DOI: 10.1111/jcpt.12768 PMID: 30171815

Chen, C. Y. C. (2011). TCM Database@ Taiwan: The world's largest traditional Chinese medicine database for drug screening in silico. *PLoS One*, *6*(1), e15939. DOI: 10.1371/journal.pone.0015939 PMID: 21253603

Cheng, H.-Y., Wu, Y.-C., Lin, M.-H., Liu, Y.-L., Tsai, Y.-Y., Wu, J.-H., Pan, K.-H., Ke, C.-J., Chen, C.-M., Liu, D.-P., Lin, I.-F., & Chuang, J.-H. (2020). Applying Machine Learning Models with An Ensemble Approach for Accurate Real-Time Influenza Forecasting in Taiwan: Development and Validation Study. [CrossRef]. *Journal of Medical Internet Research*, *22*(8), e15394. DOI: 10.2196/15394 PMID: 32755888

Chen, H., Engkvist, O., Wang, Y., Olivecrona, M., & Blaschke, T. (2018). The rise of deep learning in drug discovery. *Drug Discovery Today*, *23*(6), 1241–1250. DOI: 10.1016/j.drudis.2018.01.039 PMID: 29366762

Chen, S., Gong, E., Kazi, D. S., Gates, A. B., Karate, K. M., Girder, N., Bai, R., Alabi, K. F., Li, C., Sun, K., Hong, L., Fu, H., Peng, W., Liu, X., Chen, L., Schwalm, J., & Yan, L. L. (2016). Development of a mobile phone-based intervention to improve adherence to secondary prevention of coronary heart disease in China. *Journal of Medical Engineering & Technology*, *40*(7–8), 372–382. DOI: 10.1080/03091902.2016.1213904 PMID: 27686107

Chen, X., He, G., Lin, S., Wang, S., Sun, F., Chen, J., & Zhang, W. (2020). Analysis of serial multiRifampicin-resistant tuberculosis strains causing treatment failure and within-host evolution by whole-genome sequencing. *MSphere*, *5*(6), e00884–e00820. DOI: 10.1128/mSphere.00884-20 PMID: 33361124

Chen, X., & Reynolds, C. H. (2002). Performance of similarity measures in 2D fragment-based similarity searching: Comparison of structural descriptors and similarity coefficients. *Journal of Chemical Information and Computer Sciences*, *42*(6), 1407–1414. DOI: 10.1021/ci025531g PMID: 12444738

Chen, Y. C. (2015). Beware of docking! *Trends in Pharmacological Sciences*, *36*(2), 78–95. DOI: 10.1016/j.tips.2014.12.001 PMID: 25543280

Chen, Y., & Kirchmair, J. (2020). Cheminformatics in Natural Product-based Drug Discovery. *Molecular Informatics*, *39*(12), e2000171. DOI: 10.1002/minf.202000171 PMID: 32725781

Chen, Z., Zhao, M., You, L., Zheng, R., Jiang, Y., Zhang, X., Qiu, R., Sun, Y., Pan, H., He, T., Wei, X., Chen, Z., Zhao, C., & Shang, H. (2022). Developing an artificial intelligence method for screening hepatotoxic compounds in traditional chinese medicine and western medicine combination. *Chinese Medicine*, *17*(1), 58. DOI: 10.1186/s13020-022-00617-4 PMID: 35581608

Chisholm-Burns, M. A., & Spivey, C. A. (2012). The "cost" of medication nonadherence: Consequences we cannot afford to accept. *Journal of the American Pharmacists Association*, *52*(6), 823–826. DOI: 10.1331/JAPhA.2012.11088 PMID: 23229971

Choudhury, A., & Asan, O. (2020). Role of Artificial Intelligence in Patient Safety Outcomes: Systematic Literature Review. *JMIR Medical Informatics*, *8*(7), e18599. DOI: 10.2196/18599 PMID: 32706688

Christie, B. D., Leland, B. A., & Nourse, J. G. (1993). Structure searching in chemical databases by direct lookup methods. *Journal of Chemical Information and Computer Sciences*, *33*(4), 545–547. DOI: 10.1021/ci00014a004

Chuang, K. V., Gunsalus, L. M., & Keiser, M. J. (2020). Learning molecular representations for medicinal chemistry: Miniperspective. *Journal of Medicinal Chemistry*, *63*(16), 8705–8722. DOI: 10.1021/acs.jmedchem.0c00385 PMID: 32366098

Chu, H., Moon, S., Park, J., Bak, S., Ko, Y., & Youn, B. Y. (2022). The use of artificial intelligence in complementary and alternative medicine: A systematic scoping review. *Frontiers in Pharmacology*, *13*, 826044. DOI: 10.3389/fphar.2022.826044 PMID: 35431917

Ciallella, H. L., & Zhu, H. (2019). Advancing computational toxicology in the big data era by artificial intelligence: Data-driven and mechanism-driven modeling for chemical toxicity. *Chemical Research in Toxicology*, *32*(4), 536–547. DOI: 10.1021/acs.chemrestox.8b00393 PMID: 30907586

Cold, K. M., Xie, S., Nielsen, A. O., Clementsen, P. F., & Konge, L. (2024). Artificial intelligence improves novices' bronchoscopy performance: A Randomized controlled trial in a simulated setting. *Chest*, *165*(2), 405–413. DOI: 10.1016/j.chest.2023.08.015 PMID: 37619664

Colombo, S., Zeng, X., Ragelle, H., & Foged, C. (2014). Complexity in the Therapeutic Delivery of RNAi Medicines: An Analytical Challenge. *Expert Opinion on Drug Delivery*, *11*(9), 1481–1495. DOI: 10.1517/17425247.2014.927439 PMID: 24950005

Conn, V. S., Enriquez, M., Ropar, T. M., & Chan, K. C. (2016). Meta-analyses of Theory Use in Medication Adherence Intervention Research. *American Journal of Health Behavior*, *40*(2), 155–171. DOI: 10.5993/AJHB.40.2.1 PMID: 26931748

Conn, V. S., & Ruppar, T. M. (2017). Medication adherence outcomes of 771 intervention trials: Systematic review and meta-analysis. *Preventive Medicine*, *99*, 269–276. DOI: 10.1016/j.ypmed.2017.03.008 PMID: 28315760

Conn, V. S., Ruppar, T. M., Rn, M. E., & Cooper, P. S. (2016). Patient-Centered Outcomes of Medication Adherence Interventions: Systematic Review and Meta-Analysis. *Value in Health*, *19*(2), 277–285. DOI: 10.1016/j.jval.2015.12.001 PMID: 27021763

Corley, D. G., & Durley, R. C. (1994). Strategies for database dereplication of natural products. *Journal of Natural Products*, *57*(11), 1484–1490. DOI: 10.1021/np50113a002

Cornejo-Báez, A. A., Peña-Rodríguez, L. M., Álvarez-Zapata, R., Vázquez-Hernández, M., & Sánchez-Medina, A. (2020). Chemometrics: A complementary tool to guide the isolation of pharmacologically active natural products. *Drug Discovery Today*, *25*(1), 27–37. DOI: 10.1016/j.drudis.2019.09.016 PMID: 31600581

Coskun, B. N., Yagiz, B., Ocakoglu, G., Dalkilic, E., & Pehlivan, Y. (2024). Assessing the accuracy and completeness of artificial intelligence language models in providing information on methotrexate use. *Rheumatology International*, *44*(3), 509–515. DOI: 10.1007/s00296-023-05473-5 PMID: 37747564

Costa, M. S., Dória, F. A., Alves, T. G., Queiroz, F. M., & Nascimento Year, R. L. H.: 2022 Title: "Automated Identification of Medicinal Plants using Machine Learning Techniques" DOI: 10.3390/cells10113139 PMID: 34831362

Cox, H., Goig, G. A., Salaam-Dreyer, Z., Dippenaar, A., Reuter, A., Mohr-Holland, E., Daniels, J., Cudahy, P. G. T., Nicol, M. P., Borrell, S., Reinhard, M., Doetsch, A., Beisel, C., Gagneux, S., Warren, R. M., & Furin, J. (2022). Whole-genome sequencing has the potential to improve treatment for rifampicin-resistant tuberculosis in high-burden settings: A retrospective cohort study. *Journal of Clinical Microbiology*, *60*(3), e0236221. DOI: 10.1128/jcm.02362-21 PMID: 35170980

Cutler, R. L., Fernandez-Llimos, F., Frommer, M., Benrimoj, C., & Garcia-Cardenas, V. (2018). The economic impact of medication non-adherence by disease groups: A systematic review. *BMJ Open*, *8*(1), e016982. DOI: 10.1136/bmjopen-2017-016982 PMID: 29358417

Daina, A., Michielin, O., & Zoete, V. (2017). SwissADME: A free web tool to evaluate pharmacokinetics, drug-likeness and medicinal chemistry friendliness of small molecules. *Scientific Reports*, *7*(1), 42717. DOI: 10.1038/srep42717 PMID: 28256516

Daka, A., & Peer, D. (2012). RNAi-Based Nanomedicines for Targeted Personalized Therapy. *Advanced Drug Delivery Reviews*, *64*(13), 1508–1521. DOI: 10.1016/j.addr.2012.08.014 PMID: 22975009

Dale, K., Globan, M., Horan, K., Sherry, N., Ballard, S., Tay, E. L., Bittmann, S., Meagher, N., Price, D. J., Howden, B. P., Williamson, D. A., & Denholm, J. (2022). Whole genome sequencing for tuberculosis in Victoria, Australia: A genomic implementation study from 2017 to 2020. *The Lancet Regional Health. Western Pacific*, *28*, 100556. DOI: 10.1016/j.lanwpc.2022.100556 PMID: 36034164

Danker, T., & Möller, C. (2014). Early identification of hERG liability in drug discovery programs by automated patch clamp. *Frontiers in Pharmacology*, *5*, 203. DOI: 10.3389/fphar.2014.00203 PMID: 25228880

Dara, S., Dhamercherla, S., Jadav, S. S., Babu, C. M., & Ahsan, M. J. (2022). Machine learning in drug discovery: A review. *Artificial Intelligence Review*, *55*(3), 1947–1999. DOI: 10.1007/s10462-021-10058-4

Darwich, A. S., Polasek, T. M., Aronson, J. K., Ogungbenro, K., Wright, D. F., Achour, B., Reny, J.-L., Daali, Y., Eiermann, B., Cook, J., Lesko, L., McLachlan, A. J., & Rostami-Hodjegan, A. (2021). Model-informed precision dosing: Background, requirements, validation, implementation, and forward trajectory of individualizing drug therapy. [diva-portal.org]. *Annual Review of Pharmacology and Toxicology*, *61*(1), 225–245. DOI: 10.1146/annurev-pharmtox-033020-113257 PMID: 33035445

Dasarathy, S., Tu, W., Bellar, A., Welch, N., Kettler, C., Tang, Q., Liangpunsakul, S., Gawrieh, S., Radaeva, S., & Mitchell, M. (2024). Development and evaluation of objective trial performance metrics for multisite clinical studies: Experience from the AlcHep Network. *Contemporary Clinical Trials*, *138*, 107437. DOI: 10.1016/j.cct.2024.107437 PMID: 38215876

David, B., Wolfender, J. L., & Dias, D. A. (2015). The pharmaceutical industry and natural products: Historical status and new trends. *Phytochemistry Reviews*, *14*(2), 299–315. DOI: 10.1007/s11101-014-9367-z

David, C. (2023). "Just the Facts Ma'am": Moral and Ethical Considerations for Artificial Intelligence in Medicine and its Potential to Impact Patient Autonomy and Hope. *The Linacre Quarterly*, *90*(4), 375–394. Advance online publication. DOI: 10.1177/00243639231162431

Davison, E. K., & Brimble, M. A. (2019). Natural product derived privileged scaffolds in drug discovery. *Current Opinion in Chemical Biology*, *52*, 1–8. DOI: 10.1016/j.cbpa.2018.12.007 PMID: 30682725

De Cesco, S., Davis, J. B., & Brennan, P. E. (2020). TargetDB: A target information aggregation tool and tractability predictor. *PLoS One*, *15*(9), e0232644. DOI: 10.1371/journal.pone.0232644 PMID: 32877430

De Maria Marchiano, R., Di Sante, G., Piro, G., Carbone, C., Tortora, G., Boldrini, L., Pietragalla, A., Daniele, G., Tredicine, M., Cesario, A., Valentini, V., Gallo, D., Babini, G., D'Oria, M., & Scambia, G. (2021). Translational research in the era of precision medicine: Where we are and where we will go. [mdpi.com]. *Journal of Personalized Medicine*, *11*(3), 216. DOI: 10.3390/jpm11030216 PMID: 33803592

Dean, J., & Ghemawat, S. (2008). MapReduce: Simplified data processing on large clusters. *Communications of the ACM*, *51*(1), 107–113. DOI: 10.1145/1327452.1327492

Denck, J., Ozkirimli, E., & Wang, K. (2023). Machine-learning-based adverse drug event prediction from observational health data: A review. *Drug Discovery Today*, *28*(9), 103715. DOI: 10.1016/j.drudis.2023.103715 PMID: 37467879

Deng, S., Li, C., Cao, J., Cui, Z., Du, J., Fu, Z., Yang, H., & Chen, P. (2023). Organ-on-a-chip meets artificial intelligence in drug evaluation. In *Theranostics* (Vol. 13, Issue 13, pp. 4526–4558). Ivyspring International Publisher. DOI: 10.7150/thno.87266

Desai, N., Pande, S., Gholap, A. D., Rana, D., Salave, S., & Vora, L. K. (2024). Regulatory processes involved in clinical trials and intellectual property rights around vaccine development. In *Advanced Vaccination Technologies for Infectious and Chronic Diseases* (279–309). Academic Press.DOI: 10.1016/B978-0-443-18564-9.00008-4

Devlin, J., Chang, M.-W., Lee, K., & Toutanova, K. (2018, October 11). *BERT: Pre-training of Deep Bidirectional Transformers for Language Understanding*. ArXiv.org. https://arxiv.org/abs/1810.04805

Dhanwe, S. S., (2024). AI-driven IoT in Robotics: A Review. *Journal of Mechanisms and Robotics*, *9*(1), 41–48.

Dhillon, A., & Singh, A. (2018). Biology and Today's World Machine Learning in Healthcare Data Analysis: A Survey. *Journal of Biology and Today's World*, *8*(2), 1–10. DOI: 10.15412/J.JBTW.01070206

Dhiman, P., Malik, N., & Khatkar, A. (2018). 3D-QSAR and in-silico studies of natural products and related derivatives as monoamine oxidase inhibitors. *Current Neuropharmacology*, *16*(6), 881–900. DOI: 10.2174/1570159X15666171128143650 PMID: 29189167

Díaz-Rodríguez, N., Del Ser, J., Coeckelbergh, M., de Prado, M. L., Herrera-Viedma, E., & Herrera, F. (2023). Connecting the dots in trustworthy Artificial Intelligence: From AI principles, ethics, and key requirements to responsible AI systems and regulation. *Information Fusion*, *99*, 101896. DOI: 10.1016/j.inffus.2023.101896

Dill, K. A., & MacCallum, J. L. (2012). The protein-folding problem, 50 years on. [DOI:10.1126/science.1219021] [PMID]. *Science*, *338*(6110), 1042–1046. DOI: 10.1126/science.1219021 PMID: 23180855

Dima, A., Allemann, S., & Dediu, D. (2019). AdhereR: An Open Science Approach to Estimating Adherence to Medications Using Electronic Healthcare Databases. *PubMed*, *264*, 1451–1452. DOI: 10.3233/shti190479 PMID: 31438176

DiMatteo, M. R., Giordani, P. J., Lepper, H. S., & Croghan, T. W. (2002). Patient Adherence and Medical Treatment Outcomes. *Medical Care*, *40*(9), 794–811. DOI: 10.1097/00005650-200209000-00009 PMID: 12218770

Dippenaar, A., Goossens, S. N., Grobbelaar, M., Oostvogels, S., Cuypers, B., Laukens, K., Meehan, C. J., Warren, R. M., & van Rie, A. (2022). Nanopore sequencing for *Mycobacterium tuberculosis*: A critical review of the literature, new developments, and future opportunities. *Journal of Clinical Microbiology*, *60*(1), e0064621. DOI: 10.1128/JCM.00646-21 PMID: 34133895

Driggers, E. M., Hale, S. P., Lee, J., & Terrett, N. K. (2008). The exploration of macrocycles for drug discovery—An underexploited structural class. *Nature Reviews. Drug Discovery*, *7*(7), 608–624. DOI: 10.1038/nrd2590 PMID: 18591981

Drummond, M. F., Sculpher, M. J., Claxton, K., Stoddart, G. L., & Torrance, G. W. (2015). *Methods for the economic evaluation of health care programs* (4th ed.). Oxford University Press.

Durant, J. L., Leland, B. A., Henry, D. R., & Nourse, J. G. (2002). Reoptimization of MDL keys for use in drug discovery. *Journal of Chemical Information and Computer Sciences*, *42*(6), 1273–1280. DOI: 10.1021/ci010132r PMID: 12444722

Ebhohimen, I. E., Edemhanria, L., Awojide, S., Onyijen, O. H., & Anywar, G. (2020). Advances in computer-aided drug discovery. In *Phytochemicals as Lead Compounds for New Drug Discovery* (pp. 25–37). Elsevier. DOI: 10.1016/B978-0-12-817890-4.00003-2

Elasan, S., & Ateş, Y. (2023). Artificial Intelligence (AI) and Ethics in Medicine at a Global Level: Benefits and Risks. In: Karaman, E. & Önder, G. Ö. (eds.), *Current Researches in Health Sciences-II.* Özgür Publications. DOI: https://doi.org/10.58830/ozgur.pub128.c508

Ellen, J. G., Matos, J., Viola, M., Gallifant, J., Quion, J., Anthony Celi, L., & Abu Hussein, N. S. (2024). Participant flow diagrams for health equity in AI. *Journal of Biomedical Informatics, 152*, 104631. DOI: 10.1016/j.jbi.2024.104631 PMID: 38548006

Elton, D. C., Boukouvalas, Z., Fuge, M. D., & Chung, P. W. (2019). Deep learning for molecular design—A review of the state of the art. *Molecular Systems Design & Engineering, 4*(4), 828-849.

Erlina, L., Paramita, R. I., Kusuma, W. A., Fadilah, F., Tedjo, A., Pratomo, I. P., Ramadhanti, N. S., Nasution, A. K., Surado, F. K., Fitriawan, A., Istiadi, K. A., & Yanuar, A. (2022). Virtual screening of indonesian herbal compounds as COVID-19 supportive therapy: Machine learning and pharmacophore modeling approaches. *BMC Complementary Medicine and Therapies, 22*(1), 207. DOI: 10.1186/s12906-022-03686-y PMID: 35922786

Ernst, P., Siu, A., & Weikum, G. (2015). Knowlife: A versatile approach for constructing a large knowledge graph for biomedical sciences. *BMC Bioinformatics, 16*(1), 1–13. DOI: 10.1186/s12859-015-0549-5 PMID: 25971816

Eskandar, K. (2023). Revolutionizing biotechnology and bioengineering: unleashing the power of innovation. *Journal of Applied Biotechnology and Bioengineering. 10*(3):81–88.

Esmaeilzadeh, P. (2020). Use of AI-based tools for healthcare purposes: A consumer survey study. *BMC Medical Informatics and Decision Making, 20*(1). Advance online publication. DOI: 10.1186/s12911-020-01191-1 PMID: 32698869

Esteva, A., Kuprel, B., Novoa, R. A., Ko, J., Swetter, S. M., Blau, H. M., & Thrun, S. (2017). Dermatologist-level classification of skin cancer with deep neural networks. *Nature, 542*(7639), 115–118. DOI: 10.1038/nature21056 PMID: 28117445

Estrada, C. A., Naranjo, S. S., Toasa, V. J., & Yoo, S. G. 2024. A Systematic Literature Review of Blockchain Technology: Applications Fields, Platforms, and Consensus Protocols. In *Proceedings of the 2023 7th International Conference on Computer Science and Artificial Intelligence (CSAI '23)*. Association for Computing Machinery, New York, NY, USA, 123–131. https://doi.org/DOI: 10.1145/3638584.3638632

European Commission. (2020, April 13). *Health: Digital health and care*. European Commission. https://ec.europa.eu/health/ehealth/overview_en

Fan, B., Fan, W., Smith, C., & Garner, H. (2020). Adverse drug event detection and extraction from open data: A deep learning approach. *Information Processing & Management*, *57*(1), 102131. DOI: 10.1016/j.ipm.2019.102131

Fanti, L., Guarascio, D., & Moggi, M. (2022). From Heron of Alexandria to Amazon's Alexa: A stylized history of AI and its impact on business models, organization and work. *Economia e Politica Industriale*, *49*(3), 495–518. DOI: 10.1007/s40812-022-00222-4

Fernandez-Lazaro, C. I., Adams, D. P., Fernandez-Lazaro, D., Garcia-González, J. M., Caballero-Garcia, A., & Miron-Canelo, J. A. (2018). Medication adherence and barriers among low-income, uninsured patients with multiple chronic conditions. *Research in Social & Administrative Pharmacy*, *15*(6), 744–753. DOI: 10.1016/j.sapharm.2018.09.006 PMID: 30241872

Firth-Butterfield, K. (2023, January 18). 2022 was a big year for AI development. In 2023, we must decide how best to use it. *Asia News Network*. https://asianews.network/2022-was-a-big-year-for-ai-developmentin-2023-we-must-decide-how-best-to-use-it

Fischer, M. A., Stedman, M. R., Lii, J., Vogeli, C., Shrank, W. H., Brookhart, M. A., & Weissman, J. S. (2011). Primary medication non-adherence: Analysis of 195,930 electronic prescriptions. *Journal of General Internal Medicine*, *25*(4), 284–290. DOI: 10.1007/s11606-010-1253-9 PMID: 20131023

Fogel, A. L., & Kvedar, J. C. (2018). Artificial intelligence powers digital medicine. *NPJ Digital Medicine*, *1*(1), 5. Advance online publication. DOI: 10.1038/s41746-017-0012-2 PMID: 31304291

Fogel, D. B. (2000). What is evolutionary computation? *IEEE Spectrum*, *37*(5), 26–32. DOI: 10.1109/6.819926

Fong, S. J., Li, G., Dey, N., Gonzalez-Crespo, R., & Herrera-Viedma, E. (2020). Finding an Accurate Early Forecasting Model from Small Dataset: A Case of 2019-nCoV Novel Coronavirus Outbreak. [CrossRef]. *International Journal of Interactive Multimedia and Artificial Intelligence*, *6*(1), 132. DOI: 10.9781/ijimai.2020.02.002

Fountoulakis, K. N., & Stahl, S. M. (2021). Precision and personalized assessment, diagnosis and treatment in psychiatry. [HTML]. *CNS Spectrums*, *26*(4), 326–332. DOI: 10.1017/S1092852920000139 PMID: 32228728

Freifeld, C. C., Brownstein, J. S., Menone, C. M., Bao, W., Filice, R., Kass-Hout, T., & Dasgupta, N. (2014). Digital Drug Safety Surveillance: Monitoring Pharmaceutical Products in Twitter. *Drug Safety*, *37*(5), 343–350. DOI: 10.1007/s40264-014-0155-x PMID: 24777653

Friedman, C., Shagina, L., Lussier, Y., & Hripcsak, G. (2004). Automated Encoding of Clinical Documents Based on Natural Language Processing. *Journal of the American Medical Informatics Association : JAMIA*, *11*(5), 392–402. DOI: 10.1197/jamia.M1552 PMID: 15187068

Gadade, D. D., Kulkarni, D. A., Raj, R., Patil, S. G., & Modi, A. (2024). Pushing Boundaries: The Landscape of AI-Driven Drug Discovery and Development with Insights Into Regulatory Aspects. In Khanna, A., El Barachi, M., Jain, S., Kumar, M., & Nayyar, A. (Eds.), *Artificial Intelligence and Machine Learning in Drug Design and Development* (533-561). https://doi.org/10.1002/9781394234196.ch17

Gadkari, A. S., & McHorney, C. A. (2012). Unintentional non-adherence to chronic prescription medications: How unintentional is it? *BMC Health Services Research*, *12*(1), 98. Advance online publication. DOI: 10.1186/1472-6963-12-98 PMID: 22510235

Gamieldien, J., Fielding, B. C., & Berry, M. (2015). Potential broad spectrum inhibitors of the coronavirus 3clpro: a virtual screening and structure-based drug design study.

Gandomi, A., & Haider, M. (2015). Beyond the Hype: Big Data Concepts, Methods, and Analytics. *International Journal of Information Management*, *35*(2), 137–144. DOI: 10.1016/j.ijinfomgt.2014.10.007

Gao, C. X., Dwyer, D., Zhu, Y., Smith, C. L., Du, L., Filia, K. M., Bayer, J., Menssink, J. M., Wang, T., Bergmeir, C., Wood, S., & Cotton, S. M. (2023). An overview of clustering methods with guidelines for application in mental health research. *Psychiatry Research*, *327*, 115265. DOI: 10.1016/j.psychres.2023.115265 PMID: 37348404

Geldof, T., Huys, I., & Van Dyck, W. (2019). Real-World Evidence Gathering in Oncology: The Need for a Biomedical Big Data Insight-Providing Federated Network. *Frontiers in Medicine*, *6*, 43. Advance online publication. DOI: 10.3389/fmed.2019.00043 PMID: 30906740

Gellad, W. F., Grenard, J. L., & Marcum, Z. A. (2011). A Systematic Review of Barriers to Medication Adherence in the Elderly. *The American Journal of Geriatric Pharmacotherapy*, *9*(1), 11–23. DOI: 10.1016/j.amjopharm.2011.02.004 PMID: 21459305

Ghadge, A., Bourlakis, M., Kamble, S., & Seuring, S. (2023). Blockchain implementation in pharmaceutical supply chains: A review and conceptual framework. *International Journal of Production Research*, *61*(19), 6633–6651. DOI: 10.1080/00207543.2022.2125595

Ghassemi, M., Naumann, T., Schulam, P., Beam, A. L., Chen, I. Y., & Ranganath, R. (2019, December 5). *A Review of Challenges and Opportunities in Machine Learning for Health*. ArXiv.org. https://doi.org//arXiv.1806.00388DOI: 10.48550

Giordanetto, F., & Kihlberg, J. (2014). Macrocyclic drugs and clinical candidates: What can medicinal chemists learn from their properties? *Journal of Medicinal Chemistry*, *57*(2), 278–295. DOI: 10.1021/jm400887j PMID: 24044773

Godyn, M., Kedziora, M., Ren, Y., Liu, Y., & Song, H. H. (2022). Analysis of solutions for a blockchain compliance with GDPR. *Scientific Reports*, *12*(1), 15021. DOI: 10.1038/s41598-022-19341-y PMID: 36056166

Gohil, S., Vuik, S., & Darzi, A. (2018). Sentiment Analysis of Health Care Tweets: Review of the Methods Used. *JMIR Public Health and Surveillance*, *4*(2), e43. DOI: 10.2196/publichealth.5789 PMID: 29685871

Goldsack, J. (2019). Synthetic control arms can save time and money in clinical trials. *STAT News*.https://www.statnews.com/2019/02/05/synthetic-control-arms-clinical-trials/ (accessed November 5, 2021)

Gopinath, N. (2021). Artificial intelligence: Potential tool to subside SARS-CoV-2 pandemic. [CrossRef]. *Process Biochemistry (Barking, London, England)*, *110*, 94–99. DOI: 10.1016/j.procbio.2021.08.001 PMID: 34366689

Gornet, M. & Maxwell, W. (2024). The European approach to regulating AI through technical standards. *Internet Policy Review*.

Gouiza, N., Jebari, H., & Reklaoui, K. (2024). INTEGRATION OF IOT-ENABLED TECHNOLOGIES AND ARTIFICIAL INTELLIGENCE IN DIVERSE DOMAINS: RECENT ADVANCEMENTS AND FUTURE TRENDS. *Journal of Theoretical and Applied Information Technology*, *102*, 1975–2029.

Grant, R. M. (2018). *Contemporary Strategy Analysis* (10th ed.). Wiley.

Greaves, F., Ramirez-Cano, D., Millett, C., Darzi, A., & Donaldson, L. (2013). Use of Sentiment Analysis for Capturing Patient Experience From Free-Text Comments Posted Online. *Journal of Medical Internet Research*, *15*(11), e239. DOI: 10.2196/jmir.2721 PMID: 24184993

Greenstein, S. (2001). The commercialization of the Internet: The interaction. *Innovation Policy and the Economy*, *1*, 151–186. DOI: 10.1086/ipe.1.25056144

Grigalunas, M., Burhop, A., Christoforow, A., & Waldmann, H. (2020). Pseudo-natural products and natural product-inspired methods in chemical biology and drug discovery. *Current Opinion in Chemical Biology*, *56*, 111–118. DOI: 10.1016/j.cbpa.2019.10.005 PMID: 32362382

Grilo, A. L., & Mantalaris, A. (2019). The Increasingly Human and Profitable Monoclonal Antibody Market. *Trends in Biotechnology*, *37*(1), 9–16. DOI: 10.1016/j.tibtech.2018.05.014 PMID: 29945725

Grinnan, D., Trankle, C., Andruska, A., Bloom, B., & Spiekerkoetter, E. (2019). Drug repositioning in pulmonary arterial hypertension: Challenges and opportunities. *Pulmonary Circulation*, *9*(1), 1–18. Advance online publication. DOI: 10.1177/2045894019832226 PMID: 30729869

Grisoni, F., Consonni, V., & Todeschini, R. (2018). Impact of molecular descriptors on computational models. *Computational chemogenomics*, 171-209.

Gruchmann, T., Elgazzar, S., & Ali, A. H. (2023). Blockchain technology in pharmaceutical supply chains: A transaction cost perspective. *Modern Supply Chain Research and Applications*, *5*(2), 115–133. DOI: 10.1108/MSCRA-10-2022-0023

Grys, B. T., Lo, D. S., Sahin, N., Kraus, O. Z., Morris, Q., Boone, C., & Andrews, B. J. (2017). Machine learning and computer vision approaches for phenotypic profiling. *The Journal of Cell Biology*, *216*(1), 65–71. DOI: 10.1083/jcb.201610026 PMID: 27940887

Gulshan, V., Peng, L., Coram, M., Stumpe, M. C., Wu, D., Narayanaswamy, A., Venugopalan, S., Widner, K., Madams, T., Cuadros, J., Kim, R., Raman, R., Nelson, P. C., Mega, J. L., & Webster, D. R. (2016). Development and Validation of a Deep Learning Algorithm for Detection of Diabetic Retinopathy in Retinal Fundus Photographs. *Journal of the American Medical Association*, *316*(22), 2402. DOI: 10.1001/jama.2016.17216 PMID: 27898976

Guo, P., Liu, T., Zhang, Q., Wang, L., Xiao, J., Zhang, Q., Luo, G., Li, Z., He, J., Zhang, Y., & Ma, W. (2017). Developing a dengue forecast model using machine learning: A case study in China. [CrossRef] [PubMed]. *PLoS Neglected Tropical Diseases*, *11*(10), e0005973. DOI: 10.1371/journal.pntd.0005973 PMID: 29036169

Gupta, R., Srivastava, D., Sahu, M., Tiwari, S., Ambasta, R. K., & Kumar, P. (2021). Artificial intelligence to deep learning: Machine intelligence approach for drug discovery. *Molecular Diversity*, *25*(3), 1315–1360. DOI: 10.1007/s11030-021-10217-3 PMID: 33844136

Gupta, S., & Singh, R., and A. SharmaYear: 2024Title: "Enhanced Medicinal Plant Identification Using Deep Learning Architectures" DOI: 10.1002/sim.4417 PMID: 22161304

Gurulingappa, H., Rajput, A. M., Roberts, A., Fluck, J., Hofmann-Apitius, M., & Toldo, L. (2012). Development of a benchmark corpus to support the automatic extraction of drug-related adverse effects from medical case reports. *Journal of Biomedical Informatics*, *45*(5), 885–892. DOI: 10.1016/j.jbi.2012.04.008 PMID: 22554702

Habib, G., Sharma, S., Ibrahim, S., Ahmad, I., Qureshi, S., & Ishfaq, M. (2022). Blockchain Technology: Benefits, Challenges, Applications, and Integration of Blockchain Technology with Cloud Computing. *Future Internet*, *14*(11), 341. DOI: 10.3390/fi14110341

Haelterman, H. (2022). Breaking Silos of Legal and Regulatory Risks to Outperform Traditional Compliance Approaches. *European Journal on Criminal Policy and Research*, *28*(1), 19–36. DOI: 10.1007/s10610-020-09468-x

Haenlein, M., & Kaplan, A. M. (2019). A brief history of artificial intelligence: On artificial intelligence's past, present, and future. *California Management Review*, *61*(4), 5–14. DOI: 10.1177/0008125619864925

Hafen, E., Kossmann, D., & Brand, A. (2014). Health data cooperatives - citizen empowerment. *Methods of Information in Medicine*, *53*(2), 82–86. DOI: 10.3414/ME13-02-0051 PMID: 24514946

Halli, U. M. (2022). Nanotechnology in IoT Security, *Journal of Nanoscience. Nanoengineering & Applications*, *12*(3), 11–16.

Han, R., Yoon, H., Kim, G., Lee, H., & Lee, Y. (2023). Revolutionizing medicinal chemistry: the application of artificial intelligence (AI) in early drug discovery. *Pharmaceuticals*, *16*(9):1259. 10.3390/ph16091259

Han, K., Zhang, L., Wang, M., Zhang, R., Wang, C., & Zhang, C. (2018). Prediction methods of herbal compounds in Chinese medicinal herbs. *Molecules (Basel, Switzerland)*, *23*(9), 2303. DOI: 10.3390/molecules23092303 PMID: 30201875

Han, R., Acosta, J. N., Shakeri, Z., Ioannidis, J. P. A., Topol, E. J., & Rajpurkar, P. (2024). Randomized controlled trials evaluating artificial intelligence in clinical practice: A scoping review. *The Lancet. Digital Health*, *6*(5), e367–e373. DOI: 10.1016/S2589-7500(24)00047-5 PMID: 38670745

Han, S. M., Greenfield, G., Majeed, A., & Hayhoe, B. (2020). Impact of Remote Consultations on Antibiotic Prescribing in Primary Health Care: Systematic Review. *Journal of Medical Internet Research*, *22*(11), e23482. DOI: 10.2196/23482 PMID: 33031045

Hanson, C. W.III, & Marshall, B. E. (2001). Artificial intelligence applications in the intensive care unit. *Critical Care Medicine*, *29*(4), 427–435. DOI: 10.1097/00003246-200102000-00038 PMID: 11269246

Harrer, S., Menard, J., Rivers, M., Green, D. V. S., Karpiak, J., Jeliazkov, J. R., & Sternke, M. C. (2024). Artificial intelligence drives the digital transformation of pharma. In Krittanawong, C. (Ed.), *Artificial Intelligence in Clinical Practice* (pp. 345–372). Academic Press., DOI: 10.1016/B978-0-443-15688-5.00049-8

Harrer, S., Shah, P., Antony, B., & Hu, J. (2019). Artificial intelligence for clinical trial design. *Trends in Pharmacological Sciences*, *40*(8), 577–591. DOI: 10.1016/j.tips.2019.05.005 PMID: 31326235

Harrison, C. (2014). Patenting natural products just got harder. *Nature Biotechnology*, *32*(5), 403–405. DOI: 10.1038/nbt0514-403a PMID: 24811496

Hartl, D., de Luca, V., Kostikova, A., Laramie, J., Kennedy, S., Ferrero, E., Siegel, R., Fink, M., Ahmed, S., Millholland, J., Schuhmacher, A., Hinder, M., Piali, L., & Roth, A. (2021). Translational precision medicine: an industry perspective. In *Journal of Translational Medicine* (Vol. 19, Issue 1). BioMed Central Ltd. DOI: 10.1186/s12967-021-02910-6

Hassan, M., Awan, F. M., Naz, A., deAndrés-Galiana, E. J., Alvarez, O., Cernea, A., Fernández-Brillet, L., Fernández-Martínez, J. L., & Kloczkowski, A. (2022). Innovations in genomics and big data analytics for personalized medicine and health care: A review. [mdpi.com]. *International Journal of Molecular Sciences*, *23*(9), 4645. DOI: 10.3390/ijms23094645 PMID: 35563034

Haynes, R. B., Taylor, D. W., & Sackett, D. L. (1979). *Compliance in health care* (1st ed.). The John Hopkins University Press.

Haynes, R., McDonald, H., Garg, A., & Montague, P. (2002). Interventions for helping patients to follow prescriptions for medications. *The Cochrane Library*. Advance online publication. DOI: 10.1002/14651858.CD000011 PMID: 12076376

Heller, S. R., McNaught, A., Pletnev, I., Stein, S., & Tchekhovskoi, D. (2015). InChI, the IUPAC international chemical identifier. *Journal of Cheminformatics*, *7*(1), 1–34. DOI: 10.1186/s13321-015-0068-4 PMID: 26136848

Hemedan, A. A., Abd Elaziz, M., Jiao, P., Alavi, A. H., Bahgat, M., Ostaszewski, M., Schneider, R., Ghazy, H. A., Ewees, A. A., & Lu, S. (2020). Prediction of the Vaccine-derived Poliovirus Outbreak Incidence: A Hybrid Machine Learning Approach. [CrossRef] [PubMed]. *Scientific Reports*, *10*(1), 5058. DOI: 10.1038/s41598-020-61853-y PMID: 32193487

Henderson, R. M., & Clark, K. B. (1990). Architectural innovation: The reconfiguration of existing. *Administrative Science Quarterly*, *35*(1), 9. DOI: 10.2307/2393549

Henkemans, O. B., Bierman, B. P., Janssen, J., Neerincx, M. A., Looije, R., Van Der Bosch, H., & Van Der Giessen, J. A. (2013). Using a robot to personalize health education for children with diabetes type 1: A pilot study. *Patient Education and Counseling*, *92*(2), 174–181. DOI: 10.1016/j.pec.2013.04.012 PMID: 23684366

Hisang, Jen. (2019). *Hsieh*. Chung-Chih, Lin. Intelligent Medicinal Plant Factory., DOI: 10.1109/PHM-Paris.2019.00047

Hong, N., Li, D., Yu, Y., Xiu, Q., Liu, H., & Jiang, G. (2016). A computational framework for converting textual clinical diagnostic criteria into the quality data model. *Journal of Biomedical Informatics*, *63*, 11–21. DOI: 10.1016/j.jbi.2016.07.016 PMID: 27444185

Ho, P. M., Magid, D. J., Masoudi, F. A., McClure, D. L., & Rumsfeld, J. S. (2006). Adherence to cardioprotective medications and mortality among patients with diabetes and ischemic heart disease. *BMC Cardiovascular Disorders*, *6*(1), 48. Advance online publication. DOI: 10.1186/1471-2261-6-48 PMID: 17173679

Ho, P. M., Rumsfeld, J. S., Masoudi, F. A., McClure, D. L., Plomondon, M. E., Steiner, J. F., & Magid, D. J. (2006). Effect of Medication Nonadherence on Hospitalization and Mortality Among Patients with Diabetes Mellitus. *Archives of Internal Medicine*, *166*(17), 1836. DOI: 10.1001/archinte.166.17.1836 PMID: 17000939

Horne, R., Weinman, J., Barber, N., Elliott, R., & Morgan, M. (2005). *Concordance, adherence, and compliance in medicine taking*. National Coordinating Centre for NHS Service Delivery and Organisation R&D. https://www.ahpo.net/assets/NCCSDo%20Compliance%202005.pdf

Horne, R., Weinman, J., Barber, N., Elliott, R., & Morgan, M. (2005). *Concordance, adherence, and compliance in medicine taking*. National Coordinating Centre for NHS Service Delivery and Organisation R&D. https://www.ahpo.net/assets/NCCSDO%20Compliance%202005.pdf

Hossain, E., Rana, R., Higgins, N., Soar, J., Barua, P. D., Pisani, A. R., & Turner, K. (2023). Use of ai/ml-enabled state-of-the-art method in electronic medical records: A systematic review. *Computers in Biology and Medicine*, *155*, 106649. DOI: 10.1016/j.compbiomed.2023.106649 PMID: 36805219

Hripcsak, G., & Albers, D. J. (2012). Next-generation phenotyping of electronic health records. *Journal of the American Medical Informatics Association : JAMIA*, *20*(1), 117–121. DOI: 10.1136/amiajnl-2012-001145 PMID: 22955496

Hripcsak, G., Duke, J. D., Shah, N. H., Reich, C. G., Huser, V., Schuemie, M. J., Suchard, M. A., Park, R. W., Wong, I. C. K., Rijnbeek, P. R., van der Lei, J., Pratt, N., Norén, G. N., Li, Y.-C., Stang, P. E., Madigan, D., & Ryan, P. B. (2015). Observational Health Data Sciences and Informatics (OHDSI): Opportunities for Observational Researchers. *Studies in Health Technology and Informatics*, *216*, 574–578. https://pubmed.ncbi.nlm.nih.gov/26262116/. DOI: 10.3233/978-1-61499-564-7-574 PMID: 26262116

Huang, D., Yang, M., Wen, X., Xia, S., & Yuan, B. (2024). AI-Driven Drug Discovery: Accelerating The Development Of Novel Therapeutics In Biopharmaceuticals. *Journal of Knowledge Learning and Science Technology, 3*(3), 206-224.

Huang, C. J., Chen, Y. H., Ma, Y., & Kuo, P. H. (2020). Multiple-input deep convolutional neural network model for COVID-19 forecasting in China. *medRxiv*. DOI: 10.1101/2020.03.23.20041608

Hubert, J., Nuzillard, J. M., & Renault, J. H. (2017). Dereplication strategies in natural product research: How many tools and methodologies behind the same concept? *Phytochemistry Reviews*, *16*(1), 55–95. DOI: 10.1007/s11101-015-9448-7

Hughes, D. A. (2012). Pharmacoeconomics. In *British Journal of Clinical Pharmacology* (Vol. 73, Issue 6, pp. 968–972). DOI: 10.1111/j.1365-2125.2012.04247.x

Huigens, R. W.III, Morrison, K. C., Hicklin, R. W., Flood, T. A.Jr, Richter, M. F., & Hergenrother, P. J. (2013). A ring-distortion strategy to construct stereochemically complex and structurally diverse compounds from natural products. *Nature Chemistry*, *5*(3), 195–202. DOI: 10.1038/nchem.1549 PMID: 23422561

Huss, R. (2016, October 3). The high price of failed clinical trials: Time to rethink the model. *Clinical Leader.*https://www.clinicalleader.com/doc/the-high-price-of-failed-clinical-trials-time-to-rethink-the-model-0001 (accessed November 10, 2022)

Hussain, M. I., Raziq, A., Ahmed, A., Iqbal, M. W., Tian, R., Li, J., Liu, L., & Liu, Y. (2023). Recent progress in CRISPR-based bioengineering of microbial cell factories for important nutraceuticals synthesis. *Journal of Applied Microbiology*, *134*(6), lxad114. DOI: 10.1093/jambio/lxad114 PMID: 37279904

Hu, Z., Ge, Q., Li, S., Jin, S., & Xiong, M. (2020). Artificial intelligence forecasting of COVID-19 in China. *arXiv*. https://arxiv.org/abs/2002.07112

Imam, S. S., & Gilani, S. J. (2017). Computer aided drug design: A novel loom to drug discovery. *Organ Med Chem Int J*, *1*, 113–118.

Infulata, R., Wilczynski, N., Navarro, T., Hobson, N., Jeffery, R., Keepanasseril, A., Agoritsas, T., Mistry, N., Iorio, A., Jack, S., Sivaramalingam, B., Iserman, E., Mustafa, R. A., Jedraszewski, D., Cotoi, C., & Haynes, R. B. (2014). Interventions for enhancing medication adherence. *Cochrane Database of Systematic Reviews*, *11*(11), CD000011. Advance online publication. DOI: 10.1002/14651858.CD000011.pub4 PMID: 25412402

Ioakeim-Skoufa, I., Poblador-Plou, B., Carmona-Pírez, J., Díez-Manglano, J., Navickas, R., Gimeno-Feliu, L. A., González-Rubio, F., Jureviciene, E., Dambrauskas, L., Prados-Torres, A., & Gimeno-Miguel, A. (2020). Multimorbidity Patterns in the General Population: Results from the EpiChron Cohort Study. *International Journal of Environmental Research and Public Health*, *17*(12), 4242. DOI: 10.3390/ijerph17124242 PMID: 32545876

Iorio, F., Bosotti, R., Scacheri, E., Belcastro, V., Mithbaokar, P., Ferriero, R., Murino, L., Tagliaferri, R., Brunetti-Pierri, N., & Isacchi, A.. (2010). Discovery of Rifampicin Mode of Action and Rifampicin Repositioning from Transcriptional Responses. *Proceedings of the National Academy of Sciences of the United States of America*, *107*, 14621–14626. DOI: 10.1073/pnas.1000138107 PMID: 20679242

Iqbal, J., Cortés Jaimes, D. C., Makineni, P., Subramani, S., Hemaida, S., Thugu, T. R., Butt, A. N., Sikto, J. T., Kaur, P., Lak, M. A., Augustine, M., Shahzad, R., & Arain, M. (2023). Reimagining Healthcare: Unleashing the Power of Artificial Intelligence in Medicine. *Cureus*. Advance online publication. DOI: 10.7759/cureus.44658 PMID: 37799217

ISO. (2015). *ISO/HL7 10781:2015 Health informatics — HL7 electronic health records-system functional model, Release 2 (EHR FM)*. ISO. https://www.iso.org/standard/57757.html

ISO. (2019). *ISO 13606-1:2019 Health Informatics Electronic Health Record Communication Part 1: Reference model*. ISO. https://www.iso.org/standard/67868.html

Jain, A. N., & Nicholls, A. (2008). Recommendations for evaluation of computational methods. *Journal of Computer-Aided Molecular Design*, *22*(3-4), 133–139. DOI: 10.1007/s10822-008-9196-5 PMID: 18338228

Jain, A., Mao, J., & Mohiuddin, K. (1996). Artificial neural networks: A tutorial. *Computer*, *29*(3), 31–44. DOI: 10.1109/2.485891

Janosevic, D., De Luca, T., Project, K. P. M., & Eadon, M. T. (2024). The Kidney Precision Medicine Project and Single-Cell Biology of the Injured Proximal Tubule. *The American Journal of Pathology*.

Jee, K., & Kim, G.-H. (2013). Potentiality of Big Data in the Medical Sector: Focus on How to Reshape the Healthcare System. *Healthcare Informatics Research*, *19*(2), 79. DOI: 10.4258/hir.2013.19.2.79 PMID: 23882412

Jena, A., Singh, A. K., Kumar-M, P., Sharma, V., & Sebastian, S. (2020). Systematic review on failure to adhere to IBD therapies during the COVID-19 pandemic: Correct information is crucial. *Digestive and Liver Disease*, *52*(11), 1254–1256. DOI: 10.1016/j.dld.2020.09.012 PMID: 33011089

Jenkins, J. L., Bender, A., & Davies, J. W. (2006). In Silico Target Fishing: Predicting Biological Targets from Chemical Structure. *Drug Discovery Today. Technologies*, *3*(4), 413–421. DOI: 10.1016/j.ddtec.2006.12.008

Jiang, M., Chen, Y., Liu, M., Rosenbloom, S. T., Mani, S., Denny, J. C., & Xu, H. (2011). A study of machine-learning-based approaches to extract clinical entities and their assertions from discharge summaries. *Journal of the American Medical Informatics Association : JAMIA*, *18*(5), 601–606. DOI: 10.1136/amiajnl-2011-000163 PMID: 21508414

Jiménez-Luna, J., Grisoni, F., Weskamp, N., & Schneider, G. (2021). Artificial intelligence in drug discovery: Recent advances and future perspectives. *Expert Opinion on Drug Discovery*, *16*(9), 949–959. DOI: 10.1080/17460441.2021.1909567 PMID: 33779453

Johnson, J. A., & Cavallari, L. H. (2013). Pharmacogenetics and Cardiovascular Disease—Implications for Personalized Medicine. *Pharmacological Reviews*, *65*(3), 987–1009. DOI: 10.1124/pr.112.007252 PMID: 23686351

Johnston, C. W., Skinnider, M. A., Wyatt, M. A., Li, X., Ranieri, M. R., Yang, L., Zechel, D. L., Ma, B., & Magarvey, N. A. (2015). An automated Genomes-to-Natural Products platform (GNP) for the discovery of modular natural products. *Nature Communications*, *6*(1), 8421. DOI: 10.1038/ncomms9421 PMID: 26412281

Jordan, M. I., & Mitchell, T. M. (2015). Machine learning: Trends, perspectives, and prospects. *Science*, *349*(6245), 255–260. DOI: 10.1126/science.aaa8415 PMID: 26185243

José, L., Medina-Franco. (2013). Advances in computational approaches for drug discovery based on natural products. *Revista Latinoamericana de Química*, *41*(2), 95–110.

Jung, K., LePendu, P., & Shah, N. (2013). Automated Detection of Systematic Off-label Drug Use in Free Text of Electronic Medical Records. *AMIA Joint Summits on Translational Science Proceedings AMIA Summit on Translational Science*, *2013*, 94–98. https://www.ncbi.nlm.nih.gov/pmc/articles/PMC3814472/ PMID: 24303308

Kahn, C. E.Jr, Heilbrun, M. E., & Applegate, K. E. (2013). From Guidelines to Practice: How Reporting Templates Promote the Use of Radiology Practice Guidelines. *Journal of the American College of Radiology*, *10*(4), 268–273. DOI: 10.1016/j.jacr.2012.09.025 PMID: 23332496

Kalepu, S., & Nekkanti, V. (2015). Insoluble Rifampicin Delivery Strategies. *Review of Recent Advances and Business Prospects. Acta Pharm. Sin. B.*, *5*, 442–453. DOI: 10.1016/j.apsb.2015.07.003 PMID: 26579474

Kamel, I. (2024). Artificial intelligence in medicine. *Journal of Medical Artificial Intelligence*, *7*, 4. DOI: 10.21037/jmai-24-12

Kang, S. N., Hong, S.-S., Lee, M.-K., & Lim, S.-J. (2012). Dual function of tributyrin emulsion: Solubilization and enhancement of anticancer effect of celecoxib. *International Journal of Pharmaceutics*, *428*(1-2), 76–81. DOI: 10.1016/j.ijpharm.2012.02.037 PMID: 22405988

Kaplan, A. M. (2022). *Artificial intelligence, business, and civilization: Our fate made in machines*. Routledge. DOI: 10.4324/9781003244554

Kaplan, A. M., & Haenlein, M. (2019). Siri, Siri, in my hand: Who is the fairest in the land? On the interpretations, illustrations, and implications of artificial intelligence. *Business Horizons*, *62*(1), 15–25. DOI: 10.1016/j.bushor.2018.08.004

Karageorgis, G., Foley, D. J., Laraia, L., & Waldmann, H. (2020). Principle and design of pseudo-natural products. *Nature Chemistry*, *12*(3), 227–235. DOI: 10.1038/s41557-019-0411-x PMID: 32015480

Karageorgis, G., Reckzeh, E. S., Ceballos, J., Schwalfenberg, M., Sievers, S., Ostermann, C., Pahl, A., Ziegler, S., & Waldmann, H. (2018). Chromopynones are pseudo natural product glucose uptake inhibitors targeting glucose transporters GLUT-1 and-3. *Nature Chemistry*, *10*(11), 1103–1111. DOI: 10.1038/s41557-018-0132-6 PMID: 30202104

Kardas, P., Cieszyński, J., Czech, M., Banaś, I., & Lewek, P. (2020). Primary nonadherence to medication and its drivers in Poland: The electronic prescription pilot analysis findings. *Polish Archives of Internal Medicine*, *130*(1), 8–16. DOI: 10.20452/pamw.14994 PMID: 31559971

Kasaraneni, R. K. (2021). AI-enhanced pharmacoeconomics: Evaluating cost-effectiveness and budget impact of new pharmaceuticals. *Australian Journal of Machine Learning Research & Applications*, *1*(1), 291–327. https://sydneyacademics.com/index.php/ajmlra/article/view/136

Kasat, K., Shaikh, N., Rayabharapu, V. K., & Nayak, M. (2023). Implementation and Recognition of Waste Management System with Mobility Solution in Smart Cities using Internet of Things, *2023 Second International Conference on Augmented Intelligence and Sustainable Systems (ICAISS)*, Trichy, India, 2023, pp. 1661-1665, DOI: 10.1109/ICAISS58487.2023.10250690

Kaur, S., & Kaur, P. (2019). Plant species identification based on plant leaf using computer vision and machine learning techniques. *J. Multim. Inform. Syst.*, *6*(2), 49–60. DOI: 10.33851/JMIS.2019.6.2.49

Kazi, K. (2024). Modelling and Simulation of Electric Vehicle for Performance Analysis: BEV and HEV Electrical Vehicle Implementation Using Simulink for E-Mobility Ecosystems. In L. D., N. Nagpal, N. Kassarwani, V. Varthanan G., & P. Siano (Eds.), E-Mobility in Electrical Energy Systems for Sustainability (pp. 295-320). IGI Global. Available at: https://www.igi-global.com/gateway/chapter/full-text-pdf/341172DOI: 10.4018/979-8-3693-2611-4.ch014

Kazi, K. (2024). Complications with Malware Identification in IoT and an Overview of Artificial Immune Approaches. *Research & Reviews. The Journal of Immunology : Official Journal of the American Association of Immunologists, 14*(01), 54–62.

Kazi, K. (2024a). IoT Technologies for the Intelligent Dairy Industry: A New Challenge. In Thandekkattu, S. G., & Vajjhala, N. R. (Eds.), *Designing Sustainable Internet of Things Solutions for Smart Industries*. IGI Global. DOI: 10.4018/979-8-3693-5498-8.ch012

Kazi, K. (2024a). Machine Learning (ML)-Based Braille Lippi Characters and Numbers Detection and Announcement System for Blind Children in Learning. In Sart, G. (Ed.), *Social Reflections of Human-Computer Interaction in Education, Management, and Economics*. IGI Global., DOI: 10.4018/979-8-3693-3033-3.ch002

Kazi, K. (2024b). Machine Learning-Driven-Internet of Things(MLIoT) Based Healthcare Monitoring System. In Wickramasinghe, N. (Ed.), *Impact of Digital Solutions for Improved Healthcare Delivery*. IGI Global.

Kazi, K. (2024c). Moonlighting in Carrier. In Tunio, M. N. (Ed.), *Applications of Career Transitions and Entrepreneurship*. IGI Global.

Kazi, K. (2024d). Heart Health Monitoring Using IoT and Machine Learning Methods. In Shaik, A. (Ed.), *AI-Powered Advances in Pharmacology*. IGI Global.

Kazi, K. S. (2017). Significance And Usage Of Face Recognition System. *Scholarly Journal For Humanity Science and English Language, 4*(20), 4764–4772.

Kazi, K. S. (2024). Artificial Intelligence (AI)-Driven IoT (AIIoT)-Based Agriculture Automation. In Satapathy, S., & Muduli, K. (Eds.), *Advanced Computational Methods for Agri-Business Sustainability* (pp. 72–94). IGI Global., DOI: 10.4018/979-8-3693-3583-3.ch005

Kazi, K. S. (2024). Computer-Aided Diagnosis in Ophthalmology: A Technical Review of Deep Learning Applications. In Garcia, M., & de Almeida, R. (Eds.), *Transformative Approaches to Patient Literacy and Healthcare Innovation* (pp. 112–135). IGI Global., Available at https://www.igi-global.com/chapter/computer-aided-diagnosis-in-ophthalmology/342823, DOI: 10.4018/979-8-3693-3661-8.ch006

Kazi, K. S. (2024). Machine Learning-Based Pomegranate Disease Detection and Treatment. In Zia Ul Haq, M., & Ali, I. (Eds.), *Revolutionizing Pest Management for Sustainable Agriculture* (pp. 469–498). IGI Global., DOI: 10.4018/979-8-3693-3061-6.ch019

Kazi, K. S. (2024b). IoT Driven by Machine Learning (MLIoT) for the Retail Apparel Sector. In Tarnanidis, T., Papachristou, E., Karypidis, M., & Ismyrlis, V. (Eds.), *Driving Green Marketing in Fashion and Retail* (pp. 63–81). IGI Global., DOI: 10.4018/979-8-3693-3049-4.ch004

Kazi, K. S. L. (2018). Significance of Projection and Rotation of Image in Color Matching for High-Quality Panoramic Images used for Aquatic study. *International Journal of Aquatic Science*, *09*(02), 130–145.

Kazi, K. S. L. (2024). IoT and Sensor-based Smart Agriculturing Driven by NodeMCU. *Research & Review: Electronics and Communication Engineering*, *1*(2), 25–33.

Kazi, K. S. L. (2024). Nanotechnology in BattleField: A Study. *Journal of Nanoscience. Nanoengineering & Applications.*, *14*(2), 18–30p.

Kazi, K. S. L. (2024). Smart Agriculture based on AI-Driven-IoT(AIIoT): A KSK Approach, *Advance Research in Communication Engineering and its. Innovations*, *1*(2), 23–32.

Kazi, K., & Sayyad, L., (2024). Explainable AI in Healthcare. In Anitha Kamaraj, A. (Ed.), *Explainable Artificial Intelligence in healthcare System*. Debi Prasanna Acharjya., DOI: 10.52305/GOMR8163

Keskinbora, K. H. (2019). Medical ethics considerations on artificial intelligence. *Journal of Clinical Neuroscience*, *64*, 277–282. DOI: 10.1016/j.jocn.2019.03.001 PMID: 30878282

Khalighi, S., Reddy, K., Midya, A., Pandav, K. B., Madabhushi, A., & Abedalthagafi, M. (2024). Artificial intelligence in neuro-oncology: advances and challenges in brain tumor diagnosis, prognosis, and precision treatment. *npj Precision Oncology*, *8*(1), 80. DOI: 10.1038/s41698-024-00575-0

Khan, M. T., Kaushik, A. C., Ji, L., Malik, S. I., Ali, S., & Wei, D.-Q. (2019). Artificial Neural Networks for Prediction of Tuberculosis Disease. [CrossRef]. *Frontiers in Microbiology*, *10*, 395. DOI: 10.3389/fmicb.2019.00395 PMID: 30886608

Kim, E., Choi, A. S., & Nam, H. (2019). Drug repositioning of herbal compounds via a machine-learning approach. *BMC Bioinformatics*, *20*(S10, Suppl. 10), 247. DOI: 10.1186/s12859-019-2811-8 PMID: 31138103

Kim, J. H., Lim, J. W., Lee, S. W., Kim, K., & No, K. T. (2011). Ligand supported homology modeling and docking evaluation of CCR2: Docked pose selection by consensus scoring. *Journal of Molecular Modeling*, *17*(10), 2707–2716. DOI: 10.1007/s00894-010-0943-x PMID: 21213000

Kiss, P., Carcel, C., Hockham, C., & Peters, S. A. E. (2020). The impact of the COVID-19 pandemic on the care and management of patients with acute cardiovascular disease: A systematic review. *European Heart Journal. Quality of Care & Clinical Outcomes*, *7*(1), 18–27. DOI: 10.1093/ehjqcco/qcaa084 PMID: 33151274

Koch, M. A., Schuffenhauer, A., Scheck, M., Wetzel, S., Casaulta, M., Odermatt, A., Ertl, P., & Waldmann, H. (2005). Charting biologically relevant chemical space: A structural classification of natural products (SCONP). *Proceedings of the National Academy of Sciences of the United States of America*, *102*(48), 17272–17277. DOI: 10.1073/pnas.0503647102 PMID: 16301544

Koehn, F. E., & Carter, G. T. (2005). The evolving role of natural products in drug discovery. *Nature Reviews. Drug Discovery*, *4*(3), 206–220. DOI: 10.1038/nrd1657 PMID: 15729362

Kokla, M., Virtanen, J., Kolehmainen, M., Paananen, J., & Hanhineva, K. (2019). Random forest-based imputation outperforms other methods for imputing LC-MS metabolomics data: A comparative study. *BMC Bioinformatics*, *20*(1), 1–11. DOI: 10.1186/s12859-019-3110-0 PMID: 31601178

Kolluri, S., Lin, J., Liu, R., Zhang, Y., & Zhang, W. (2022). Machine Learning and Artificial Intelligence in Pharmaceutical Research and Development: a Review. In *AAPS Journal* (Vol. 24, Issue 1). Springer Science and Business Media Deutschland GmbH. DOI: 10.1208/s12248-021-00644-3

Koohy, H. (2017). The rise and fall of machine learning methods in biomedical research. *F1000 Research*, *6*, 2012. Advance online publication. DOI: 10.12688/f1000research.13016.1 PMID: 29375816

Kostkova, P., Pinheiro dos Santos, W., & Massoni, T. (2019). ZIKA: Improved surveillance and forecast of Zika virus in Brazil. [CrossRef]. *European Journal of Public Health*, *29*(Suppl. 4), ckz186–ckz085. DOI: 10.1093/eurpub/ckz186.085

Kourou, K., Exarchos, T. P., Exarchos, K. P., Karamouzis, M. V., & Fotiadis, D. I. (2015). Machine learning applications in cancer prognosis and prediction. *Computational and Structural Biotechnology Journal*, *13*(13), 8–17. DOI: 10.1016/j.csbj.2014.11.005 PMID: 25750696

KPMG. (2020). *Living in an AI world 2020 report: Healthcare insiders: Taking the temperature of artificial intelligence in healthcare*. KPMG. https://advisory.kpmg.us/content/dam/advisory/en/pdfs/2020/healthcare-living-in-an-ai-world.pdf

KPMG. (2020). *Living in an AI world 2020: Healthcare insiders.* KPMG. https://advisory.kpmg.us/content/dam/advisory/en/pdfs/2020/healthcare-living-in-an-ai-world.pdf

Krallinger, M., Rabal, O., Lourenco, A., Oyarzabal, J., & Valencia, A. (2017). Information retrieval and text mining technologies for chemistry. *Chemical reviews, 117*(12), 7673-7761. 62

Kreimeyer, K., Foster, M., Pandey, A., Arya, N., Halford, G., Jones, S. F., Forshee, R., Walderhaug, M., & Botsis, T. (2017). Natural language processing systems for capturing and standardizing unstructured clinical information: A systematic review. *Journal of Biomedical Informatics, 73*, 14–29. DOI: 10.1016/j.jbi.2017.07.012 PMID: 28729030

Krenn, M., Häse, F., Nigam, A., Friederich, P., & Aspuru-Guzik, A. (2020). Self-referencing embedded strings (SELFIES): A 100% robust molecular string representation. *Machine Learning: Science and Technology, 1*(4), 045024. DOI: 10.1088/2632-2153/aba947

Kreps, G. L., & Neuhauser, L. (2013). Artificial intelligence and immediacy: Designing health communication to engage consumers and providers personally. *Patient Education and Counseling, 92*(2), 205–210. DOI: 10.1016/j.pec.2013.04.014 PMID: 23683341

Kripalani, S., Yao, X., & Haynes, R. B. (2007). Interventions to Enhance Medication Adherence in Chronic Medical Conditions. *Archives of Internal Medicine, 167*(6), 540. DOI: 10.1001/archinte.167.6.540 PMID: 17389285

Krizhevsky, A., Sutskever, I., & Hinton, G. E. (2012). Imagenet classification with deep convolutional neural networks. *Advances in neural information processing systems, 25*.

Kruse, C. S., Goswamy, R., Raval, Y., & Marawi, S. (2016). Challenges and Opportunities of Big Data in Health Care: A Systematic Review. *JMIR Medical Informatics, 4*(4), e38. DOI: 10.2196/medinform.5359 PMID: 27872036

Kumar, P., Dwivedi, Y. K., & Anand, A. (2023). Responsible artificial intelligence (AI) for value formation and market performance in healthcare: The mediating role of patient's cognitive engagement. *Information Systems Frontiers*.

Kumar, A., & Kumar, B. (2017). Automatic recognition of medicinal plants using machine learning techniques. *International Journal of Advanced Computer Science and Applications, 8*(4), 166–175. DOI: 10.14569/IJACSA.2017.080424

Kumar, K. P. V., Lakshmi, B., & Sai Kumar, S. M. V, N. R. Sai and V. Nagamalleswara, "Blockchain Technology: A Comprehensive Review and Future Directions," *2023 Second International Conference on Augmented Intelligence and Sustainable Systems (ICAISS)*, Trichy, India, 2023, pp. 1362-1368, DOI: 10.1109/ICAISS58487.2023.10250707

Kumar, M. S., Ganesh, D., Turukmane, A. V., Batta, U., & Sayyadliyakat, K. K. (2022). Deep convolution neural network based solution for detecting plant diseases. *Journal of Pharmaceutical Negative Results*, *13*, 464–471.

Kutubuddin, K. (2024c). Vehicle Health Monitoring System (VHMS) by Employing IoT and Sensors, *Grenze International Journal of Engineering and Technology,* Vol 10, Issue 2, pp- 5367-5374. Available at: https://thegrenze.com/index.php?display=page&view=journalabstract&absid=3371&id=8

Kutubuddin, K. (2024e). A Novel Approach on ML based Palmistry, *Grenze International Journal of Engineering and Technology,* Vol 10, Issue 2, pp- 5186-5193. Available at: https://thegrenze.com/index.php?display=page&view=journalabstract&absid=3344&id=8

Kutubuddin, K. (2024e). IoT based Boiler Health Monitoring for Sugar Industries, *Grenze. IACSIT International Journal of Engineering and Technology*, *10*(2), 5178–5185. https://thegrenze.com/index.php?display=page&view=journalabstract&absid=3343&id=8

Labovitz, D. L., Shafner, L., Reyes Gil, M., Virmani, D., & Hanina, A. (2017). Using artificial intelligence to reduce the risk of nonadherence in patients on anticoagulation therapy. *Stroke*, *48*(5), 1416–1419. DOI: 10.1161/STROKEAHA.116.016281 PMID: 28386037

Laius, O., Pisarev, H., Maasalu, K., Kõks, S., & Märtson, A. (2017). Adherence to osteoporosis medicines in Estonia—A 15-year retrospective prescriptions database study. *Archives of Osteoporosis*, *12*(1), 59. Advance online publication. DOI: 10.1007/s11657-017-0354-z PMID: 28643266

Lal, J. C., Mao, C., Zhou, Y., Gore-Panter, S. R., Rennison, J. H., Lovano, B. S., Castel, L., Shin, J., Gillinov, A. M., Smith, J. D., Barnard, J., Wagoner, D. R. V., Luo, Y., Cheng, F., & Chung, M. K. (2022). Transcriptomics-based network medicine approach identifies metformin as a repurposable drug for atrial fibrillation. *Cell Reports Medicine*, *3*(10), 100749. Advance online publication. DOI: 10.1016/j.xcrm.2022.100749 PMID: 36223777

Lam, B. D., Dodge, L. E., Zerbey, S., Robertson, W., Rosovsky, R. P., Lake, L., Datta, S., Elavakanar, P., Adamski, A., Reyes, N., Abe, K., Vlachos, I. S., Zwicker, J. I., & Patell, R. (2024). The potential use of artificial intelligence for venous thromboembolism prophylaxis and management: Clinician and healthcare informatician perspectives. *Scientific Reports*, *14*(1), 12010. DOI: 10.1038/s41598-024-62535-9 PMID: 38796561

Lamberti, M. J., Wilkinson, M., Donzanti, B. A., Wohlhieter, G. E., Parikh, S., Wilkins, R. G., & Getz, K. (2019). A study on the application and use of artificial intelligence to support drug development. *Clinical Therapeutics*, *41*(8), 1414–1426. DOI: 10.1016/j.clinthera.2019.05.018 PMID: 31248680

Lamsal, R. (2020). Design and analysis of a large-scale COVID-19 tweets dataset. *Applied Intelligence*. Advance online publication. DOI: 10.1007/s10489-020-02029-z PMID: 34764561

Larson, D. B., Harvey, H., Rubin, D. L., Irani, N., Justin, R. T., & Langlotz, C. P. (2021). Regulatory frameworks for development and evaluation of artificial intelligence–based diagnostic imaging algorithms: Summary and recommendations. *Journal of the American College of Radiology*, *18*(3), 413–424. DOI: 10.1016/j.jacr.2020.09.060 PMID: 33096088

Lavecchia, A. (2015). Machine-learning approaches in drug discovery: Methods and applications. *Drug Discovery Today*, *20*(3), 318–331. DOI: 10.1016/j.drudis.2014.10.012 PMID: 25448759

Lee, D. D., & Seung, H. S. (1999). Learning the parts of objects by non-negative matrix factorization. *Nature*, *401*(6755), 788–791. DOI: 10.1038/44565 PMID: 10548103

Lee, J.-G., Jun, S., Cho, Y.-W., Lee, H., Kim, G. B., Seo, J. B., & Kim, N. (2017). Deep learning in medical imaging: General overview. *Korean Journal of Radiology*, *18*(4), 570–584. DOI: 10.3348/kjr.2017.18.4.570 PMID: 28670152

Lee, M. C. M., Parker, C. H., Liu, L. W. C., Farahvash, A., & Jeyalingam, T. (2024). Impact of study design on adenoma detection in the evaluation of artificial intelligence–aided colonoscopy: A systematic review and meta-analysis. *Gastrointestinal Endoscopy*, *99*(5), 676–687.e616. DOI: 10.1016/j.gie.2024.01.021 PMID: 38272274

Lehmann, A., Aslani, P., Ahmed, R., Celio, J., Gauchet, A., Bedouch, P., Bugnon, O., Allenet, B., & Schneider, M. P. (2013). Assessing medication adherence: Options to consider. *International Journal of Clinical Pharmacy*, *36*(1), 55–69. DOI: 10.1007/s11096-013-9865-x PMID: 24166659

Liebal, U. W., Phan, A. N., Sudhakar, M., Raman, K., & Blank, L. M. (2020). Machine learning applications for mass spectrometry-based metabolomics. *Metabolites*, *10*(6), 243. DOI: 10.3390/metabo10060243 PMID: 32545768

Li, L. (2021). Xianghao, Zhan., Rumeng, Wu., Xiaoqing, Guan., Zhan, Wang., Wei, Zhang., Mert, Pilanci., You, Wang., Zhiyuan, Luo., Guang, Li. Boost AI Power: Data Augmentation Strategies with Unlabelled Data and Conformal Prediction, a Case in Alternative Herbal Medicine Discrimination with Electronic Nose. *IEEE Sensors Journal*. Advance online publication. DOI: 10.1109/JSEN.2021.3102488

Li, M., Liu, R., Lin, J., Bunn, V., & Zhao, H. (2020). Bayesian semi-parametric design (BSD) for adaptive dose-finding with multiple strata. *Journal of Biopharmaceutical Statistics*, *30*(5), 806–820. DOI: 10.1080/10543406.2020.1730870 PMID: 32129133

Lin, C., Liu, W.-T., Chang, C.-H., Lee, C.-C., Hsing, S.-C., Fang, W.-H., . . . Cheng, C.-C. (2024). Artificial intelligence–powered rapid identification of ST-elevation myocardial infarction via electrocardiogram (ARISE)—A pragmatic randomized controlled trial. *NEJM AI*, *1*(7), DOI: 10.1056/AIoa2400190

Lipinski, C. A., Lombardo, F., Dominy, B. W., & Feeney, P. J. (1997). Experimental and computational approaches to estimate solubility and permeability in drug discovery and development settings. *Advanced Drug Delivery Reviews*, *23*(1-3), 3–25. DOI: 10.1016/S0169-409X(96)00423-1 PMID: 11259830

Little, R. J. A., & Rubin, D. B. (2020). *Statistical analysis with missing data* (3rd ed.). John Wiley & Sons, Inc.

Liu, R., Lin, J., & Li, P. (2020). Design considerations for phase I/II dose-finding clinical trials in immuno-oncology and cell therapy. *Contemporary Clinical Trials*, *96*, 106083. DOI: 10.1016/j.cct.2020.106083 PMID: 32659438

Liu, Y., Chen, P.-H. C., Krause, J., & Peng, L. (2019). How to Read Articles That Use Machine Learning: Users' Guides to the Medical Literature. *Journal of the American Medical Association*, *322*(18), 1806–1816. DOI: 10.1001/jama.2019.16489 PMID: 31714992

Liyakat Kazi, K. S. (2024). ChatGPT: An Automated Teacher's Guide to Learning. In Bansal, R., Chakir, A., Hafaz Ngah, A., Rabby, F., & Jain, A. (Eds.), *AI Algorithms and ChatGPT for Student Engagement in Online Learning* (pp. 1–20). IGI Global., DOI: 10.4018/979-8-3693-4268-8.ch001

Liyakat, K. K. S. (2023). Machine Learning Approach Using Artificial Neural Networks to Detect Malicious Nodes in IoT Networks. In Shukla, P. K., Mittal, H., & Engelbrecht, A. (Eds.), *Computer Vision and Robotics. CVR 2023. Algorithms for Intelligent Systems*. Springer., DOI: 10.1007/978-981-99-4577-1_3

Liyakat, K. K. S. (2023).Detecting Malicious Nodes in IoT Networks Using Machine Learning and Artificial Neural Networks, *2023 International Conference on Emerging Smart Computing and Informatics (ESCI)*, Pune, India, 2023, pp. 1-5, DOI: 10.1109/ESCI56872.2023.10099544

Liyakat, K. K. S. (2024). Explainable AI in healthcare. *Explainable Artificial Intelligence in Healthcare Systems, 2024*, 271–284.

Liyakat, K. K. S. (2024). Machine Learning Approach Using Artificial Neural Networks to Detect Malicious Nodes in IoT Networks. In Udgata, S. K., Sethi, S., & Gao, X. Z. (Eds.), *Intelligent Systems. ICMIB 2023. Lecture Notes in Networks and Systems* (Vol. 728). Springer., available at https://link.springer.com/chapter/10.1007/978-981-99-3932-9_12, DOI: 10.1007/978-981-99-3932-9_12

Liyakat, K. S. (2023). Intelligent Watering System (IWS) for Agricultural Land Utilising Raspberry Pi. *Recent Trends in Fluid Mechanics.*, *10*(2), 26–31.

Liyakat, S. S. (2023a). Nanomedicine as a Potential Therapeutic Approach to COVID-19. *International Journal of Applied Nanotechnology*, *9*(2), 27–35p.

Liyakat, S. S. (2023b). IoT Changing the Electronics Manufacturing Industry. *Journal of Analog and Digital Communications*, *8*(3), 13–17. DOI: 10.46610/JoADC.2023.v08i03.003

Liyakat, S. S. (2023c). IoT in the Electric Power Industry. *Journal of Controller and Converters*, *8*(3), 1–7.

Liyakat, S. S. (2024). IoT-based Alcohol Detector using Blynk. *Journal of Electronics Design and Technology*, *1*(1), 10–15.

Lomenick, B., Olsen, R. W., & Huang, J. (2011). Identification of Direct Protein Targets of Small Molecules. *ACS Chemical Biology*, *6*(1), 34–46. DOI: 10.1021/cb100294v PMID: 21077692

Long, J., Yuan, M. J., & Poonawala, R. (2016). An Observational Study to Evaluate the Usability and Intent to Adopt an Artificial Intelligence–Powered Medication Reconciliation Tool. *Interactive Journal of Medical Research*, *5*(2), e14. DOI: 10.2196/ijmr.5462 PMID: 27185210

Loomans, B. A. C., Mendes, F. M., Vinayahalingam, S., Xi, T., Opdam, N. J. M., Kreulen, C. M., Pereira-Cenci, T., & Cenci, M. S. (2024). Challenges in conducting clinical research in primary care dentistry. *Journal of Dentistry*, *144*, 104958. DOI: 10.1016/j.jdent.2024.104958 PMID: 38522408

López-López, E., Bajorath, J., & Medina-Franco, J. L. (2020). Informatics for chemistry, biology, and biomedical sciences. *Journal of Chemical Information and Modeling*, *61*(1), 26–35. DOI: 10.1021/acs.jcim.0c01301 PMID: 33382611

Lou, N., Cui, X., Lin, X., Gao, R., Xu, C., Qiao, N., Jiang, J., Wang, L., Wang, W., Wang, S., Shen, W., Zheng, X., & Han, X. (2024). Development and validation of a deep learning-based model to predict response and survival of T790M mutant non-small cell lung cancer patients in early clinical phase trials using electronic medical record and pharmacokinetic data. *Translational Lung Cancer Research*, *13*(4), 706–720. DOI: 10.21037/tlcr-23-737 PMID: 38736496

Luo, J., Wu, M., Gopukumar, D., & Zhao, Y. (2016). Big Data Application in Biomedical Research and Health Care: A Literature Review. *Biomedical Informatics Insights, 8*. *Biomedical Informatics Insights*, *S31559*, BII.S31559. Advance online publication. DOI: 10.4137/BII.S31559 PMID: 26843812

Lu, X., Ma, W., Fan, B., Li, P., Gao, J., Liu, Q., Hu, C., Li, Y., Yao, M., Ning, H., & Xing, L. (2021). Integrating network pharmacology, transcriptome and artificial intelligence for investigating into the effect and mechanism of Ning Fei Ping Xue decoction against the acute respiratory distress syndrome. *Frontiers in Pharmacology*, *12*, 731377. DOI: 10.3389/fphar.2021.731377 PMID: 34803679

MacKay, E. J., Stubna, M. D., Chivers, C., Draugelis, M. E., Hanson, W. J., Desai, N. D., & Groeneveld, P. W. (2021). Application of machine learning approaches to administrative claims data to predict clinical outcomes in medical and surgical patient populations. *PLoS One*, *16*(6), e0252585. DOI: 10.1371/journal.pone.0252585 PMID: 34081720

Madhav, N., Oppenheim, B., Gallivan, M., Mulembakani, P., Rubin, E., & Wolfe, N. (2017). Pandemics: Risks, impacts, and mitigation. In *Disease control priorities: Improving health and reducing poverty* (3rd ed., Vol. 9, pp. 315–345). The International Bank for Reconstruction and Development/The World Bank.

Madhavi Sastry, G., Adzhigirey, M., Day, T., Annabhimoju, R., & Sherman, W. (2013). Protein and ligand preparation: Parameters, protocols, and influence on virtual screening enrichments. *Journal of Computer-Aided Molecular Design*, *27*(3), 221–234. DOI: 10.1007/s10822-013-9644-8 PMID: 23579614

Ma, J., Sheridan, R. P., Liaw, A., Dahl, G. E., & Svetnik, V. (2015). Deep neural nets as a method for quantitative structure–activity relationships. *Journal of Chemical Information and Modeling*, *55*(2), 263–274. DOI: 10.1021/ci500747n PMID: 25635324

Mak, K. K., Wong, Y. H., & Pichika, M. R. (2024). Artificial intelligence in drug discovery and development. In *Drug discovery and evaluation: safety and pharmacokinetic assays* (1461-1498). doi.org/10.1007/978-3-030-73317-9_92-1

Mak, K.-K., & Pichika, M. R. (2019). Artificial intelligence in drug development: Present status and future prospects. *Drug Discovery Today*, *24*(3), 773–780. DOI: 10.1016/j.drudis.2018.11.014 PMID: 30472429

Mandal, L., & Jana, N. D. (2019). Prediction of active drug molecule using backpropagation neural network. In *Proceedings of the 8th International Conference System Modeling and Advancement in Research Trends (SMART)* (pp. 22–26). Moradabad, India DOI: 10.1109/SMART46866.2019.9117378

Maniyar, D. M., Nabney, I. T., Williams, B. S., & Sewing, A. (2006). Data visualization during the early stages of drug discovery. *Journal of Chemical Information and Modeling*, *46*(4), 1806–1818. DOI: 10.1021/ci050471a PMID: 16859312

Manta, C., Patrick-Lake, B., & Goldsack, J. C. (2020). Digital measures that matter to patients: a framework to guide the selection and development of digital measures of health. Digital Biomarkers. karger.comDOI: 10.1186/s13054-021-03822-z PMID: 34814925

Marcus, J. L., Sewell, W. C., Balzer, L. B., & Krakower, D. S. (2020). Artificial Intelligence and Machine Learning for HIV Prevention: Emerging Approaches to Ending the Epidemic. [CrossRef]. *Current HIV/AIDS Reports*, *17*(3), 171–179. DOI: 10.1007/s11904-020-00490-6 PMID: 32347446

Marini, M., Chokani, N., & Abhari, R. S. COVID-19 Epidemic in Switzerland: Growth Prediction and Containment Strategy Using Artificial Intelligence and Big Data. *medRxiv* 2020. *medRxiv*:2020.03.30.20047472. DOI: 10.1101/2020.03.30.20047472

Marino, M., Lucas, J., Latour, E., & Heintzman, J. D. (2021). Missing data in primary care research: Importance, implications and approaches. *Family Practice*, *38*(2), 199–202. DOI: 10.1093/fampra/cmaa134 PMID: 33480404

Master Grid of Standards. Health Level Seven International. URL: https://www.hl7.org/implement/standards/product_brief.cfm?product_id=7V [accessed 2020-04-13]

Mater, A. C., & Coote, M. L. (2019). Deep learning in chemistry. *Journal of Chemical Information and Modeling*, *59*(6), 2545–2559. DOI: 10.1021/acs.jcim.9b00266 PMID: 31194543

May, B. H., Zhang, A., Lu, Y., Lu, C., & Xue, C. C. (2014). The systematic assessment of traditional evidence from the premodern Chinese medical literature: A text-mining approach. *Journal of Alternative and Complementary Medicine (New York, N.Y.)*, *20*(12), 937–942. DOI: 10.1089/acm.2013.0372 PMID: 25389563

Mayr, A., Klambauer, G., Unterthiner, T., & Hochreiter, S. (2016). DeepTox: Toxicity prediction using deep learning. *Frontiers in Environmental Science, 3*, 80.57

Medina-Franco, J. L., Naveja, J. J., & López-López, E. (2019). Reaching for the bright StARs in chemical space. *Drug Discovery Today*, *24*(11), 2162–2169. DOI: 10.1016/j.drudis.2019.09.013 PMID: 31557448

Medina-Franco, J. L., & Saldívar-González, F. I. (2020). Cheminformatics to characterize pharmacologically active natural products. *Biomolecules*, *10*(11), 1566. DOI: 10.3390/biom10111566 PMID: 33213003

Mercado, , RRastemo, , TLindelöf, , EKlambauer, , GEngkvist, , OChen, , HBjerrum, , E. J. (2020). Practical notes on building molecular graph generative models. *Applied AI Letters*, *1*(2).

Merk, D., Grisoni, F., Friedrich, L., & Schneider, G. (2018). Tuning artificial intelligence on the de novo design of natural-product-inspired retinoid X receptor modulators. *Communications Chemistry*, *1*(1), 68. DOI: 10.1038/s42004-018-0068-1

Meskó, B. & Topol, E. J. (2023). The imperative for regulatory oversight of large language models (or generative AI) in healthcare. *NPJ digital medicine.*

Meystre, S. M., Savova, G. K., Kipper-Schuler, K. C., & Hurdle, J. F. (2008). Extracting information from textual documents in the electronic health record: A review of recent research. *Yearbook of Medical Informatics*, •••, 128–144. https://pubmed.ncbi.nlm.nih.gov/18660887/ PMID: 18660887

Mhlanga, D. (2021). Artificial intelligence in the industry 4.0, and its impact on poverty, innovation, infrastructure development, and the sustainable development goals: Lessons from emerging economies? *Sustainability*. 10.3390/su13115788

Miles, J., & Walker, A. The potential application of artificial intelligence in transport. IEE Proc.-Intell. Transport Syst. 2006; 153:183–198 DOI: 10.1049/ip-its:20060014

Miller, M. I., Shih, L. C., & Kolachalama, V. B. (2023). Machine learning in clinical trials: A primer with applications to neurology. *Neurotherapeutics; the Journal of the American Society for Experimental NeuroTherapeutics, 20*(4), 1066–1080. DOI: 10.1007/s13311-023-01384-2 PMID: 37249836

Miotto, R., Wang, F., Wang, S., Jiang, X., & Dudley, J. T. (2018). Deep Learning for healthcare: Review, Opportunities and Challenges. *Briefings in Bioinformatics, 19*(6), 1236–1246. DOI: 10.1093/bib/bbx044 PMID: 28481991

Mirakhori, F., & Niazi, S. K. (2025). Harnessing the AI/ML in Drug and Biological Products Discovery and Development: The Regulatory Perspective. *Pharmaceuticals, 18*(1), 47. https://doi.org/10.3390/ph18010047

Mishra Sunil, B.. (2024). AI-Driven IoT (AI IoT) in Thermodynamic Engineering. *Journal of Modern Thermodynamics in Mechanical System, 6*(1), 1–8.

Mohsen, A., Tripathi, L. P., & Mizuguchi, K. (2021). Deep Learning Prediction of Adverse Drug Reactions in Drug Discovery Using Open TG–GATEs and FAERS Databases. *Frontiers in Drug Discovery, 1*, 768792. Advance online publication. DOI: 10.3389/fddsv.2021.768792

Mohsin, N. A., Aslam, S., Ahmad, M., Irfan, M., Al-Hussain, S. A., & Zaki, M. E. A.Mohsin NuA. (2022). Aslam S, Ahmad M, Irfan M, Al-Hussain SA, Zaki MEA. Cyclooxygenase-2 (COX-2) as a Target of Anticancer Agents: A Review of Novel Synthesized Scaffolds Having Anticancer and COX-2 Inhibitory Potentialities. *Pharmaceuticals (Basel, Switzerland), 15*(12), 1471. DOI: 10.3390/ph15121471 PMID: 36558921

Mongkhon, P., Ashcroft, D. M., Scholfield, C. N., & Kongkaew, C. (2018). Hospital admissions associated with medication non-adherence: A systematic review of prospective observational studies. *BMJ Quality & Safety, 27*(11), 902–914. DOI: 10.1136/bmjqs-2017-007453 PMID: 29666309

Moosivand, A., Rajabzadeh Ghatari, A., & Rasekh, H. R. (2019, Spring). Supply Chain Challenges in Pharmaceutical Manufacturing Companies: Using Qualitative System Dynamics Methodology. *Iranian Journal of Pharmaceutical Research : IJPR, 18*(2), 1103–1116. DOI: 10.22037/ijpr.2019.2389 PMID: 31531092

Morris, G. M., Huey, R., & Olson, A. J. (2008). Using autodock for ligand-receptor docking. *Current Protocols in Bioinformatics, 24*(1), 8–14. DOI: 10.1002/0471250953.bi0814s24 PMID: 19085980

Mozayan, A., Fabbri, A. R., Maneevese, M., Tocino, I., & Chheang, S. (2021). Practical Guide to Natural Language Processing for Radiology. *Radiographics, 41*(5), 1446–1453. DOI: 10.1148/rg.2021200113 PMID: 34469212

Muehlematter, U. J., Daniore, P., & Vokinger, K. N. (2021). Approval of artificial intelligence and machine learning-based medical devices in the USA and Europe (2015-20): A comparative analysis. [DOI:10.1016/ S2589-7500(20)30292-2] [PMID]. *The Lancet. Digital Health, 3*(3), e195–e203. DOI: 10.1016/S2589-7500(20)30292-2 PMID: 33478929

Müller, R. (2008). Junghanns Nanocrystal Technology, Rifampicin Delivery and Clinical Applications. *International Journal of Nanomedicine, 3*, 295–310. DOI: 10.2147/IJN.S595 PMID: 18990939

Mullowney, M. W., Duncan, K. R., Elsayed, S. S., Garg, N., van der Hooft, J. J. J., Martin, N. I., Meijer, D., Terlouw, B. R., Biermann, F., Blin, K., Durairaj, J., Gorostiola González, M., Helfrich, E. J. N., Huber, F., Leopold-Messer, S., Rajan, K., de Rond, T., van Santen, J. A., Sorokina, M., . . . Medema, M. H. (2023). Artificial intelligence for natural product drug discovery. In *Nature Reviews Drug Discovery* (Vol. 22, Issue 11, pp. 895–916). Nature Research. DOI: 10.1038/s41573-023-00774-7

Muratov, E. N., Bajorath, J., Sheridan, R. P., Tetko, I. V., Filimonov, D., Poroikov, V., Oprea, T. I., Baskin, I. I., Varnek, A., Roitberg, A., Isayev, O., Curtalolo, S., Fourches, D., Cohen, Y., Aspuru-Guzik, A., Winkler, D. A., Agrafiotis, D., Cherkasov, A., & Tropsha, A. (2020). QSAR without borders. *Chemical Society Reviews, 49*(11), 3525–3564. DOI: 10.1039/D0CS00098A PMID: 32356548

Murdoch, T. B., & Detsky, A. S. (2013). The Inevitable Application of Big Data to Health Care. *Journal of the American Medical Association, 309*(13), 1351. DOI: 10.1001/jama.2013.393 PMID: 23549579

Murff, H. J., FitzHenry, F., Matheny, M. E., Gentry, N., Kotter, K. L., Crimin, K., Dittus, R. S., Rosen, A. K., Elkin, P. L., Brown, S. H., & Speroff, T. (2011). Automated Identification of Postoperative Complications Within an Electronic Medical Record Using Natural Language Processing. *Journal of the American Medical Association, 306*(8). Advance online publication. DOI: 10.1001/jama.2011.1204 PMID: 21862746

Murphy, S. N., Morgan, M. M., Barnett, G. O., & Chueh, H. C. (1999). Optimizing healthcare research data warehouse design through past COSTAR query analysis. *Proceedings. AMIA Symposium*, 892–896. https://pubmed.ncbi.nlm.nih.gov/10566489/

Murphy, R. M., Klopotowska, J. E., de Keizer, N. F., Jager, K. J., Leopold, J. H., Dongelmans, D. A., Abu-Hanna, A., & Schut, M. C. (2023). Adverse drug event detection using natural language processing: A scoping review of supervised learning methods. *PLoS One*, *18*(1), e0279842. DOI: 10.1371/journal.pone.0279842 PMID: 36595517

Murphy, S. N., Mendis, M., Hackett, K., Kuttan, R., Pan, W., Phillips, L. C., Gainer, V., Berkowicz, D., Glaser, J. P., Kohane, I., & Chueh, H. C. (2007). Architecture of the Open-source Clinical Research Chart from Informatics for Integrating Biology and the Bedside. *AMIA ... Annual Symposium Proceedings - AMIA Symposium. AMIA Symposium*, *2007*, 548–552. https://www.ncbi.nlm.nih.gov/pmc/articles/PMC2655844/ PMID: 18693896

Nadarzynski, T., Miles, O., Cowie, A., & Ridge, D. (2019). Acceptability of artificial intelligence (AI)-led chatbot services in healthcare: A mixed-methods study. *Digital Health*, *5*, 205520761987180. DOI: 10.1177/2055207619871808 PMID: 31467682

Naderi, S. H., Bestwick, J. P., & Wald, D. S. (2012). Adherence to Drugs That Prevent Cardiovascular Disease: Meta-analysis on 376,162 Patients. *The American Journal of Medicine*, *125*(9), 882–887.e1. DOI: 10.1016/j.amjmed.2011.12.013 PMID: 22748400

Nagrale, M., Pol, R. S., Birajadar, G. B., & Mulani, A. O. (2024). Internet of Robotic Things in Cardiac Surgery: An Innovative Approach. *African Journal of Biological Sciences*, *6*(6), 709–725. DOI: 10.33472/AFJBS.6.6.2024.709-725

Naman, S., Sharma, S., Jain, A., Jindal, S., & Baldi, A. (2023). Artificial Intelligence-based Machine Learning Model for Identification of Spices and Herbs. *Systematic Reviews*.

Nashwan, A. J., & Hani, S. B. (2023). Transforming cancer clinical trials: The integral role of artificial intelligence in electronic health records for efficient patient recruitment. *Contemporary Clinical Trials Communications, 36*, 101223, 101223. DOI: 10.1016/j.conctc.2023.101223

Nassif, A. B., Talib, M. A., Nasir, Q., & Dakalbab, F. M. (2021). Machine Learning for Anomaly Detection: A Systematic Review. *IEEE Access : Practical Innovations, Open Solutions*, *9*, 78658–78700. DOI: 10.1109/ACCESS.2021.3083060

National Association of Community Health Centers. (2019). *Research fact sheets and infographics*. https://nachc.org/research-and-data/research-fact-sheets-and-infographics/

Nawab, K., Ramsey, G., & Schreiber, R. (2020). Natural Language Processing to Extract Meaningful Information from Patient Experience Feedback. *Applied Clinical Informatics*, *11*(02), 242–252. DOI: 10.1055/s-0040-1708049 PMID: 32236917

Nayarisseri, A., Khandelwal, R., Tanwar, P., Madhavi, M., Sharma, D., Thakur, G., & Singh, S. K. (2021). Artificial intelligence, big data and machine learning approaches in precision medicine & drug discovery. *Current Drug Targets*, *22*(6), 631–655. DOI: 10.2174/18735592MTEzsMDMnz PMID: 33397265

Nebeker, C., Torous, J., & Ellis, R. J. B. (2019b). Building the case for actionable ethics in digital health research supported by artificial intelligence. *BMC Medicine*, *17*(1), 137. Advance online publication. DOI: 10.1186/s12916-019-1377-7 PMID: 31311535

Neeraja, P., Kumar, R. G., Kumar, M. S., Liyakat, K. K. S., & Vani, M. S. (2024, February). DL-based somnolence detection for improved driver safety and alertness monitoring. In 2024 IEEE International Conference on Computing, Power and Communication Technologies (IC2PCT) (Vol. 5, pp. 589-594). IEEE.

Nene, L., Flepisi, B. T., Brand, S. J., Basson, C., & Balmith, M. (2024). Evolution of drug development and regulatory affairs: The demonstrated power of artificial intelligence. *Clinical Therapeutics*. DOI: 10.1016/j.clinthera.2024.05.012 PMID: 38981791

Nerkar, P. M., & Dhaware, B. U. (2023). Predictive Data Analytics Framework Based on Heart Healthcare System (HHS) Using Machine Learning, Journal of Advanced Zoology, 2023, Volume 44, Special Issue -2. *Page*, *3673*, 3686.

Newman, D. J., & Cragg, G. M. (2020). Natural products as sources of new drugs over the nearly four decades from 01/1981 to 09/2019. *Journal of Natural Products*, *83*(3), 770–803. DOI: 10.1021/acs.jnatprod.9b01285 PMID: 32162523

Ngiam, K. Y., & Khor, I. W. (2019). Big data and machine learning algorithms for healthcare delivery. *The Lancet. Oncology*, *20*(5), e262–e273. DOI: 10.1016/S1470-2045(19)30149-4 PMID: 31044724

Nguyen, A., Lamouri, S., Pellerin, R., & Giraldo, T. (2021). Data analytics in pharmaceutical supply chains: State of the art, opportunities, and challenges. *International Journal of Production Research*, *60*(22), 6888–6907. Advance online publication. DOI: 10.1080/00207543.2021.1950937

Nguyen, L., Bellucci, E., & Nguyen, L. T. (2014). Electronic health records implementation: An evaluation of information system impact and contingency factors. *International Journal of Medical Informatics*, *83*(11), 779–796. DOI: 10.1016/j.ijmedinf.2014.06.011 PMID: 25085286

Ni, Y., Wright, J., Perentesis, J., Lingren, T., Deleger, L., Kaiser, M., Solti, I. (2015). Increasing the efficiency of trial-patient matching: Automated clinical trial eligibility prescreening for pediatric oncology patients clinical decision-making, knowledge support systems, and theory. *BMC Medical Informatics and Decision Making, 15*(1), 28, 28. DOI: 10.1186/s12911-015-0149-3

Niazi, S. K., & Mariam, Z. (2024). Computer-Aided Drug Design and Drug Discovery: A Prospective Analysis. In *Pharmaceuticals* (Vol. 17, Issue 1). Multidisciplinary Digital Publishing Institute (MDPI). DOI: 10.3390/ph17010022

Nilsson, N. J. (2010). *The quest for artificial intelligence: A history of ideas and achievements*. Cambridge University Press.

Nomura, A., Noguchi, M., Kometani, M., Furukawa, K., & Yoneda, T. (2021). Artificial Intelligence in Current Diabetes Management and Prediction. In *Current Diabetes Reports* (Vol. 21, Issue 12). Springer. DOI: 10.1007/s11892-021-01423-2

Nugroho, A. E., & Morita, H. (2019). Computationally-assisted discovery and structure elucidation of natural products. *Journal of Natural Medicines*, *73*(4), 687–695. DOI: 10.1007/s11418-019-01321-8 PMID: 31093833

O'Sullivan, S., Nevejans, N., Allen, C., Blyth, A., Leonard, S., Pagallo, U., Holzinger, K., Holzinger, A., Sajid, M. I., & Ashrafian, H. (2019). Legal, regulatory, and ethical frameworks for developing standards in artificial intelligence (AI)and autonomous robotic surgery. [DOI:10.1002/rcs.1968] [PMID]. *International Journal of Medical Robotics and Computer Assisted Surgery*, *15*(1), e1968. DOI: 10.1002/rcs.1968 PMID: 30397993

Obermeyer, Z., & Emanuel, E. J. (2016). Predicting the Future — Big Data, Machine Learning, and Clinical Medicine. *The New England Journal of Medicine*, *375*(13), 1216–1219. DOI: 10.1056/NEJMp1606181 PMID: 27682033

O'Boyle, N., & Dalke, A. (2018). DeepSMILES: an adaptation of SMILES for use in machine-learning of chemical structures.

Obschonka, M., & Audretsch, D. B. (2020). Artificial intelligence and big data in entrepreneurship: A new era has begun. *Small Business Economics*, *55*(3), 529–539. DOI: 10.1007/s11187-019-00202-4

OECD. (2018).. . *Health at a Glance. Europe, 2018,* •••. https://www.oecd.org/health/health-at-a-glance-europe-23056088.htm

OECD. (2019). *Artificial Intelligence in Society*. OECD.

OECD. (2019). Health in the 21st Century: Putting Data to Work for Stronger Health System. In *OECD Health Policy Studies*. OECD Publishing.

Oladoyinbo, T. O., Olabanji, S. O., Olaniyi, O. O., Adebiyi, O. O., Okunleye, O. J., & Ismaila Alao, A. (2024). Exploring the challenges of artificial intelligence in data integrity and its influence on social dynamics. *Asian Journal of Advanced Research and Reports*, *18*(2), 1–23. DOI: 10.9734/ajarr/2024/v18i2601

Osasona, F., Amoo, O. O., Atadoga, A., Abrahams, T. O., Farayola, O. A., & Ayinla, B. S. (2024). Reviewing the ethical implications of AI in decision making processes. *International Journal of Management & Entrepreneurship Research*, *6*(2), 322–335. DOI: 10.51594/ijmer.v6i2.773

Osolodkin, D. I., Radchenko, E. V., Orlov, A. A., Voronkov, A. E., Palyulin, V. A., & Zefirov, N. S. (2015). Progress in visual representations of chemical space. *Expert Opinion on Drug Discovery*, *10*(9), 959–973. DOI: 10.1517/17460441.2015.1060216 PMID: 26094796

Ozcelik, F., Dundar, M. S., Yildirim, A. B., Henehan, G., Vicente, O., Sánchez-Alcázar, J. A., Gokce, N., Yildirim, D. T., Bingol, N. N., Karanfilska, D. P., Bertelli, M., Pojskic, L., Ercan, M., Kellermayer, M., Sahin, I. O., Greiner-Tollersrud, O. K., Tan, B., Martin, D., Marks, R., & Dundar, M. (2024). The impact and future of artificial intelligence in medical genetics and molecular medicine: An ongoing revolution. *Functional & Integrative Genomics*, *24*(4), 138. DOI: 10.1007/s10142-024-01417-9 PMID: 39147901

Öztürk, H., Özgür, A., Schwaller, P., Laino, T., & Ozkirimli, E. (2020). Exploring chemical space using natural language processing methodologies for drug discovery. *Drug Discovery Today*, *25*(4), 689–705. DOI: 10.1016/j.drudis.2020.01.020 PMID: 32027969

Padmanaban, H. (2023). Navigating the intricacies of regulations: Leveraging AI/ML for Accurate Reporting. *Journal of Knowledge Learning and Science Technology, 2*(3), 401-412.

Palmer, K., Marengoni, A., Forjaz, M. J., Jureviciene, E., Laatikainen, T., Mammarella, F., Muth, C., Navickas, R., Prados-Torres, A., Rijken, M., Rothe, U., Souchet, L., Valderas, J., Vontetsianos, T., Zaletel, J., & Onder, G. (2017). Multimorbidity care model: Recommendations from the consensus meeting of the Joint Action on Chronic Diseases and Promoting Healthy Ageing across the Life Cycle (JA-CHRODIS). *Health Policy (Amsterdam), 122*(1), 4–11. DOI: 10.1016/j.healthpol.2017.09.006 PMID: 28967492

Pandey, M., Fernandez, M., Gentile, F., Isayev, O., Tropsha, A., Stern, A. C., & Cherkasov, A. (2022). The transformational role of GPU computing and deep learning in drug discovery. *Nature Machine Intelligence*, *4*(3), 211–221.

Pang, B., Lee, L., & Vaithyanathan, S. (2002). Thumbs up? Sentiment Classification using Machine Learning Techniques. *Proceedings of the ACL-02 Conference on Empirical Methods in Natural Language Processing - EMNLP '02, 10*. DOI: 10.3115/1118693.1118704

Pang, X. C., Kang, D., Fang, J. S., Zhao, Y., Xu, L. J., Lian, W. W., Liu, A.-L., & Du, G.-H. (2018). Network Pharmacology-Based Analysis of Chinese Herbal Naodesheng Formula for Application to Alzheimer's Disease. *Chinese Journal of Natural Medicines*, *16*(1), 53–62. DOI: 10.1016/S1875-5364(18)30029-3 PMID: 29425590

Paolini, G. V., Shapland, R. H., van Hoorn, W. P., Mason, J. S., & Hopkins, A. L. (2006). Global mapping of pharmacological space. *Nature Biotechnology*, *24*(7), 805–815. DOI: 10.1038/nbt1228 PMID: 16841068

Papanikolaou, N., Pavlopoulos, G. A., Theodosiou, T., & Iliopoulos, I. (2015). Protein–protein interaction predictions using text mining methods. *Methods (San Diego, Calif.)*, *74*, 47–53. DOI: 10.1016/j.ymeth.2014.10.026 PMID: 25448298

Park, S., Ock, C.-Y., Kim, H., Pereira, S., Park, S., Ma, M., Choi, S., Kim, S., Shin, S., Aum, B. J., Paeng, K., Yoo, D., Cha, H., Park, S., Suh, K. J., Jung, H. A., Kim, S. H., Kim, Y. J., Sun, J.-M., & Lee, S.-H. (2022). Artificial Intelligence-Powered Spatial Analysis of Tumor-Infiltrating Lymphocytes as Complementary Biomarker for Immune Checkpoint Inhibition in Non-Small-Cell Lung Cancer. *Journal of Clinical Oncology*, *40*(17), 1916–1928. DOI: 10.1200/JCO.21.02010 PMID: 35271299

Patel, V. & Shah, M. (2022). Artificial intelligence and machine learning in drug discovery and development. *Intelligent Medicine*.

Patel, S. J., Yousuf, S., Padala, J. V., Reddy, S., Saraf, P., Nooh, A., Fernandez Gutierrez, L. M. A., Abdirahman, A. H., Tanveer, R., & Rai, M. (2024). Advancements in artificial intelligence for precision diagnosis and treatment of myocardial infarction: A comprehensive review of clinical trials and randomized controlled trials. *Cureus*, *16*(5), e60119. DOI: 10.7759/cureus.60119 PMID: 38864061

Paul, D., Sanap, G., Shenoy, S., Kalyane, D., Kalia, K., & Tekade, R. K. (2021). Artificial intelligence in drug discovery and development. In *Drug Discovery Today* (Vol. 26, Issue 1, pp. 80–93). Elsevier Ltd. DOI: 10.1016/j.drudis.2020.10.010

Pedersen, M., Pardoe, H. R., de Weger, A., Hutchison, D., Abbott, D., Verspoor, K., & Jackson, G. D. (2023). Artificial intelligence is changing the ethics of medicine: Reflections from the Australian Epilepsy Project.

Peng, J., Jury, E. C., Dönnes, P., & Ciurtin, C. (2021). Machine Learning Techniques for Personalised Medicine Approaches in Immune-Mediated Chronic Inflammatory Diseases: Applications and Challenges. *Frontiers in Pharmacology*, *12*(1), 720694. Advance online publication. DOI: 10.3389/fphar.2021.720694 PMID: 34658859

Peng, Y., Wang, H., Fang, Q., Xie, L., Shu, L., Sun, W., & Liu, Q. (2020). Effectiveness of Mobile Applications on Medication Adherence in Adults with Chronic Diseases: A Systematic Review and Meta-Analysis. *Journal of Managed Care & Specialty Pharmacy*, *26*(4), 550–561. DOI: 10.18553/jmcp.2020.26.4.550 PMID: 32223596

Pereira, F., & Aires-de-Sousa, J. (2018). Computational methodologies in the exploration of marine natural product leads. *Marine Drugs*, *16*(7), 236. DOI: 10.3390/md16070236 PMID: 30011882

Perera, M. G. M., Karunarathna, A. N., & Wijewardana Year, K. P. (2023). "Machine learning-based identification of medicinal plants. *RE:view*.

Platt, R., Carnahan, R. M., Brown, J. S., Chrischilles, E., Curtis, L. H., Hennessy, S., Nelson, J. C., Racoosin, J. A., Robb, M., Schneeweiss, S., Toh, S., & Weiner, M. G. (2012). The U.S. Food and Drug Administration's Mini-Sentinel program: Status and direction. *Pharmacoepidemiology and Drug Safety*, *21*(S1), 1–8. DOI: 10.1002/pds.2343 PMID: 22262586

Porras, G., Chassagne, F., Lyles, J. T., Marquez, L., Dettweiler, M., Salam, A. M., Samarakoon, T., Shabih, S., Farrokhi, D. R., & Quave, C. L. (2020). Ethnobotany and the role of plant natural products in antibiotic drug discovery. *Chemical Reviews*, *121*(6), 3495–3560. DOI: 10.1021/acs.chemrev.0c00922 PMID: 33164487

Pradeepa, M., ... (2022). Student Health Detection using a Machine Learning Approach and IoT, 2022 IEEE 2nd Mysore sub section International Conference (MysuruCon), 2022.

Prasad, K. R., Karanam, S. R., Ganesh, D., Liyakat, K. K. S., Talasila, V., & Purushotham, P. (2024, May). AI in public-private partnership for IT infrastructure development. *The Journal of High Technology Management Research*, *35*(1), 100496. DOI: 10.1016/j.hitech.2024.100496

Prayaga, R. B., Jeong, E. W., Feger, E., Noble, H. K., Kmiec, M., & Prayaga, R. S. (2018b). Improving Refill Adherence in Medicare Patients with Tailored and Interactive Mobile Text Messaging: Pilot Study. *JMIR mHealth and uHealth*, *6*(1), e30. DOI: 10.2196/mhealth.8930 PMID: 29382623

Prayag, R. B., Agrawal, R., Nguyen, B., Jeong, E. W., Noble, H. K., Paster, A., & Prayaga, R. S. (2019). Impact of Social Determinants of Health and Demographics on Refill Requests by Medicare Patients Using a Conversational Artificial Intelligence Text Messaging Solution: Cross-Sectional Study. *JMIR mHealth and uHealth*, *7*(11), e15771. DOI: 10.2196/15771 PMID: 31738170

Rafferty, R. J., Hicklin, R. W., Maloof, K. A., & Hergenrother, P. J. (2014). Synthesis of complex and diverse compounds through ring distortion of abietic acid. *Angewandte Chemie*, *126*(1), 224–228. DOI: 10.1002/ange.201308743 PMID: 24273016

Raghupathi, W., & Raghupathi, V. (2014). Big data analytics in healthcare: Promise and potential. *Health Information Science and Systems*, *2*(1), 1–10. DOI: 10.1186/2047-2501-2-3 PMID: 25825667

Raghu, S. A., Kavitha, P., & Suma Year, M. C.: 2018 Title: "Medicinal plant leaf identification using texture and shape features with machine learning algorithms" DOI: 10.1039/D1SC04471K PMID: 35282622

Rahim, A. (2022). M., M., Al-Amidi., Hamed, Mohammadi., Mehmet, Çifci., Avat, Daryab., Eugenio, Cavallo. An AI Based Approach for Medicinal Plant Identification Using Deep CNN Based on Global Average Pooling. *Agronomy (Basel)*, *12*(11), 2723. Advance online publication. DOI: 10.3390/agronomy12112723

Raja, D. B., Mallol, R., Ting, C. Y., Kamaludin, F., Ahmad, R., Ismail, S., Jayaraj, V. J., & Sundaram, B. M. (2019). Artificial intelligence model as a predictor for dengue outbreaks. *Malaysian Journal of Public Health Medicine*, *19*(2), 103–108. DOI: 10.37268/mjphm/vol.19/no.2/art.176

Rajan, K., Zielesny, A., & Steinbeck, C. J. (2020). *Cheminf* 12:65. [PMC free article] [PubMed] [Google Scholar]

Rajkomar, A., Oren, E., Chen, K., Dai, A. M., Hajaj, N., Hardt, M., Liu, P. J., Liu, X., Marcus, J., Sun, M., Sundberg, P., Yee, H., Zhang, K., Zhang, Y., Flores, G., Duggan, G. E., Irvine, J., Le, Q., Litsch, K., & Dean, J. (2018). Scalable and accurate deep learning with electronic health records. *NPJ Digital Medicine*, *1*(1), 18. Advance online publication. DOI: 10.1038/s41746-018-0029-1 PMID: 31304302

Rakočević, T., & Markovic, M. (2024). Assessing the impact of AI: The case of the pharmaceutical industry. *European Journal of Business and Management Research*, *9*(5), 70–75. DOI: 10.24018/ejbmr.2024.9.5.1124

Rakočević, T., & Markovic, M. (2024). Assessing the Impact of AI: The Case of the Pharmaceutical Industry. *European Journal of Business and Management Research, 9*5), 70-75.)

Ralhan, K., & Person. (2024, January 18). *Ai's emerging role in natural product drug discovery*. RSS. https://www.cas.org/resources/cas-insights/ais-emerging-role-in-natural-product-drug-discovery

Ramesh, A. N., Kambhampati, C., Monson, J. R., & Drew, P. J. (2004). Artificial intelligence in medicine. *Annals of the Royal College of Surgeons of England*, *86*(5), 334–338. DOI: 10.1308/147870804290 PMID: 15333167

Raparthi, M., Gayam, S. R., Nimmagadda, V. S. P., Sahu, M. K., Putha, S., Pattyam, S. P., & Kuna, S. S. (2022). AI assisted drug discovery: Emphasizing its role in accelerating precision medicine initiatives and improving treatment outcomes. *Human-Computer Interaction Perspectives*, *2*(2), 1–10.

Rasmussen, J. N., Chong, A., & Alter, D. A. (2007). Relationship Between Adherence to Evidence-Based Pharmacotherapy and Long-term Mortality After Acute Myocardial Infarction. *Journal of the American Medical Association*, *297*(2), 177. DOI: 10.1001/jama.297.2.177 PMID: 17213401

Rasool, S., Ali, M., Shahroz, H. M., Hussain, H. K., & Gill, A. Y. (2024). Innovations in AI-Powered Healthcare: Transforming Cancer Treatment with Innovative Methods. *BULLET: Jurnal Multidisiplin Ilmu*, *3*(1), 118–128.

Ravali, R. S., Auguskani, J. P. L., Reddy, L. K. V., Narapureddy, B. R., Chellathurai, A., & Mavaluru, D. (2023). Pioneering ethical boundaries: Empowering AI governance for the future of pharmaceutical and nursing sectors. *Latin American Journal of Pharmacy*, *42*(3), 695–701.

Rawat, W., & Wang, Z. (2017). Deep convolutional neural networks for image classification: A comprehensive review. *Neural Computation*, *29*(9), 2352–2449. DOI: 10.1162/neco_a_00990 PMID: 28599112

Rebholz-Schuhmann, D., Oellrich, A., & Hoehndorf, R. (2012). Text-mining solutions for biomedical research: Enabling integrative biology. *Nature Reviews. Genetics*, *13*(12), 829–839. DOI: 10.1038/nrg3337 PMID: 23150036

Renner, S., Van Otterlo, W. A., Dominguez Seoane, M., Möcklinghoff, S., Hofmann, B., Wetzel, S., Schuffenhauer, A., Ertl, P., Oprea, T. I., Steinhilber, D., Brunsveld, L., Rauh, D., & Waldmann, H. (2009). Bioactivity-guided mapping and navigation of chemical space. *Nature Chemical Biology*, *5*(8), 585–592. DOI: 10.1038/nchembio.188 PMID: 19561619

Ren, Y. S., Lei, L., Deng, X., Zheng, Y., Li, Y., Li, J., & Mei, Z. N. (2019). Novel application of neural network modelling for multicomponent herbal medicine optimization. *Scientific Reports*, *9*(1), 15442. DOI: 10.1038/s41598-019-51956-6 PMID: 31659222

Reutlinger, M., & Schneider, G. (2012). Nonlinear dimensionality reduction and mapping of compound libraries for drug discovery. *Journal of Molecular Graphics & Modelling*, *34*, 108–117. DOI: 10.1016/j.jmgm.2011.12.006 PMID: 22326864

Rijal, Syamsu, Saranani, Fajar, & Joseph, Amal & C, Midhun & Ajibade, Samuel & Salvia, Vijay & Nazir, Mamona. (2023). Block chain Technology: Challenges, Opportunities and Future Direction. *European Chemical Bulletin*, *12*, 3494–3515.

Rikap, C., & Lundvall, B. (2021). *The Digital Innovation Race*. Springer Books. DOI: 10.1007/978-3-030-89443-6

Risum, A. B., & Bro, R. (2019). Using deep learning to evaluate peaks in chromatographic data. *Talanta*, *204*, 255–260. DOI: 10.1016/j.talanta.2019.05.053 PMID: 31357290

Rodrigues, T. (2017). Harnessing the potential of natural products in drug discovery from a cheminformatics vantage point. *Organic & Biomolecular Chemistry*, *15*(44), 9275–9282. DOI: 10.1039/C7OB02193C PMID: 29085945

Rodrigues, T., Reker, D., Schneider, P., & Schneider, G. (2016). Counting on natural products for drug design. *Nature Chemistry*, *8*(6), 531–541. DOI: 10.1038/nchem.2479 PMID: 27219696

Rogers, D., & Hahn, M. (2010). Extended-connectivity fingerprints. *Journal of Chemical Information and Modeling*, *50*(5), 742–754. DOI: 10.1021/ci100050t PMID: 20426451

Rolnick, S. J., Pawloski, P. A., Hedblom, B. D., Asche, S. E., & Bruzek, R. J. (2013). Patient Characteristics Associated with Medication Adherence. *Clinical Medicine & Research*, *11*(2), 54–65. DOI: 10.3121/cmr.2013.1113 PMID: 23580788

Romagnoli, A., Ferrara, F., Langella, R., & Zovi, A. (2024). Healthcare systems and artificial intelligence: Focus on challenges and the international regulatory framework. *Pharmaceutical Research*, *41*(4), 721–730. DOI: 10.1007/s11095-024-03685-3 PMID: 38443632

Romano, J. D., & Tatonetti, N. P. (2019). Informatics and computational methods in natural product drug discovery: A review and perspectives. *Frontiers in Genetics*, *10*, 368. DOI: 10.3389/fgene.2019.00368 PMID: 31114606

Rosén, J., Gottfries, J., Muresan, S., Backlund, A., & Oprea, T. I. (2009). Novel chemical space exploration via natural products. *Journal of Medicinal Chemistry*, *52*(7), 1953–1962. DOI: 10.1021/jm801514w PMID: 19265440

Rubeis, G. (2020). The disruptive power of Artificial Intelligence. Ethical aspects of gerontechnology in elderly care. *Archives of Gerontology and Geriatrics*, *91*, 104186. DOI: 10.1016/j.archger.2020.104186 PMID: 32688106

Rutz, A., Sorokina, M., Galgonek, J., Mietchen, D., Willighagen, E., Gaudry, A., . . . Allard, P. M. (2021). The LOTUS initiative for open natural products research: knowledge management through Wikidata. BioRxiv, 2021-02.

Ryan, D. K., Maclean, R. H., Balston, A., Scourfield, A., Shah, A. D., & Ross, J. (2024). Artificial intelligence and machine learning for clinical pharmacology. *British Journal of Clinical Pharmacology*, *90*(3), 629–639. DOI: 10.1111/bcp.15930 PMID: 37845024

Ryan, P., Zhang, Y., Liu, F., Gao, J., Bigger, J. T., Hripcsak, G., Weng, C., & Li, Y. (2014). A Distribution-based Method for Assessing The Differences between Clinical Trial Target Populations and Patient Populations in Electronic Health Records. *Applied Clinical Informatics*, *05*(02), 463–479. DOI: 10.4338/ACI-2013-12-RA-0105 PMID: 25024761

Sabaté, E. (2003). Adherence to long-term therapies: Evidence for action. *World Health Organization*. Retrieved from https://apps.who.int/iris/handle/10665/42682

Sadee, W., Wang, D., Hartmann, K., & Toland, A. E. (2023). Pharmacogenomics: Driving Personalized Medicine. In *Pharmacological Reviews* (Vol. 75, Issue 4, pp. 789–814). American Society for Pharmacology and Experimental Therapy (ASPET). DOI: 10.1124/pharmrev.122.000810

Sáez, M. (2020). Blockchain-Enabled Platforms: Challenges and Recommendations. *International Journal of Interactive Multimedia and Artificial Intelligence*, *6*(3), 73. DOI: 10.9781/ijimai.2020.08.005

Saldívar-González, F. I., Pilón-Jiménez, B. A., & Medina-Franco, J. L. (2019). Chemical space of naturally occurring compounds. *Physical Sciences Reviews*, *4*(5), 20180103.

Salim, N. A. M., Wah, Y. B., Reeves, C., Smith, M., Yaacob, W. F. W., Mudin, R. N., Dapari, R., Sapri, N. N. F. F., & Haque, U. (2021). Sapri, NNFF; Haque, U. Prediction of dengue outbreak in Selangor Malaysia using machine learning techniques. [CrossRef]. *Scientific Reports*, *11*(1), 939. DOI: 10.1038/s41598-020-79193-2 PMID: 33441678

Sanchez-Lengeling, B., Wei, J. N., Lee, B. K., Gerkin, R. C., Aspuru-Guzik, A., & Wiltschko, A. B. (2019). Machine learning for scent: Learning generalizable perceptual representations of small molecules. *arXiv preprint arXiv:1910.10685*.

Sarpatwari, A., Barenie, R., Curfman, G., Darrow, J. J., & Kesselheim, A. S. (2019). The US Biosimilar Market: Stunted Growth and Possible Reforms. *Clinical Pharmacology and Therapeutics*, *105*(1), 92–100. DOI: 10.1002/cpt.1285 PMID: 30415479

Savova, G. K., Masanz, J. J., Ogren, P. V., Zheng, J., Sohn, S., Kipper-Schuler, K. C., & Chute, C. G. (2010). Mayo clinical Text Analysis and Knowledge Extraction System (cTAKES): Architecture, component evaluation and applications. *Journal of the American Medical Informatics Association : JAMIA*, *17*(5), 507–513. DOI: 10.1136/jamia.2009.001560 PMID: 20819853

Schäfer, T., Kriege, N., Humbeck, L., Klein, K., Koch, O., & Mutzel, P. (2017). Scaffold Hunter: A comprehensive visual analytics framework for drug discovery. *Journal of Cheminformatics*, *9*(1), 28. DOI: 10.1186/s13321-017-0213-3 PMID: 29086162

Schepps, M. A., Wong, W. K., Austin, M., & Anisimov, V. (2024). Optimizing patient recruitment in global clinical trials using nature-inspired metaheuristics. *Statistics in Biopharmaceutical Research*, 1–15. DOI: 10.1080/19466315.2024.2308882

Schlander, M., Hernandez-Villafuerte, K., Cheng, C. Y., Mestre-Ferrandiz, J., & Baumann, M. (2021). How much does it cost to research and develop a new drug? A systematic review and assessment. *PharmacoEconomics*, *39*(11), 1243–1269. DOI: 10.1007/s40273-021-01065-y PMID: 34368939

Schneider, G. (2018). Automating drug discovery. *Nature Reviews. Drug Discovery*, *17*(2), 97–113. DOI: 10.1038/nrd.2017.232 PMID: 29242609

Schneider, P., Walters, W. P., Plowright, A. T., Sieroka, N., Listgarten, J., Goodnow, R. A.Jr, Fisher, J., Jansen, J. M., Duca, J. S., Rush, T. S., Zentgraf, M., Hill, J. E., Krutoholow, E., Kohler, M., Blaney, J., Funatsu, K., Luebkemann, C., & Schneider, G. (2020). Rethinking drug design in the artificial intelligence era. *Nature Reviews. Drug Discovery*, *19*(5), 353–364. DOI: 10.1038/s41573-019-0050-3 PMID: 31801986

Schreiber, S. L. (2000). Target-oriented and diversity-oriented organic synthesis in drug discovery. *Science*, *287*(5460), 1964–1969. DOI: 10.1126/science.287.5460.1964 PMID: 10720315

Schwendicke, F., Samek, W., & Krois, J. (2020). Artificial intelligence in dentistry: Chances and challenges. [DOI:10.1177/0022034520915714] [PMID]. *Journal of Dental Research*, *99*(7), 769–774. DOI: 10.1177/0022034520915714 PMID: 32315260

Sellwood, M. A. (2018). Artificial intelligence in drug discovery. *Fut. Sci.*, *10*, 2025–2028. PMID: 30101607

Selvaraj, C., Chandra, I., & Singh, S. K. (2021). Artificial intelligence and machine learning approaches for drug design: challenges and opportunities for the pharmaceutical industries. In *Molecular diversity*. doi.org/10.1007/s11030-021-10326-z

Sezgin, E., Hussain, S.-A., Rust, S., & Huang, Y. (2022). Extracting Medical Information from Free-text and Unstructured Patient-Generated Health Data using Natural Language Processing Methods: A Feasibility Study with Real-world Data (Preprint). *JMIR Formative Research*. Advance online publication. DOI: 10.2196/43014 PMID: 36881467

Shah, H., & the Bioinformatics Tools for Pharmaceutical Rifampicin Product Development. Wiley; Hoboken, NJ, USA: 2023. Applications of Bioinformatics Tools in Medicinal Biology and Biotechnology; pp. 95–116.

Shameer, K., Johnson, K. W., Glicksberg, B. S., Dudley, J. T., & Sengupta, P. P. (2018). Machine learning in cardiovascular medicine: Are we there yet? *Heart (British Cardiac Society)*, *104*(14), 1156–1164. DOI: 10.1136/heartjnl-2017-311198 PMID: 29352006

Sharma, S., Naman, S., Dwivedi, J., & Baldi, A. Artificial Intelligence-Based Smart Identification System Using Herbal Images: Decision Making Using Various Machine Learning Models. In *Applications of Optimization and Machine Learning in Image Processing and IoT* (pp. 123-155). Chapman and Hall/CRC.

Sharma, P., Jindal, R., & Borah, M. D. (2022). A Review of Blockchain-Based Applications and Challenges. *Wireless Personal Communications*, *123*(2), 1201–1243. DOI: 10.1007/s11277-021-09176-7

Sharma, R., Shishodia, A., Gunasekaran, A., Min, H., & Munim, Z. H. (2022). The Role of Artificial Intelligence in Supply Chain Management: Mapping the Territory. *International Journal of Production Research*, *60*(24), 7527–7550. DOI: 10.1080/00207543.2022.2029611

Sharma, V., Law, W., Balick, M. J., & Sarkar, I. N. (2018, April). Harnessing biomedical natural language processing tools to identify medicinal plant knowledge from historical texts. *AMIA ... Annual Symposium Proceedings - AMIA Symposium. AMIA Symposium*, *2017*, 1537. PMID: 29854223

Shaw, J., Ali, J., Atuire, C. A., Cheah, P. Y., Español, A. G., Gichoya, J. W., Hunt, A., Jjingo, D., Littler, K!., Paolotti, D., & Vayena, E. (2024). Research ethics and artificial intelligence for global health: Perspectives from the global forum on bioethics in research. *BMC Medical Ethics*, *25*(1), 46. DOI: 10.1186/s12910-024-01044-w PMID: 38637857

Shefali, A. (2023). Sukanya, Chettri., V., Percha., Deepak, Kumar., Mamta, Latwal. Artificial intelligence: A virtual chemist for natural product drug discovery. *Journal of Biomolecular Structure & Dynamics*, •••, 1–10. DOI: 10.1080/07391102.2023.2216295

Sheikhalishahi, S., Miotto, R., Dudley, J. T., Lavelli, A., Rinaldi, F., & Osmani, V. (2019). Natural Language Processing of Clinical Notes on Chronic Diseases: Systematic Review. *JMIR Medical Informatics*, *7*(2), e12239. DOI: 10.2196/12239 PMID: 31066697

Sheng, Y., Xue, Y., Wang, J., Liu, S., & Jiang, Y. (2023). Fast screening and identification of illegal adulteration in dietary supplements and herbal medicines using molecular networking with deep-learning-based similarity algorithms. *Analytical and Bioanalytical Chemistry*, *415*(16), 3285–3293. DOI: 10.1007/s00216-023-04708-5 PMID: 37119358

Shergis, J. L., Wu, L., May, B. H., Zhang, A. L., Guo, X., Lu, C., & Xue, C. C. (2015). Natural products for chronic cough: Text mining the East Asian historical literature for future therapeutics. *Chronic Respiratory Disease*, *12*(3), 204–211. DOI: 10.1177/1479972315583043 PMID: 25901012

Shi, X., Chen, Z., Wang, H., Yeung, D. Y., Wong, W. K., & Woo, W. C. (2015). Convolutional LSTM network: A machine learning approach for precipitation nowcasting. *Advances in Neural Information Processing Systems, 28*. https://dl.acm.org/doi/10.5555/2969239.2969329

Shickel, B., Tighe, P. J., Bihorac, A., & Rashidi, P. (2018). Deep EHR: A Survey of Recent Advances in Deep Learning Techniques for Electronic Health Record (EHR) Analysis. *IEEE Journal of Biomedical and Health Informatics*, *22*(5), 1589–1604. DOI: 10.1109/JBHI.2017.2767063 PMID: 29989977

Shi, Y., Yao, X., Xu, J., Hu, X., Tu, L., Lan, F., Cui, J., Cui, L., Huang, J., Li, J., Bi, Z., & Li, J. (2022). A new approach of fatigue classification based on data of tongue and pulse with machine learning. *Frontiers in Physiology*, *12*, 708742. DOI: 10.3389/fphys.2021.708742 PMID: 35197858

Shi, Z., Hu, B., Lu, M., Chen, Z., Zhang, M., Yu, Y., Zhou, C., Zhong, J., Wu, B., Zhang, X., Wei, Y., & Zhang, L. J.China Aneurysm. (2024). Assessing the impact of an artificial intelligence-based model for intracranial aneurysm detection in CT angiography on patient diagnosis and outcomes (IDEAL Study)—A protocol for a multicenter, double-blinded randomized controlled trial. *Trials*, *25*(1), 358. DOI: 10.1186/s13063-024-08184-9 PMID: 38835091

Shortreed, S. M., Cook, A. J., Coley, R. Y., Bobb, J. F., & Nelson, J. C. (2019). Challenges and opportunities for using big healthcare data to advance medical science and public health. *American Journal of Epidemiology*, *188*(5), 851–861. DOI: 10.1093/aje/kwy292 PMID: 30877288

Sim, J., Huang, X., Horan, M. R., Stewart, C. M., Robison, L. L., Hudson, M. M., Baker, J. N., & Huang, I.-C. (2023). Natural language processing with machine learning methods to analyze unstructured patient-reported outcomes derived from electronic health records: A systematic review. *Artificial Intelligence in Medicine*, *146*, 102701–102701. DOI: 10.1016/j.artmed.2023.102701 PMID: 38042599

Simpson, S. H., Eurich, D. T., Majumdar, S. R., Padwal, R. S., Tsuyuki, R. T., Varney, J., & Johnson, J. A. (2006). A meta-analysis of the association between adherence to drug therapy and mortality. *BMJ (Clinical Research Ed.)*, *333*(7557), 15. DOI: 10.1136/bmj.38875.675486.55 PMID: 16790458

Sinha, A., & Rathi, M. (2021). COVID-19 prediction using AI analytics for South Korea. [CrossRef] [PubMed]. *Applied Intelligence*, *51*(12), 8579–8597. DOI: 10.1007/s10489-021-02352-z PMID: 34764592

Size, D. I. M., & Growth, D. I. M. S. (2018). Share & trends analysis report by product (titanium implants, zirconium implants), by region (north america, europe, asia pacific, latin america, mea), and segment forecasts, 2018-2024. *Personalized Medicine Market Analysis By Product And Segment Forecasts To*, *2022*, 5.

Smith, R. G., & Farquhar, A. (2000). The road ahead for knowledge management: An AI perspective. *AI Magazine*, *21*, 17–17.

Solat, S., Calvez, P., & Naït-Abdesselam, F. (2020). Permissioned vs. Permissionless Blockchain: How and Why There Is Only One Right Choice. *Journal of Software, 16*, 95–106. DOI: 10.17706/jsw.16.3.95-106

Solomon, D. H., Avorn, J., Katz, J. N., Weinblatt, M. E., Setoguchi, S., Levin, R., & Schneeweiss, S. (2008). Compliance with osteoporosis medications. *Archives of Internal Medicine, 165*(20), 2414–2419. DOI: 10.1001/archinte.165.20.2414 PMID: 16287772

Soni, U., Gupta, N., & Sakshi, . (2021). Sakshi. An Artificial Intelligence Approach for Forecasting Ebola Disease. [CrossRef]. *Journal of Physics: Conference Series, 1950*(1), 012038. DOI: 10.1088/1742-6596/1950/1/012038

Sorokina, M., Merseburger, P., Rajan, K., Yirik, M. A., & Steinbeck, C. (2021). COCONUT online: Collection of open natural products database. *Journal of Cheminformatics, 13*(1), 2. DOI: 10.1186/s13321-020-00478-9 PMID: 33423696

Srija, K., Prithvi, P. P. R., Saxena, A., Grover, A., Chandra, S., & Jain, S. J. (2021). Artificial Intelligence in Personalized Medicine. *Artificial Intelligence and Machine Learning in Healthcare*, 57-69.

Srinivasan, N. S., Babu, K. S., & Kumar Year, P.: 2021 Title: "Medicinal Plant Recognition using Convolutional Neural Networks and Genetic Algorithms"

Steele, L., Orefuwa, E., Bino, S., Singer, S. R., Lutwama, J., & Dickmann, P. (2020). Earlier outbreak detection—A generic model and novel methodology to guide earlier detection supported by data from low- and mid-income countries. *Frontiers in Public Health, 8*, 452. DOI: 10.3389/fpubh.2020.00452 PMID: 33014967

Stokes, J. M., Yang, K., Swanson, K., Jin, W., Cubillos-Ruiz, A., Donghia, N. M., MacNair, C. R., French, S., Carfrae, L. A., Bloom-Ackermann, Z., Tran, V. M., Chiappino-Pepe, A., Badran, A. H., Andrews, I. W., Chory, E. J., Church, G. M., Brown, E. D., Jaakkola, T. S., Barzilay, R., & Collins, J. J. (2020). A deep learning approach to antibiotic discovery. *Cell, 180*(4), 688–702. DOI: 10.1016/j.cell.2020.01.021 PMID: 32084340

Strianese, O., Rizzo, F., Ciccarelli, M., Galasso, G., D'Agostino, Y., Salvati, A., Del Giudice, C., Tesorio, P., & Rusciano, M. R. (2020). Precision and personalized medicine: How genomic approach improves the management of cardiovascular and neurodegenerative disease. [mdpi.com]. *Genes, 11*(7), 747. DOI: 10.3390/genes11070747 PMID: 32640513

Strohl, W. R. (2000). The role of natural products in a modern drug discovery program. *Drug Discovery Today*, *5*(2), 39–41. DOI: 10.1016/S1359-6446(99)01443-9 PMID: 10652450

Su, K., Xu, L., Li, G., Ruan, X., Li, X., Deng, P., Li, X., Li, Q., Chen, X., Xiong, Y., Lu, S., Qi, L., Shen, C., Tang, W., Rong, R., Hong, B., Ning, Y., Long, D., Xu, J., & Li, Y. (2019). Forecasting influenza activity using a self-adaptive AI model and multi-source data in Chongqing, China. [CrossRef]. *EBioMedicine*, *47*, 284–292. DOI: 10.1016/j.ebiom.2019.08.024 PMID: 31477561

Sun, J., Ni, Q., Jiang, F., Liu, B., Wang, J., Zhang, L., & Huang, J. (2023). Discovery and validation of traditional chinese and western medicine combination antirheumatoid arthritis drugs based on machine learning (random forest model). *BioMed Research International*, *6086388*(1), 6086388. Advance online publication. DOI: 10.1155/2023/6086388 PMID: 36845640

Sun, M., Zhao, S., Gilvary, C., Elemento, O., Zhou, J., & Wang, F. (2020). Graph convolutional networks for computational drug development and discovery. *Briefings in Bioinformatics*, *21*(3), 919–935. DOI: 10.1093/bib/bbz042 PMID: 31155636

Suriyaamporn, P., Pamornpathomkul, B., Patrojanasophon, P., Ngawhirunpat, T., Rojanarata, T., & Opanasopit, P. (2024). The artificial intelligence-powered new era in pharmaceutical research and development: A review. *AAPS PharmSciTech*, *25*(6), 188. DOI: 10.1208/s12249-024-02901-y PMID: 39147952

Sur, S., Sharma, P., & Dave, V. (2022). AI in Pharmacy, Herbal Medicine and Drug Delivery: A Sci-fi or a Reality. *Advanced Pharmaceutical and Herbal Nanoscience for Targeted Drug Delivery Systems*, *1*, 259. DOI: 10.2174/9789815036541122010016

Svensson, E., Nielsen, R. B., Hasvold, P., Lund, J. L., & Thomsen, R. W. (2015). Statin use and discontinuation in Denmark: A nationwide drug utilization study. *British Journal of Clinical Pharmacology*, *80*(6), 1444–1452. DOI: 10.1111/bcp.12704

Swathi, N. L., & Kumar, A. (2024). Advanced technologies in clinical research and drug development. In Kumar, R., Joshi, A., Sharan, H., Peng, S., & Dudhagara, C. (Eds.), *The Ethical Frontier of AI and Data Analysis* (pp. 1–17). IGI Global., DOI: 10.4018/979-8-3693-2964-1.ch001

Swendeman, D., Rotheram-Borus, M. J., Arnold, E. M., Fernández, M. I., Comulada, W. S., Lee, S.-J., Ocasio, M. A., Ishimoto, K., Gertsch, W., Duan, N., Reback, C. J., Murphy, D. A., Lewis, K. A., Abdalian, S. E., Bolan, R., Bryson, Y., Cortado, R., Flynn, R., Kerin, T., & Weiss, R. E. (2024). Optimal strategies to improve uptake of and adherence to HIV prevention among young people at risk for HIV acquisition in the USA (ATN 149): A randomized, controlled, factorial trial. *The Lancet. Digital Health, 6*(3), e187–e200. DOI: 10.1016/S2589-7500(23)00252-2 PMID: 38395539

Sydow, D., Burggraaff, L., Szengel, A., van Vlijmen, H. W., IJzerman, A. P., van Westen, G. J., & Volkamer, A. (2019). Advances and challenges in computational target prediction. *Journal of Chemical Information and Modeling, 59*(5), 1728–1742. DOI: 10.1021/acs.jcim.8b00832 PMID: 30817146

Tan, D. S. (2005). Diversity-oriented synthesis: Exploring the intersections between chemistry and biology. *Nature Chemical Biology, 1*(2), 74–84. DOI: 10.1038/nchembio0705-74 PMID: 16408003

Tenenbaum, J. D. (2016). Translational Bioinformatics: Past, Present, and Future. *Genomics, Proteomics & Bioinformatics, 14*(1), 31–41. DOI: 10.1016/j.gpb.2016.01.003 PMID: 26876718

Thorlund, K., Haggstrom, J., Park, J. J., & Mills, E. J. (2018). Key design considerations for adaptive clinical trials: A primer for clinicians. [CrossRef]. *BMJ (Clinical Research Ed.), 360*, k698. DOI: 10.1136/bmj.k698 PMID: 29519932

Tibshirani, R. (1996). Regression Shrinkage and Selection Via the Lasso. *Journal of the Royal Statistical Society. Series B, Statistical Methodology, 58*(1), 267–288. DOI: 10.1111/j.2517-6161.1996.tb02080.x

Tiwari, N., Chhipa, A., Shukla, S., Patel, S., Balar, P., Paiva-Santos, A., & Patravale, V. (2023). Conventional and Novel Diagnostic Tools for the Diagnosis of Emerging SARS-CoV-2 Variants. *Vaccines, 11*(2), 374. DOI: 10.3390/vaccines11020374 PMID: 36851252

Todeschini, R., Consonni, V., Xiang, H., Holliday, J., Buscema, M., & Willett, P. (2012). Similarity coefficients for binary chemoinformatics data: Overview and extended comparison using simulated and real data sets. *Journal of Chemical Information and Modeling, 52*(11), 2884–2901. DOI: 10.1021/ci300261r PMID: 23078167

Topol, E. J. (2019). High-performance medicine: The convergence of human and artificial intelligence. *Nature Medicine, 25*(1), 44–56. https://www.nature.com/articles/s41591-018-0300-7. DOI: 10.1038/s41591-018-0300-7 PMID: 30617339

Truchon, J. F., & Bayly, C. I. (2007). Evaluating virtual screening methods: Good and bad metrics for the "early recognition" problem. *Journal of Chemical Information and Modeling*, *47*(2), 488–508. DOI: 10.1021/ci600426e PMID: 17288412

Tshitoyan, V., Dagdelen, J., Weston, L., Dunn, A., Rong, Z., Kononova, O., Persson, K. A., Ceder, G., & Jain, A. (2019). Unsupervised word embeddings capture latent knowledge from materials science literature. *Nature*, *571*(7763), 95–98. DOI: 10.1038/s41586-019-1335-8 PMID: 31270483

Tufts Center for the Study of Drug Development. (2014). *The cost of developing a new drug*. Tufts University. https://csdd.tufts.edu

Tushman, M. L., & Anderson, P. (1986). Technological discontinuities and organizational environments. *Administrative Science Quarterly*, *31*(3), 439–465. DOI: 10.2307/2392832

Tu, Y. (2011). The discovery of artemisinin (qinghaosu) and gifts from Chinese medicine. [DOI] [PubMed] [Google Scholar]. *Nature Medicine*, *17*(10), 1217–1220. DOI: 10.1038/nm.2471 PMID: 21989013

Tyson, L. D., & Zysman, J. (2022). Automation, AI, and work. *Daedalus*, *151*(2), 256–271. https://www.jstor.org/stable/48662040. DOI: 10.1162/daed_a_01914

Tyson, R. J., Park, C. C., Powell, J. R., Patterson, J. H., Weiner, D., Watkins, P. B., & Gonzalez, D. (2020). Precision dosing priority criteria: Drug, disease, and patient population variables. [frontiersin.org]. *Frontiers in Pharmacology*, *11*, 420. DOI: 10.3389/fphar.2020.00420 PMID: 32390828

UNCTAD. (2021). *Digital Economy Report. Cross-Border Data Flows and Development: For Whom the Data Flows*. United Nations Publication.

Unger, J. M. (2019). Vaidya, R.; Hershman, D.L.; Minasian, L.M.; E Fleury, M. Systematic Review and Meta-Analysis of the Magnitude of Structural, Clinical, and Physician and Patient Barriers to Cancer Clinical Trial Participation. [CrossRef]. *Gynecologic Oncology*, *111*, 245–255. PMID: 30856272

Uzzan, M., Bouhnik, Y., Abreu, M., Ahmad, H. A., Adsul, S., Carlier, H., Dubinsky, M., Germinaro, M., Jairath, V., Modesto, I., Mortensen, E., Narula, N., Neimark, E., Oortwijn, A., Protic, M., Rubin, D. T., Oh, Y. S., Wichary, J., Peyrin-Biroulet, L., & Reinisch, W. (2023). Declining enrolment and other challenges in IBD clinical trials: Causes and potential solutions. *Journal of Crohn's and Colitis*, *17*(7), 1066–1078. DOI: 10.1093/ecco-jcc/jjad020 PMID: 36738443

Vamathevan, J., Clark, D., Czodrowski, P., Dunham, I., Ferran, E., Lee, G., Li, B., Madabhushi, A., Shah, P., Spitzer, M., & Zhao, S. (2019). Applications of machine learning in drug discovery and development. *Nature Reviews. Drug Discovery, 18*(6), 463–477. DOI: 10.1038/s41573-019-0024-5 PMID: 30976107

van Dam, P. M. E. L., van Doorn, W. P. T. M., van Gils, F., Sevenich, L., Lambriks, L., Meex, S. J. R., Cals, J. W. L., & Stassen, P. M. (2024). Machine learning for risk stratification in the emergency department (MARS-ED) study protocol for a randomized controlled pilot trial on the implementation of a prediction model based on machine learning technology predicting 31-day mortality in the emergency department. *Scandinavian Journal of Trauma, Resuscitation and Emergency Medicine, 32*(1), 5. DOI: 10.1186/s13049-024-01177-2 PMID: 38263188

Varma, A., Dixit, N., Ray, S., & Kaur, J. (2024). Blockchain technology for sustainable supply chains: A comprehensive review and future prospects. *World Journal of Advanced Research and Reviews., 21*(3), 980–994. DOI: 10.30574/wjarr.2024.21.3.0804

Vasey, B., Nagendran, M., Campbell, B., Clifton, D. A., Collins, G. S., Denaxas, S., & McCulloch, P. (2022). Reporting guideline for the early stage clinical evaluation of decision support systems driven by artificial intelligence: DECIDE-AI. 10.1136/bmj-2022-070904

Vatansever, S., Schlessinger, A., Wacker, D., Kaniskan, H. Ü., Jin, J., Zhou, M. M., & Zhang, B. (2021). Artificial intelligence and machine learning-aided drug discovery in central nervous system diseases: State-of-the-arts and future directions. *Medicinal Research Reviews, 41*(3), 1427–1473. DOI: 10.1002/med.21764 PMID: 33295676

Veena, C., Sridevi, M., Liyakat, K. K. S., Saha, B., Reddy, S. R., & Shirisha, N. (2023). *"HEECCNB: An Efficient IoT-Cloud Architecture for Secure Patient Data Transmission and Accurate Disease Prediction in Healthcare Systems," 2023 Seventh International Conference on Image Information Processing*. ICIIP., Available at https://ieeexplore.ieee.org/document/10537627, DOI: 10.1109/ICIIP61524.2023.10537627

Venkatramanan, S., Sadilek, A., Fadikar, A., Barrett, C. L., Biggerstaff, M., Chen, J., Dotiwalla, X., Eastham, P., Gipson, B., Higdon, D., Kucuktunc, O., Lieber, A., Lewis, B. L., Reynolds, Z., Vullikanti, A. K., Wang, L., & Marathe, M. (2021). Forecasting Influenza Activity Using Machine-Learned Mobility Map. [CrossRef] [PubMed]. *Nature Communications, 12*(1), 726. DOI: 10.1038/s41467-021-21018-5 PMID: 33563980

Vijayan, R. S. K., Kihlberg, J., Cross, J. B., & Poongavanam, V. (2022). Enhancing preclinical drug discovery with artificial intelligence. *Drug Discovery Today*, *27*(4), 967–984. DOI: 10.1016/j.drudis.2021.11.023 PMID: 34838731

Viraswami-Appanna, K., Buenconsejo, J., Baidoo, C., Chan, I., Li, D., Micsinai-Balan, M., Tiwari, R., Yang, L., & Sethuraman, V. (2024). Accelerating drug development at Bristol Myers Squibb through innovation. *Drug Discovery Today*, *29*(5), 103952. DOI: 10.1016/j.drudis.2024.103952 PMID: 38508230

Vora, L. K., Gholap, A. D., Jetha, K., Thakur, R. R. S., Solanki, H. K., & Chavda, V. P. (2023). Artificial Intelligence in Pharmaceutical Technology and Drug Delivery Design. In *Pharmaceutics* (Vol. 15, Issue 7). Multidisciplinary Digital Publishing Institute (MDPI). DOI: 10.3390/pharmaceutics15071916

Vosooghi, M., & Amini, M. (2014). The discovery and development of cyclooxygenase-2 inhibitors as potential anticancer therapies. *Expert Opinion on Drug Discovery*, *9*(3), 255–267. DOI: 10.1517/17460441.2014.883377 PMID: 24483845

Vrijens, B., De Geest, S., Hughes, D. A., Przemyslaw, K., Demonceau, J., Ruppar, T., Dobbels, F., Fargher, E., Morrison, V., Lewek, P., Matyjaszczyk, M., Mshelia, C., Clyne, W., Aronson, J. K., & Urquhart, J. (2012). A new taxonomy for describing and defining adherence to medications. *British Journal of Clinical Pharmacology*, *73*(5), 691–705. DOI: 10.1111/j.1365-2125.2012.04167.x PMID: 22486599

Vyas, M. (2018). Artificial intelligence: The beginning of a new era in pharmacy profession. *Asian Journal of Pharmaceutics*, *12*, 72–76.

Wahida, A., Buschhorn, L., Fröhling, S., Jost, P. J., Schneeweiss, A., Lichter, P., & Kurzrock, R. (2023). The coming decade in precision oncology: Six riddles. [HTML]. *Nature Reviews. Cancer*, *23*(1), 43–54. DOI: 10.1038/s41568-022-00529-3 PMID: 36434139

Wale, A. D., & Dipali, R.. (2019). Smart Agriculture System using IoT. *International Journal of Innovative Research In Technology*, *5*(10), 493–497.

Wallace, B. C., Paul, M. J., Sarkar, U., Trikalinos, T. A., & Dredze, M. (2014). A large-scale quantitative analysis of latent factors and sentiment in online doctor reviews. *Journal of the American Medical Informatics Association : JAMIA*, *21*(6), 1098–1103. DOI: 10.1136/amiajnl-2014-002711 PMID: 24918109

Walsh, C. A., Cahir, C., Mecklenburg, S., Byrne, C., Culbertson, M. A., & Bennett, K. E. (2019). The association between medication non-adherence and adverse health outcomes in aging populations: A systematic review and meta-analysis. *British Journal of Clinical Pharmacology*, *85*(11), 2464–2478. DOI: 10.1111/bcp.14075 PMID: 31486099

Walters, W. P., & Murcko, M. (2020). Assessing the impact of generative AI on medicinal chemistry. *Nature Biotechnology*, *38*(2), 143–145. DOI: 10.1038/s41587-020-0418-2 PMID: 32001834

Wang, H., Chen, Y., Wang, L., Liu, Q., Yang, S., & Wang, C. (2023). Advancing herbal medicine: Enhancing product quality and safety through robust quality control practices. *Frontiers in Pharmacology*, *14*, 1265178. DOI: 10.3389/fphar.2023.1265178 PMID: 37818188

Wang, K., Cui, H., Zhu, Y., Hu, X., Hong, C., Guo, Y., An, L., Zhang, Q., & Liu, L. (2024). Evaluation of an artificial intelligence-based clinical trial matching system in Chinese patients with hepatocellular carcinoma: A retrospective study. *BMC Cancer*, *24*(1), 246. DOI: 10.1186/s12885-024-11959-7 PMID: 38388861

Wang, L., Jiang, L., Pan, D., Wang, Q., Yin, Z., Kang, Z., Tian, H., Geng, X., Shao, J., Pan, W., Yin, J., Fang, L., Wang, Y., Zhang, W., Li, Z., Zheng, J., Hu, W., Pan, Y., Yu, D., & Xu, H. (2022). Novel approach by natural language processing for COVID-19 knowledge discovery. *Biomedical Journal*, *45*(3), 472–481. Advance online publication. DOI: 10.1016/j.bj.2022.03.011 PMID: 35367669

Wang, L., & Xie, X.-Q. (2014). Computational Target Fishing: What Should Chemogenomics Researchers Expect for the Future of in Silico Rifampicin Design and Discovery? *Future Medicinal Chemistry*, *6*(3), 247–249. DOI: 10.4155/fmc.14.5 PMID: 24575960

Wang, L., Zhou, G. B., Liu, P., Song, J. H., Liang, Y., Yan, X. J., Xu, F., Wang, B.-S., Mao, J.-H., Shen, Z.-X., Chen, S.-J., & Chen, Z. (2008). Dissection of mechanisms of chinese medicinal formula realgar-indigo naturalis as an effective treatment for promyelocytic leukemia. [DOI] [PMC free article] [PubMed] [Google Scholar]. *Proceedings of the National Academy of Sciences of the United States of America*, *105*(12), 4826–4831. DOI: 10.1073/pnas.0712365105 PMID: 18344322

Wang, M., Qian, Y., Yang, Y., Chen, H., & Rao, W.-F. (2024). Improved stacking ensemble learning based on feature selection to accurately predict warfarin dose. *Frontiers in Cardiovascular Medicine*, *10*, 1320938. DOI: 10.3389/fcvm.2023.1320938 PMID: 38312950

Wang, Y., Kung, L., & Byrd, T. A. (2018). Big data analytics: Understanding its capabilities and potential benefits for healthcare organizations. *Technological Forecasting and Social Change*, *126*(1), 3–13. DOI: 10.1016/j.techfore.2015.12.019

Wang, Y., Wang, L., Rastegar-Mojarad, M., Moon, S., Shen, F., Afzal, N., Liu, S., Zeng, Y., Mehrabi, S., Sohn, S., & Liu, H. (2018). Clinical information extraction applications: A literature review. *Journal of Biomedical Informatics*, *77*, 34–49. DOI: 10.1016/j.jbi.2017.11.011 PMID: 29162496

Warrer, P., Hansen, E. H., Juhl-Jensen, L., & Aagaard, L. (2012). Using text-mining techniques in electronic patient records to identify ADRs from medicine use. *British Journal of Clinical Pharmacology*, *73*(5), 674–684. DOI: 10.1111/j.1365-2125.2011.04153.x PMID: 22122057

Weininger, D. (1988). SMILES, a chemical language and information system. 1. Introduction to methodology and encoding rules. *Journal of Chemical Information and Computer Sciences*, *28*(1), 31–36. DOI: 10.1021/ci00057a005

Weiskopf, N. G., & Weng, C. (2013). Methods and dimensions of electronic health record data quality assessment: Enabling reuse for clinical research. *Journal of the American Medical Informatics Association : JAMIA*, *20*(1), 144–151. DOI: 10.1136/amiajnl-2011-000681 PMID: 22733976

Wei, W. Q., Cronin, R. M., Xu, H., Lasko, T. A., Bastarache, L., & Denny, J. C. (2013). Development and evaluation of an ensemble resource linking medications to their indications. *Journal of the American Medical Informatics Association : JAMIA*, *20*(5), 954–961. DOI: 10.1136/amiajnl-2012-001431 PMID: 23576672

Welcome to FHIR. HL7. URL: https://www.hl7.org/fhir/ [accessed 2020-04-13]

Wells, T. N. (2011). Natural products as starting points for future anti-malarial therapies: Going back to our roots? *Malaria Journal*, *10*(S1), 1–12. DOI: 10.1186/1475-2875-10-S1-S3 PMID: 21411014

Wender, P. A., Quiroz, R. V., & Stevens, M. C. (2015). Function through synthesis-informed design. *Accounts of Chemical Research*, *48*(3), 752–760. DOI: 10.1021/acs.accounts.5b00004 PMID: 25742599

Wender, P. A., Verma, V. A., Paxton, T. J., & Pillow, T. H. (2008). Function-oriented synthesis, step economy, and drug design. *Accounts of Chemical Research*, *41*(1), 40–49. DOI: 10.1021/ar700155p PMID: 18159936

Wetzel, S., Klein, K., Renner, S., Rauh, D., Oprea, T. I., Mutzel, P., & Waldmann, H. (2009). Interactive exploration of chemical space with Scaffold Hunter. *Nature Chemical Biology*, *5*(8), 581–583. DOI: 10.1038/nchembio.187 PMID: 19561620

Whitley, D. (1994). A genetic algorithm tutorial. *Statistics and Computing*, *4*(1), 65–85.

Williamson, D. J., Struyven, R. R., Antaki, F., Chia, M. A., Wagner, S. K., Jhingan, M., Wu, Z., Guymer, R., Skene, S. S., Tammuz, N., Thomson, B., Chopra, R., & Keane, P. A. (2024). Artificial intelligence to facilitate clinical trial recruitment in age-related macular degeneration. *Ophthalmology Science*, (6), 100566. DOI: 10.1016/j.xops.2024.100566 PMID: 39139546

Wirtz, B. W., Weyerer, J. C., & Geyer, C. (2019). Artificial intelligence and the public sector—Applications and challenges. *International Journal of Public Administration*, *42*(7), 596–615. DOI: 10.1080/01900692.2018.1498103

Witharana, P., Chang, L., Maier, R., Ogundimu, E., Wilkinson, C., Athanasiou, T., & Akowuah, E. (2024). Feasibility study of rehabilitation for cardiac patients aided by an artificial intelligence web-based programme: A randomized controlled trial (RECAP trial)—a study protocol. *BMJ Open*, *14*(4), e079404. DOI: 10.1136/bmjopen-2023-079404 PMID: 38688664

Witting, M., & Böcker, S. (2020). Current status of retention time prediction in metabolite identification. *Journal of Separation Science*, *43*(9-10), 1746–1754. DOI: 10.1002/jssc.202000060 PMID: 32144942

Wolfender, J. L., Litaudon, M., Touboul, D., & Queiroz, E. F. (2019). Innovative omics-based approaches for prioritisation and targeted isolation of natural products–new strategies for drug discovery. *Natural Product Reports*, *36*(6), 855–868. DOI: 10.1039/C9NP00004F PMID: 31073562

Wolfer, A. M., Lozano, S., Umbdenstock, T., Croixmarie, V., Arrault, A., & Vayer, P. (2016). UPLC–MS retention time prediction: A machine learning approach to metabolite identification in untargeted profiling. *Metabolomics*, *12*(1), 8. DOI: 10.1007/s11306-015-0888-2

Wolff, J., Pauling, J., Keck, A., & Baumbach, J. (2019). Systematic Review of Economic Impact Studies of Artificial Intelligence in Health Care. *Journal of Medical Internet Research*, *22*(2), e16866. DOI: 10.2196/16866 PMID: 32130134

Wolf, R. M., Channa, R., Liu, T. Y. A., Zehra, A., Bromberger, L., Patel, D., Ananthakrishnan, A., Brown, E. A., Prichett, L., Lehmann, H. P., & Abramoff, M. D. (2024). Autonomous artificial intelligence increases screening and follow-up for diabetic retinopathy in youth: The ACCESS randomized control trial. *Nature Communications*, *15*(1), 421. DOI: 10.1038/s41467-023-44676-z PMID: 38212308

Xiang, D., & Cai, W. (2021, October 7). Privacy Protection and Secondary Use of Health Data: Strategies and Methods. *BioMed Research International*, *6967166*(1), 6967166. Advance online publication. DOI: 10.1155/2021/6967166 PMID: 34660798

Xia, X., May, B. H., Zhang, A. L., Guo, X., Lu, C., Xue, C. C., & Huang, Q. (2020). Chinese Herbal Medicines for Rheumatoid Arthritis: Text-Mining the Classical Literature for Potentially Effective Natural Products. *Evidence-Based Complementary and Alternative Medicine : eCAM*, *2020*(1), 7531967. DOI: 10.1155/2020/7531967 PMID: 32419824

Xie, X., Luo, C., Wu, S., Qiao, W., Deng, W., Jin, L., Lu, J., Bu, L., Duffau, H., Zhang, J., & Yao, Y. (2024). Recursive partitioning analysis for survival stratification and early imaging prediction of molecular biomarker in glioma patients. *BMC Cancer*, *24*(1), 818. DOI: 10.1186/s12885-024-12542-w PMID: 38982347

Xie, Z., St Clair, P., Goldman, D. P., & Joyce, G. (2019). Racial and ethnic disparities in medication adherence among privately insured patients in the United States. *PLoS One*, *14*(2), e0212117. DOI: 10.1371/journal.pone.0212117 PMID: 30763400

Xiong, Y., Ba, X., Hou, A., Zhang, K., Chen, L., & Li, T. (2018). Automatic detection of mycobacterium tuberculosis using artificial intelligence. [CrossRef]. *Journal of Thoracic Disease*, *10*(3), 1936–1940. DOI: 10.21037/jtd.2018.01.91 PMID: 29707349

Xi, Y., Miao, Y., Zhou, R., Wang, M., Zhang, F., Li, Y., Zhang, Y., Yang, H., & Guo, F. (2022). Exploration of the specific pathology of HXMM tablet against retinal injury based on drug attack model to network robustness. *Frontiers in Pharmacology*, *13*, 826535. DOI: 10.3389/fphar.2022.826535 PMID: 35401181

Xu, J., Biomedical, R., & Sciences, H. (2016). *Mapping SNOMED CT to ICD-10-CM.* https://rucore.libraries.rutgers.edu/rutgers-lib/49049/PDF/1/play/

Xue, L., Singla, R. K., He, S., Arrasate, S., González-Díaz, H., Miao, L., & Shen, B. (2024). Warfarin–A natural anticoagulant: A review of research trends for precision medication. *Phytomedicine*, *128*, 155479. DOI: 10.1016/j.phymed.2024.155479 PMID: 38493714

Xu, H., Aldrich, M. C., Chen, Q., Liu, H., Peterson, N. B., Dai, Q., Levy, M., Shah, A., Han, X., Ruan, X., Jiang, M., Li, Y., Julien, J. S., Warner, J., Friedman, C., Roden, D. M., & Denny, J. C. (2014). Validating drug repurposing signals using electronic health records: A case study of metformin associated with reduced cancer mortality. *Journal of the American Medical Informatics Association : JAMIA*, *22*(1), 179–191. DOI: 10.1136/amiajnl-2014-002649 PMID: 25053577

Xu, H.-B., Shen, F.-M., & Lv, Q.-Z. (2015). Celecoxib enhanced the cytotoxic effect of cisplatin in drug-resistant human gastric cancer cells by inhibition of cyclooxygenase-2. *European Journal of Pharmacology*, *769*, 1–7. DOI: 10.1016/j.ejphar.2015.09.025 PMID: 26407653

Xu, M., Chen, X., & Kou, G. (2019). A systematic review of blockchain. *Financial Innovation*, *5*(1), 27. DOI: 10.1186/s40854-019-0147-z

Yabuuchi, H., Hayashi, K., Shigemoto, A., Fujiwara, M., Nomura, Y., Nakashima, M., Ogusu, T., Mori, M., Tokumoto, S., & Miyai, K. (2023). Virtual screening of antimicrobial plant extracts by machine-learning classification of chemical compounds in semantic space. *PLoS One*, *18*(5), e0285716. DOI: 10.1371/journal.pone.0285716 PMID: 37186641

Yadav, S., Singh, A., Singhal, R., & Yadav, J. P. (2024). Revolutionizing drug discovery: The impact of artificial intelligence on advancements in pharmacology and the pharmaceutical industry. *Intelligent Pharmacy*.

Yang, K., Yu, Z., Su, X., He, X., Wang, N., Zheng, Q., . . . Zhou, X. (2023). A optimization framework for herbal prescription planning based on deep reinforcement learning. *arXiv preprint arXiv:2304.12828*.

Yang, L., Xue, Y., Wei, J., Dai, Q., & Li, P. (2021). Integrating metabolomic data with machine learning approach for discovery of Q-markers from jinqi jiangtang preparation against type 2 diabetes. *Chinese Medicine*, *16*(1), 1–12. DOI: 10.1186/s13020-021-00438-x PMID: 33741031

Yang, S., & Kar, S. (2023). Application of artificial intelligence and machine learning in early detection of adverse drug reactions (ADRs) and drug-induced toxicity. *Artificial Intelligence Chemistry.*, *1*(2), 100011. DOI: 10.1016/j.aichem.2023.100011

Yao, L., Li, X., Wu, Z., Wang, J., Luo, C., Chen, B., Luo, R., Zhang, L., Zhang, C., Tan, X., Lu, Z., Zhu, C., Huang, Y., Tan, T., Liu, Z., Li, Y., Li, S., & Yu, H. (2024). Effect of artificial intelligence on novice-performed colonoscopy: A multicenter randomized controlled tandem study. *Gastrointestinal Endoscopy*, *99*(1), 91–99.e99. DOI: 10.1016/j.gie.2023.07.044 PMID: 37536635

Yao, X., Attia, Z. I., Behnken, E. M., Hart, M. S., Inselman, S. A., Weber, K. C., Li, F., Stricker, N. H., Stricker, J. L., Friedman, P. A., & Noseworthy, P. A. (2024). Realtime Diagnosis from Electrocardiogram Artificial Intelligence-Guided Screening for Atrial Fibrillation with Long Follow-Up (REGAL): Rationale and design of a pragmatic, decentralized, randomized controlled trial. *American Heart Journal*, *267*, 62–69. DOI: 10.1016/j.ahj.2023.10.005 PMID: 37913853

Yeaw, J., Benner, J. S., Walt, J. G., Sian, S., & Smith, D. B. (2009). Comparing adherence and persistence across six chronic medication classes. *Journal of Managed Care Pharmacy : JMCP, 15*(9), 728–740. DOI: 10.18553/jmcp.2009.15.9.728 PMID: 19954264

Yik, M. H. Y., Wong, V. C. W. T., Wong, T. H., & Shaw, P. C. (2021). HerBChain, a blockchain-based informative platform for quality assurance and quality control of herbal products. *Journal of Traditional and Complementary Medicine, 11*(6), 598–600. DOI: 10.1016/j.jtcme.2021.07.005 PMID: 34765524

Yin, W., Ebert, S., & Schütze, H. (2016). *Attention-Based Convolutional Neural Network for Machine Comprehension*. DOI: 10.18653/v1/W16-0103

Yingngam, B. (2024). Machine Learning Applications for Drug Repurposing. In *Artificial Intelligence and Machine Learning in Drug Design and Development* (pp. 251–294). Wiley-Scrivener., DOI: 10.1002/9781394234196.ch9

Yingngam, B., Navabhatra, A., & Sillapapibool, P. (2024). AI-Driven Decision-Making Applications in Pharmaceutical Sciences. In Nguyen, T. V. T., & Vo, N. T. M. (Eds.), *Using Traditional Design Methods to Enhance AI-Driven Decision Making* (pp. 1–63). IGI Global., DOI: 10.4018/979-8-3693-0639-0.ch001

Yingngam, B., & Sethabouppha, B. (2024). Advanced AI applications for drug discovery. In *Advances in Computational Intelligence for the Healthcare Industry 4.0* (pp. 42–86). IGI Global., DOI: 10.4018/979-8-3693-2333-5.ch003

Yi, S., Varun, B. V., Choi, Y., & Park, S. B. (2018). A brief overview of two major strategies in diversity-oriented synthesis: Build/couple/pair and ring-distortion. *Frontiers in Chemistry, 6*, 507. DOI: 10.3389/fchem.2018.00507 PMID: 30406085

Yiu, N. C. K. (2021). Toward Blockchain-Enabled Supply Chain Anti-Counterfeiting and Traceability. *Future Internet, 13*(4), 86. DOI: 10.3390/fi13040086

Young, J. D., Cai, C., & Lu, X. (2017). Unsupervised deep learning reveals prognostically relevant subtypes of glioblastoma. *BMC Bioinformatics, 18*(S11), 381. DOI: 10.1186/s12859-017-1798-2 PMID: 28984190

Yu, C. S., Chang, S. S., Chang, T. H., Wu, J. L., Lin, Y. J., Chien, H. F., & Chen, R. J. A. (2021). COVID-19 Pandemic Artificial Intelligence–Based System with Deep Learning Forecasting and Automatic Statistical Data Acquisition: Development and Implementation Study. [CrossRef]. *Journal of Medical Internet Research, 23*(5), e27806. DOI: 10.2196/27806 PMID: 33900932

Zakari, N., Al-Razgan, M., Alsaadi, A., Alshareef, H., Al Saigh, H., Alashaikh, L., Alharbi, M., Alomar, R., & Alotaibi, S. (2022, March 11). Blockchain technology in the pharmaceutical industry: A systematic review. *PeerJ. Computer Science*, *8*, e840. DOI: 10.7717/peerj-cs.840 PMID: 35634106

Zeb, S., Nizamullah, F. N. U., Abbasi, N., & Fahad, M. (2024). AI in Healthcare: Revolutionizing Diagnosis and Therapy. *International Journal of Multidisciplinary Sciences and Arts*, *3*(3), 118–128. DOI: 10.47709/ijmdsa.v3i3.4546

Zhang, M., Del Fiol, G., Grout, R. W., Jonnalagadda, S., Medlin, R.Jr, Mishra, R., & Fiszman, M. (2013). Automatic identification of comparative effectiveness research from medline citations to support clinicians' treatment information needs. *Studies in Health Technology and Informatics*, *192*, 846–850. PMID: 23920677

Zhang, P., Chen, B., Ma, L., Li, Z., Song, Z., Duan, W., & Qiu, X. (2015). The Large Scale Machine Learning in an Artificial Society: Prediction of the Ebola Outbreak in Beijing. [CrossRef] [PubMed]. *Computational Intelligence and Neuroscience*, *2015*, 1–12. DOI: 10.1155/2015/531650 PMID: 26457078

Zhang, W., (2019). Blockchain-Based Distributed Compliance in Multinational Corporations' Cross-Border Intercompany Transactions. In Arai, K., Kapoor, S., & Bhatia, R. (Eds.), *Advances in Information and Communication Networks. FICC 2018. Advances in Intelligent Systems and Computing* (Vol. 887). Springer., DOI: 10.1007/978-3-030-03405-4_20

Zhavoronkov, A., Ivanenkov, Y. A., Aliper, A., Veselov, M. S., Aladinskiy, V. A., Aladinskaya, A. V., Terentiev, V. A., Polykovskiy, D. A., Kuznetsov, M. D., Asadulaev, A., Volkov, Y., Zholus, A., Shayakhmetov, R. R., Zhebrak, A., Minaeva, L. I., Zagribelnyy, B. A., Lee, L. H., Soll, R., Madge, D., & Aspuru-Guzik, A. (2019). Deep learning enables rapid identification of potent DDR1 kinase inhibitors. *Nature Biotechnology*, *37*(9), 1038–1040. DOI: 10.1038/s41587-019-0224-x PMID: 31477924

Zhou, S., Li, K., Xiao, L., Cai, J., Liang, W., & Castiglione, A. (2023). A Systematic Review of Consensus Mechanisms in Blockchain. *Mathematics*, *11*(10), 2248. DOI: 10.3390/math11102248

Zhou, X., Peng, Y., & Liu, B. (2010). Text mining for traditional Chinese medical knowledge discovery: A survey. *Journal of Biomedical Informatics*, *43*(4), 650–660. DOI: 10.1016/j.jbi.2010.01.002 PMID: 20074663

Zhu, H. (2020). Big data and artificial intelligence modeling for drug discovery. *Annual Review of Pharmacology and Toxicology*, *60*(1), 573–589. DOI: 10.1146/annurev-pharmtox-010919-023324 PMID: 31518513

Zhu, H. H., & Huang, X. J. (2014). Oral arsenic and retinoic acid for non-high-risk acute promyelocytic leukemia. [DOI] [PubMed] [Google Scholar]. *The New England Journal of Medicine*, *371*(23), 2239–2241. DOI: 10.1056/NEJMc1412035 PMID: 25470713

Zhu, Z., Heng, B. H., & Teow, K. L. (2018). Lifetime trajectory simulation of chronic disease progression and comorbidity development. *Journal of Biomedical Informatics*, *88*, 29–36. DOI: 10.1016/j.jbi.2018.11.002 PMID: 30414473

Ziavrou, K. S., Noguera, S., & Boumba, V. A. (2022, September). Trends in counterfeit drugs and pharmaceuticals before and during COVID-19 pandemic. *Forensic Science International*, *338*, 111382. DOI: 10.1016/j.forsciint.2022.111382 PMID: 35882074

About the Contributors

Miltiadis D. Lytras is a visiting researcher at Effat University. Dr Lytras is a world-class expert in the fields of cognitive computing, information systems, technology-enabled innovation, social networks, computers in human behavior, and knowledge management. He is an expert in advanced computer science and management, editor, lecturer, and research consultant, with extensive experience in academia and the business sector in Europe and Asia. He served as the Editor in Chief of the International Journal in Semantic Web and Information Systems. He has co-edited more than 110 high impact factor special issues in ISI/Scopus indexed journals and co-Edited/Authored more than 80 books in international publishers including Elsevier, Emerald, IGI-Global, Springer, etc. Dr Lytras has co-authored more than 120 high impact factor papers in Q1 and Q2, Web of Science and Scopus indexed Journals. Dr. Lytras has a 25 years' experience on Research and Development projects and grants with significant skills and competencies to the successful conceptualization, financing and implementation of R&D projects with extensive experience in Europe, Middle East, and Far East. He has involved in more than 70 R&D projects overtime. Main areas of expertis Dr. Lytras has hold various senior editorial positions in prestigious journals over time including Editor in Chief and Associate Editor positions.

Sarah Abdulrahman Alajlan is a Doctor of Pharmacy with a deep passion for research AI and pharmaceutical economics. While not currently working as a full-time researcher, Dr. Alajlan is actively engaged in exploring the intersection of AI, pharmacy, and healthcare. She has co-edited two influential books on artificial intelligence and its impact on the pharmaceutical industry. With numerous publications in high-ranking Q1 and Q2 journals, Dr. Alajlan's research interests are broad, and her work has earned both national and international recognition. Her contributions have made her a respected figure in the fields of pharmaceutical economics and healthcare systems. Beyond her academic and research interests, Dr.

Alajlan is also a financial coach, leveraging her experience in finance to help others navigate complex financial decisions. She works as a dialysis pharmacist and supply chain analyst, where she applies her expertise to optimize patient care and healthcare operations. Driven by a commitment to continuous learning and mentoring, Dr. Alajlan is dedicated to advancing knowledge in both the pharmaceutical and economic sectors.

***

G. Sowmya is an Assistant Professor in the Department of Computer Science and Engineering at MLRIT, Hyderabad, with over a decade of teaching experience. Currently pursuing a Ph.D. in CSE from JNTUH, her research focuses on the formal verification of smart contracts. Sowmya holds an M.Tech and B.Tech in CSE and has received the prestigious Prathibha Award for academic excellence. She has contributed to numerous international journals and conferences, authored several patents, and actively engages in various FDPs and certifications, particularly in Blockchain, AI, and IoT. She has also conducted workshops and webinars on cutting-edge technologies such as blockchain and machine learning

Kazi Kutubuddin Sayyad Liyakat has completed his B.E., M.E., and Ph.D. in E&TC Engineering and is nowadays working as a Professor & Head of Department, E&TC Engineering Department and was Dean R&D. He is Post-Doctoral Fellow working on "IoT in Healthcare Applications". His area of Interest is IoT, AI and ML. He has published more than 120+ papers & Book chapters in various Journals & Books. Also published 11 books in the field of Engineering. He has published 15 Indian Patents, 2 South African Grant Patent, 2 Indian Copyright Patents and 8 UK Grant Patent. He worked as a Reviewer for Scopus Conferences and Journal. Also work as Editorial Board Member for various Journals. He got 2 Best Researcher Award, Best Faculty Award and Appreciation Letter from MoE's Innovation Cell, Govt. of India.

Nur Ozturk is a distinguished academic and researcher in the field of clinical pharmacy. She served as a faculty member in the School of Pharmacy, Department of Clinical Pharmacy, where she contributes to both teaching and research.

Abdullah Saeed is a researcher, epidemiologist, biostatistician, strategist, AI developer, and healthcare leader. He is the Director of Research and Development at the Ministry of Health, Abha, Saudi Arabia, focusing on statistical analysis, biostatistics, epidemiology, and research instrument development. He previously served as Director of Public Health and Head of the Outpatient and Dental

Departments at the Ministry of Health in Aseer and as a Resident in Public Health at King Abdulaziz University. Dr. Saeed holds a Fellowship from the American College of Healthcare Executives, a Public Health certification from the National Board of Public Health Examiners (USA), an MPH in Epidemiology and Biostatistics from King Abdulaziz University, and a Bachelor of Dental Surgery from King Khalid University. He has completed specialized courses from Stanford, Emory, and the University of Virginia. His research focuses on AI in healthcare, health system performance indicators.

Bancha Yingngam is working as Associate Professor (Pharmaceutical Sciences and Technology) in the Faculty of Pharmaceutical Sciences at Ubon Ratchathani University, Ubon Ratchathani, Thailand. He received his B.Pharm. and Ph.D. (Pharmaceutical Sciences) at the Ubon Ratchathani, and postdoctoral fellowship at Institute of Pharmaceutical Sciences, University of Graz, Graz, Austria. His areas of interest include artificial intelligence, optimization methods, green chemistry, natural product chemistry, cosmeceuticals, and pharmaceutical nanotechnology. He has authored and co-authored many scientific papers published in international journals, and proceedings of international and national scientific conferences. He has also authored more than 30 book chapters and edited three textbooks.

Index

A

B

C

D

E

H

I

K

M

N

P

R

S

T

V

www.ingramcontent.com/pod-product-compliance
Lightning Source LLC
LaVergne TN
LVHW080118011026
849160LV00013B/1131

* 9 7 9 8 3 3 7 3 0 9 0 2 6 *